Palliative Care: The Nursing Role

Neither the publishers nor the authors will be liable for any loss or damage of any nature occasioned to or suffered by any person acting or refraining from acting as a result of reliance on the material contained in this publication.

For Churchill Livingstone

Senior commissioning editor: Alex Mathieson
Project manager: Ewan Halley
Project development editor: Valerie Dearing
Design direction: Judith Wright
Project controller: Jane Shanks

Palliative Care: The Nursing Role

Edited by

Jean Lugton MA MSc PhD RGN RNT HV

Health Visitor/Researcher
West Lothian NHS Trust, UK

Margaret Kindlen DipEd MPhil RGN RM HV RNT

Lecturer in Palliative Care
University of Dundee, UK

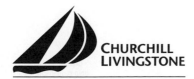

CHURCHILL
LIVINGSTONE

EDINBURGH LONDON NEW YORK PHILADELPHIA SYDNEY TORONTO

CHURCHILL LIVINGSTONE
An imprint of Harcourt Brace and Company Limited

Churchill Livingstone, Robert Stevenson House, 1–3 Baxter's Place,
Leith Walk, Edinburgh EH1 3AF, UK

© Harcourt Brace and Company Limited 1999

First published 1999

ISBN 0443 05513 0

British Library Cataloguing in Publication Data
A catalogue record for this book is available from the British Library.

Library of Congress Cataloging in Publication Data
A catalog record for this book is available from the Library of Congress.

Note
Medical knowledge is constantly changing. As new information becomes
available, changes in treatment, procedures, equipment and the use of
drugs become necessary. The editors and the publishers have, as far as
it is possible, taken care to ensure that the information given in this text
is accurate and up-to-date. However, readers are strongly advised to
confirm that the information, especially with regard to drug usage,
complies with the latest legislation and standards of practice.

The
publisher's
policy is to use
**paper manufactured
from sustainable forests**

Printed in China
NPCC/01

Contents

Contributors

Brenda Bottrill DipDY MISPA MLD MSR
Relaxation Therapist/Aromatherapist, Oncology Department and
Maggie's Centre, Western General Hospital, Edinburgh, UK
and Macmillan Centre, St John's Hospital, Livingston, UK

Dorothy E. Cyster B Mus LRAM DCM PGCE RGN RNT Dip Nursing Ethics
Formerly Lecturer in Nursing Studies, Centre for Medical Education,
University of Dundee, Dundee, UK; now Piano Instructor,
Education Department, Perth and Kinross Council, UK

Keith Farrer BA (Hons) Nursing Education RGN RNT
Clinical Nurse Specialist – Palliative Care Team, Western General
Hospital, Edinburgh, UK

Richard Gamlin MPhil DipN RGN RNT
Practitioner Lecturer, St. Benedict's Hospice, Sunderland, UK

Bridget Johnston BN (Hons) RGN FETC PGCE (FE)
Lecturer in Palliative Care, Strathcarron Hospice, Denny, UK
and part-time PhD Student, University of Glasgow, UK

Margaret Kindlen DipEd MPhil RGN RM HV RNT
Lecturer in Palliative Care, University of Dundee, UK

Ishbel Kirkwood RGN RM LLSA
Staff Nurse, Western General Hospital, Edinburgh, UK

Sally M. R. Lawton MA PhD RGN NDN RCNT RDNT
Senior Lecturer, Robert Gordon University, Aberdeen, UK

Jean Lugton MA MSc PhD RGN RNT HV
Health Visitor/Researcher, West Lothian NHS Trust, UK

Rosemary McIntyre PhD MN DipN RGN NDN RNT
Head of Studies (Scotland), Marie Curie Cancer Care, Scotland

Christine M. Pearce RGN RNT
Senior Lecturer in Palliative Care, Marie Curie Cancer Care, Ipswich, UK

Val Smith MSc RGN RM DN RNT
Lecturer, Strathcarron Hospice, Denny, UK

Margaret E. Smith BA (Hons) RGN RSCN CertEd RNT
Formerly Bradford Palliative Care Education Co-ordinator, Bradford
University Health Authority and Marie Curie Cancer Care, Bradford, UK

Norrie M. Sutherland BSc RGN CMB RHV RNT CertEd
Lecturer, The Ayrshire Hospice, Ayr, UK
Associate Lecturer, Glasgow Caledonian University, Glasgow, UK
and Associate Lecturer, Open University, UK

Sheena Walker RGN RM DN RCNT RNT
Freelance Lecturer in Palliative Care, Glasgow, UK

Preface

The quality of life of people with advanced illness depends very much on the attitudes and skills of their nurses and other professional carers. We hope that this book enables registered nurses working in hospital, community or other settings to develop their knowledge and skills to deliver high quality palliative care. We believe that nurse specialists in palliative care will also find topics of relevance. Excellent books on palliative care have been written from a medical perspective. This book focuses on palliative nursing with skills and examples derived from nursing practice.

The book explores the relationship between nurse, patient and relatives, the process of nursing and dimensions of support. We acknowledge that control of physical symptoms is paramount in palliative care. We have not included that topic here, recognising that it is very adequately covered in medical texts. Instead, the book concentrates on other aspects of holistic care where nurses have significant input, for example, the principles of needs assessment for patients and relatives. The 11 chapters provide a broad, balanced coverage of these subject areas, encompassing nursing developments in palliative care, non-specialist palliative nursing education, holistic assessment of patients' needs and the central issues of support and communication.

Spirituality is receiving increased attention in nursing and there are opportunities in this book for readers to develop their own practice applications. Extending their knowledge of issues associated with body image and sexuality will enable nurses to empower seriously ill patients to address these sensitive personal issues. The role of complementary therapies alongside medical treatments in improving the quality of life of seriously ill people and involving them in their own care is receiving increased recognition. Nurses need to be more knowledgeable about these approaches. In advanced illness, the whole family often travels a long and difficult road with the patient. Skilled and focused nursing support for family and carers during the illness journey through and beyond bereavement is therefore essential.

Ethical issues can arise every day in palliative nursing. It is important that they are not ignored and that nurses have the confidence and skills to cope with them so that they can develop respect for individuals' choices. Nurses want patients and their families to receive the highest possible quality of care, whether provided in the patient's home, in a specialist unit or hospital. Good quality care needs careful planning and auditing. Research can be used to measure and demonstrate quality in palliative care. All life-threatening illnesses have implications for the wellbeing of patient and family, and we assess nursing needs of patients with a variety of conditions, including cancer.

In the UK, most deaths occur in hospital but people will have received care in other settings during the course of their illness, many spending long periods at home being cared for by close family members. The contents of this book have application to a variety of care settings (hospital, home, nursing home and community) and especially recognise that care in the community is important. Community nurses with education in palliative care are in an excellent position to provide support for patients in the community.

The book is clinically oriented, supported by evidence of implemented research. In some chapters, the authors use examples from their own research. The book is patient centred, showing awareness of their needs and expectations and acknowledging patient choice and empowerment.

We take issues of professional accountability seriously. We would encourage readers to be aware of the different strategies appropriate to acquisition of competencies in palliative care and to be confident about how professional profiling can help them develop these competencies. Each chapter indicates the relevant dimensions of professional practice recommended by the UKCC for PREP (health problem identification, care enhancement, patient and family support, practice and education development). The activities suggested in each chapter provide opportunities for readers to increase self awareness, build their professional profiles through reflective practice and stimulate them to facilitate the learning of student nurses and care assistants. Chapters are illustrated with line drawings, boxes, tables and vignettes and contain extensive references and helpful suggestions for further reading.

The authors all have extensive experience of general palliative care as well as a special interest in their topic chapters. They have maintained contact with nursing practice through teaching, clinical involvement and research. They would like to acknowledge the help of patients and their relatives in writing this book and, in particular, their consent in allowing their experiences to be used in illustrative case studies.

Jean Lugton 1999

Overview of nursing developments in palliative care

1

Bridget Johnston

PALLIATIVE CARE: THE NURSING CONTEXT

This chapter will introduce the reader to the concept of palliative nursing by: outlining what palliative care is, discussing the development of contemporary palliative care services and outlining the role of the nurse in palliative care.

LEARNING OUTCOMES

PREP categories, patient, client and colleague support, practice development and educational development will be addressed and by the end of the chapter the reader will:

- Identify the key features of palliative care services in hospital, in hospices and in the community
- Understand the key research studies related to the role and function of the nurse in palliative care
- Distinguish the characteristics of the role of the nurse in palliative care.

PALLIATIVE CARE DEFINITION

The word 'palliative' is derived from the Latin word 'pallium', meaning a cloak or cover. The Oxford English dictionary defines palliative as 'to relieve without curing'.

In its most literal use it refers to the provision of active care for a person whose condition is not responsive to curative treatment. The development of modern day palliative care in the UK is closely bound to the development of the hospice movement.

The World Health Organisation (WHO) has defined palliative care as:

The active, total care of patients whose disease no longer responds to curative treatment. Control of pain, of other symptoms, and of psychological, social and spiritual problems is paramount. The goal of palliative care is achievement of the best possible quality of life for patients and their families.

The WHO (1990) definition states that palliative care:

- Affirms life and regards dying as a normal process
- Neither hastens nor postpones death
- Provides relief from pain and other distressing symptoms
- Integrates the psychological and spiritual aspects of patient care
- Offers a support system to help patients live as actively as possible until death
- Offers a support system to help the family cope during the patient's illness and in their own bereavement

Palliative care has been described as incorporating three essential components: symptom control, support for the family and support for the patient (Quint Benoliel 1988). Its objectives therefore are to palliate physical symptoms, alleviate disease and maintain independence for as long and as comfortably as possible; alleviate isolation, anxiety and fear associated with advancing disease; provide as dignified a death as possible; and support those who are bereaved.

The palliative care movement was born out of the hospice movement and the term was first coined by Professor Mount, a Canadian who worked with Cicely Saunders at St Christopher's Hospice in London. Since 1987, palliative medicine has been recognised as a distinct medical specialty (HMSO 1992).

Palliative nursing, as a term, was introduced by a specialist nursing group of the RCN – the Palliative Nursing Group – in 1989. It is now a widely used term in the UK and is recognised as a distinct nursing specialty with diploma, undergraduate and postgraduate degree programmes.

The premise put forward in this chapter is that all life-threatening illnesses – be they cancer, neurological, cardiac or respiratory disease – have implications for physical, social, psychological and spiritual health, for both the individual and their family. The role of palliative nursing is therefore to assess needs in each of these areas and to plan, implement and evaluate appropriate interventions. It aims to improve the quality of life and to enable a dignified death.

With the growth of palliative care as a specialty, there is now some confusion as to what specialist palliative care is and where and how this should be practised. The National Council for Hospice and Specialist Palliative Care Services (NCHSPCS, 1995) advocates the palliative care approach as a vital and integral part of all clinical practice, whatever the illness or its stage. Such an approach is informed by a knowledge and practice of palliative care principles. Palliative intervention, on the other hand, concerns intervention when the disease is not curative. Both of these are sometimes known as generic palliative care.

Specialist palliative care requires a high level of professional skills from trained staff, as well as a high staff–patient ratio. It refers to a service provided by a multiprofessional team led by clinicians with a recognised specialist palliative care training. The aim is also to support patients and their families, wherever they may be – hospital, home or hospice.

■ **REFLECTIVE PRACTICE 1.1** **Palliative care services**

- What palliative care services are available in your area?
- In your experience, what aspects of palliative care are difficult to integrate in the general care setting?
- Why do you think this is so?

HISTORY AND DEVELOPMENT OF PALLIATIVE CARE

Palliative care in hospices

Although Mme Jeanne Garnier opened the first hospice, specifically for the dying, in France during the middle of the 19th century, the founding of the modern hospice movement is attributed to Dame Cicely Saunders. Her vision arose from discussions with a Jewish patient, David Tasma, from the Warsaw Ghetto. Cicely Saunders, a former nurse, was at the time working as a social worker in London. When he died, David Tasma left a legacy to Cicely Saunders to be a 'window in your home'. This home, St Christopher's Hospice, opened for in-patient care in 1967. It was the first hospice with an academic model of integrated care that combined clinical care, research and teaching and provided a joint emphasis on medical and psychosocial enquiry. Cicely Saunders' ultimate vision for hospices was 'moving out of the NHS so that attitudes and knowledge could move back in' (Saunders 1991/2, 1993).

The modern hospice movement has proliferated since 1967. It has a worldwide philosophy, which has adapted to the needs of different cultures and settings, and is established in six continents. Hospices now often provide home care services, in-patient facilities and day care centres, and are staffed by a multidisciplinary team including nurses, doctors, physiotherapists, occupational therapists, social workers, chaplains and volunteers. Currently, there are now 288 hospice in-patient units in the UK and Ireland (see Fig. 1.1).

In the early years of the modern hospice movement there was little evaluative research on its role. Much of the existing research is American although a number of studies have now been completed in the UK. There is little research that compares how hospices differ from each other and

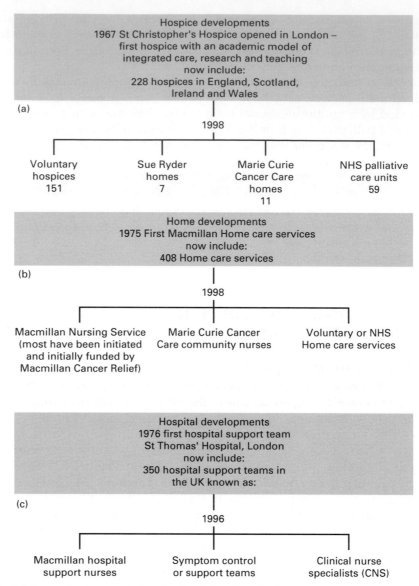

Fig. 1.1 Recent developments in hospices, hospitals and nursing homes.

whether the quality of care differs from other institutions. The role of the hospice movement in revolutionising the concept of pain control and symptom management in the care of the dying is unchallenged and widely acknowledged. The hospice movement has also paved the way in the disclosure of diagnosis, demonstrating that this can be done for the benefit of all parties concerned, although hospital doctors and GPs are now the main source of such information (Seale 1991). Despite the absence of clear research evidence, it is thought that the management of physical symptoms, in combination with attention to the person's psychosocial needs, is rarely implemented as well in other settings (Field & James 1993).

The hospice movement is not without its critics. Douglas (1992) argues the following. Why should:

- Care at the end of an illness be separate from all that has gone before and why should collective dying be a good thing?
- Only a minority of a minority (only those who die from malignancies) be singled out for special treatment?
- A large and general need be left to the 'scanty and scandalously choosy efforts of a patchwork of local charities'?

Undoubtedly, the hospice movement can no longer rest on its reputation. Harris (1991) and Doyle (1992) recommend that hospices need to open their doors to the 'disadvantaged dying', for example those suffering from life-threatening diseases, such as cardiac, respiratory and neurological diseases, those from social classes four and five and those from ethnic minorities (Hill & Penso 1995).

From a National Council for Hospice and Specialist Palliative Care Study (NCHSPCS) findings indicated a very real need for service provision for this section of the population, stating that hospices and palliative care services need to provide 'culturally sensitive services in respect of language, religion, spiritual and dietary needs and for particular attention to be given to providing appropriate and accessible information to these communities' (Hill & Penso 1995, p. 5).

■ REFLECTIVE PRACTICE 1.2   Care in hospices

What do you understand by the term disadvantaged dying? A useful article to read is that of Harris (1991) entitled 'The disadvantaged dying'.

Nursing and medical research and audit needs to evaluate the effectiveness of care and show what it is that is special about hospice care and hospice nursing. Furthermore, there is a need for education and exchange of ideas to ensure that the concept of palliative care is integrated into the mainstream of the NHS, community and private sectors.

Palliative care in hospitals

The most common place for people to die of a terminal illness is an NHS hospital, in a variety of settings within them (Cartwright 1991, Field & James 1993). Moreover, while dying is unique and highly personal to the person experiencing it and those close to them, it is part of the routine and ritual of the hospital staff caring for them (Field & James 1993, Walsh & Ford 1989). The ways in which staff define and perform their role of caring for dying patients has an important effect on patients and their relatives. According to Field (1989), care of the dying is, to a certain extent, determined by the organisational demands and routines of hospital life. Other factors that may limit the effectiveness of caring for dying people in acute settings include: inadequate and ineffective communication (Faulkner & Maguire 1994, Field 1989). Stedeford (1994) asserted that poor communication can cause more suffering than many of the symptoms of terminal disease. Other factors inhibiting the provision of effective care include the conflict between acute care and palliative care (Dunn 1992, Williams 1982). It can be difficult for staff to decide when curative care ends and palliative care begins. A number of researchers have identified caring for dying patients in acute hospitals as a major source of stress for nurses and other health care professionals (Reisseter & Thomas 1986, Vachon 1987). There is, in addition, a tendency for hospital staff to pay lip service to the multidisciplinary team rather than working within it. Often in hospital there are inadequate facilities for relatives to stay overnight and for staff to interview them and provide support (Griffin 1991, Irvine 1993). Finally, nurses often receive inadequate preparation and support for their role in caring for dying patients in acute settings (Hockley 1989, B M Irvine, unpublished work, 1990, Reisetter & Thomas 1986).

Specialist palliative care in hospitals commenced as a concept in 1976 with the first support team being established at St Thomas' Hospital in London. The idea was based on a model that originated in 1975, at St Luke's Hospital in New York (Bates et al 1981). The team initially included a chaplain, a social worker, a nurse and two part-time voluntary doctors. It operated as an advisory service and was able to facilitate a level of symptom control that enabled many patients to be discharged home earlier than anticipated. There are now 350 hospitals in the UK with support teams or support nurses. Many of these have been pump primed by the Macmillan Cancer Relief (Directory of Hospice Services 1998). Support teams, or palliative care teams (as they are sometimes known) advise and support the primary care team, usually hospital doctors and nurses, by providing support and advice on pain and symptom control, management of pain, psychosocial and spiritual needs, bereavement support and support for staff (Anstey 1993, Dunlop & Hockley 1990, Hockley et al 1988).

Palliative care in the community

At the beginning of the 20th century, the majority of people died at home. The number of people who now die at home has fallen to 23%, concurrent with the number of deaths in institutions rising to 71% (Field & James 1993). These figures relate to urban populations, as opposed to 80% of populations in rural areas who die in hospitals. In Herd's study (1990) it was noted that the further people live from hospital the greater their chance of dying at home.

The first home care team was established in 1969 as an extension to in-patient care at St Christopher's Hospice in London. This pattern continues. However, much specialist palliative care in the community is carried out by Macmillan nurses, who may or may not be attached to an in-patient hospice unit. Macmillan nurses operate specialist palliative care services. The first community Macmillan nurse post was established in 1975. The success of this venture prompted the then Cancer Relief Macmillan Fund (now Macmillan Cancer Relief) to initiate a programme whereby health authorities could apply for a 3-year grant to pump prime Macmillan nurse posts with the proviso that the health authority became responsible for continuing the service beyond the grant period. In 1996 there were over 1000 Macmillan nurses working in hospitals and the community throughout the UK. These nurses are often viewed as a model for clinical nurse specialists (CNS). The role has evolved over the years in response to a growing body of knowledge in palliative care, political changes in the health service and developments in nursing. Today, Macmillan nurses act in an advisory and supportive role to patients, professionals and the primary carer.

The debate about home death versus hospital or hospice for those dying from life-threatening illnesses has continued since the early work of Hinton (1979), Lamerton (1980) and Murray Parkes (1985). These studies contended that patients tended to choose home as a preferred place of death. More recent studies have reinforced that patients, when asked and given a choice, would prefer to die at home (Hockley et al 1988, Townsend et al 1990). Despite government policy about care in the community, the majority of people still die of terminal illness in hospital (Addington-Hall & McCarthy 1995). Studies carried out in the 1990s, however, revealed that there was a discrepancy between how patients and their carers perceive care at home (Higginson, & Wade & McCarthy 1993, Norum 1995, Spiller & Alexander 1993). The deciding factors for the families appeared to be support, co-ordination of care and respite care. Seale (1992) further identified that in order to care effectively for dying patients, home community nurses themselves need support.

Field & James (1993) indicated that the experience of patients dying in their own homes appears to vary widely, partly because homes and families differ in terms of social, psychological and spiritual make up and partly because of the nature, conduct and availability of support given to unpaid carers. Moreover, according to Cartwright (1991), Field & James (1993) and Thorpe (1993), symptom control is often less effective at home than in hospital or a hospice. In his study, Parkes (1985) proposed that people may be prepared to relinquish less than ideal physical symptom control for the social and psychological benefits of remaining in their own home.

Field & James (1993) noted that should a person choose to die at home and receive adequate support they may have up to 25 different paid carers visiting their home during the course of their terminal illness. Not surprisingly, communication and co-ordination of their care becomes inadequate, leading to fragmentation of care between health carers, e.g. doctors, nurses and home helps. These circumstances may also result in a marginalisation or exclusion of the dying person and their family from his decision-making. Field & James (1993) go on to assert that the paradox for terminal care in the community is that, at a time when professions in palliative care are being encouraged to deliver 'holistic' care, current trends in the NHS may limit the opportunity to do just that. They conclude that:

> ... the care of dying people is of such central importance to all members of our society that the manifold inadequacies are something which must be readdressed, rediscussed and improved. [Field & James 1993, p. 27]

■ REFLECTIVE PRACTICE 1.3 Care in the community

People being cared for at home very often have a multiplicity of health care personnel involved in their care.
• How can a patient's autonomy be established and maintained in such circumstances?
• Who is the advocate for patients, or indeed families, when many agencies are involved?

Day care

Day hospices are relatively new in the UK. These are units normally based in hospices where patients with advancing disease can attend on a day basis. Staff usually comprise nurses and paramedics, such as occupational therapists and physiotherapists, assisted by volunteers.

The purpose of a day hospice is to provide respite care for relatives as well as social and therapeutic benefits for the patient. These can range from craft activities to aromatherapy to direct care, such as a wound dressing or a bath. Without a doubt, the provision of day care has enhanced the care that can be offered to patients and their relatives in the community. The day centre established in 1990 at St Christopher's Hospice in London stated that its primary aim is to improve the quality of life for patients by adding a new dimension to the total package of care already in place for the patient and their family. They viewed their aims as fivefold, to provide:

• Stimulation and enjoyment through activities, focusing on the individual's needs and choices and encouraging self-esteem
• Social support and help to alleviate feelings of isolation and depression
• Respite for carers
• Basic nursing, where appropriate, to aid and improve physical well-being
• Rehabilitation by adapting the patient's physical and social environment so that independence can be maintained for as long as possible

TEAMWORK

Teamwork is central to effective palliative care (Hull et al 1989). The question arises as to who are the key members of the team? Many different health care professionals can make up a palliative care team (Box 1.1).

■ BOX 1.1

An example of a typical hospice team with integrated education and research

Hospice – 18 beds
• Director
• Administrator
• Matron

Nurses (RGN, 27 full-time equivalent, (nursing assistants, 10 full-time equivalent)
- Deputy (Matron)
- Staff nurses
- Nursing assistants (unqualified nurses)
- Home care staff (Macmillan nurses)
- Ward sister
- Day care sister

Doctors
- Two consultants
- Research fellow

Professions allied to medicine
- Social worker
- Physiotherapist
- Occupational therapist

Clergy
- Chaplain

Education department
- Two full-time lecturers
- Education secretary

Support staff
- Secretaries
- Switchboard operator
- Appeals and finance staff

Kitchen and domestic staff
- Cook
- Catering staff
- Housekeeping staff
- Gardener
- Domestic staff

Voluntary staff
- Volunteer co-ordinator
- Volunteers (190)

The key person in the team is the patient (and also his family). To exclude the patients from the team is to render them passive recipients of their care rather than partners in decision-making. Health care in modern society is often based on paternalism 'professional knows best' rather than being about partnership and patient autonomy. Palliative care seeks to redress this balance.

What then is the function of the team? Ajemain (1993) presents the argument that the primary goal of teamwork is to offer the best possible quality of life for the patient. Effective teamwork depends on good communication, effective leadership and co-ordination. Individual team members require to know their own limitations and to share in decision-making and formal review (Hull et al 1989). Ajemain (1993) presents several factors that contribute to successful team management. In addition to an individual's role within the team, shared decision-making, effective communication, common goals, certain role functions and dysfunction need close consideration. These include role expectations, ambiguity, conflict and overload.

Without a doubt the members of the team in palliative care face particular stresses and strains as a result of working with dying patients and their families. It is therefore of paramount importance to pay attention to staff support and continuing education.

■ **REFLECTIVE PRACTICE 1.4   Teamwork**

Mary is a 45-year-old lady with advanced breast cancer with a prognosis of 6–8 weeks. She is divorced, unemployed and has four school-age children. Mary is an in-patient at a hospice but wishes to have her remaining care at home.

• Which professionals might be involved in her care?
• How would they ensure that Mary's care is not duplicated and that her needs and wishes are met?
• Who do you think should co-ordinate this care?

You may wish to discuss this scenario with a district nursing sister or Macmillan nurse.

COMMUNICATION

Many authors have asserted that communication is a key aspect of the role of the nurse (Gooch 1988, Macleod Clarke 1983, Wilkinson 1991). Indeed, Buckman (1993) proposed that effective symptom control is impossible without effective communication. Patients also state that communication is key to their care being effective (B Johnston, unpublished work, 1996). Yet, despite the efforts of expert trainers, such as Faulkner & Maguire (1994), to improve communication skills, there remains evidence that these remain largely ineffective throughout the profession (Heaven & Maguire 1996, Wilkinson 1991).

A number of studies have identified the problems which professionals have with communication. These include distancing or blocking tactics, ignoring cues, false reassurance and avoidance tactics (Faulkner & Maguire 1994, Macleod Clark 1983, Wilkinson 1991).

In order to communicate effectively with patients and their families, the nurse must be supported in the workplace. This can be achieved through clinical supervision. If the nurse's morale is low or if they feel undervalued by colleagues and managers they may not have the courage or will to communicate effectively.

So what are considered effective communication skills and strategies? Most authors would agree that effective communication in palliative care incorporates effective listening skills and appropriate non-verbal communication; counselling skills, such as reflection, clarification and empathy, supportiveness, and above all, self-awareness.

Faulkner & Maguire (1994) note that in order to communicate effectively with patients, nurses need to pay attention to assessment skills, and to handling difficult questions or conflict dealing with anger denial and providing support and supervision.

■ REFLECTIVE PRACTICE 1.5   Communication

What do nurses need to do to become skilled in communication? Jot down your own thoughts before reading on.

The majority of authors assert that we gain these skills through training (Faulkner 1993, Faulkner & Maguire 1994, Heaven & Maguire 1996, Wilkinson 1991). How these skills are taught, however, is crucial. Audiotape or videotape feedback with role play, incorporated into small group teaching, have been used. Heaven & Maguire (1996) contend that simple skills training is insufficient to change clinical behaviour. They advocate that communication workshops should include handling of emotions, self-efficacy and challenging nurses' attitude and beliefs about both their communication skills and the consequences of their actions on patients. Nurses can acquire and improve their communication skills by developing their self-awareness, particularly by reflecting on their practice, by developing empathy with their patients and learning by role-modelling their peers in the clinical environment.

ROLE OF THE NURSE

Defining nursing

Despite the fact that nursing has been an occupation for several hundred years, few authors or researchers have defined it successfully. It could, however, be argued that not one definition encompasses all that nurses do, particularly when we bear in mind that nurses work in a variety of settings, adopting a variety of roles. Indeed, Florence Nightingale stated that 'I use the word nursing for want of a better' (Nightingale 1980). She went on to say that the 'very elements of nursing are all but unknown'. How far have we come in defining the role of the nurse?

Nursing is a complex activity, a practice-based, eclectic discipline. Its very essence is concerned with human nature, professional caring and the building of therapeutic relationships, with the practice of nursing involving complex decision-making processes.

Nurse–patient relationships

Nurse–patient relationships are central to the role of the nurse in palliative care and this relationship should benefit the patient. Muetzel (1988) suggested that the three concepts of partnership, intimacy and reciprocity come together in a therapeutic encounter between nurse and patient. Muetzel believed that the nurse must be self-aware, or at least growing towards that goal, for any meaningful relationship to occur. Furthermore, according to Watson (1988) a caring relationship is formed between nurse and patient when the nurse recognises the patient as an individual and is able to empathise and establish a rapport. Campbell (1984), a theologian, likens the nurse–patient relationship to a journey. Two people travel for a while together, becoming close and committed to each other, but only within defined limits. At the end of the journey they part without having formed a deep personal relationship. He called this 'moderated love'.

In a study exploring the nurse–patient relationship, Morse (1991) found that four types of nurse–patient relationship occurred. The type of relationship depended on the duration of the contact between the nurse and the patient. The four types were clinical, connected, therapeutic and over-involved relationships.

- **A clinical relationship** occurred when the patient was being treated for minor concerns. This type of relationship is normally brief, the patient's needs are not great and there is little personal emotional involvement or investment on the part of the nurse. Care is given quickly and effectively and investigations or treatments do not usually involve anything that is serious or life-threatening. In this relationship the nurse views the patient first, within their patient role and second, as a person with a life 'outside'.

- **A connected relationship** occurred when the nurse viewed the patient first as a person and second as a patient. The patient and the nurse have known each other long enough to have developed a relationship beyond the clinical relationship.

- **In a therapeutic relationship** the patient trusts the nurse. This is something we should not assume occurs in all nurse–patient encounters. The nurse here could also serve as the patient's advocate, interceding on behalf of the patient with family or medical staff. They will also try to 'protect' the patient from some of the more unpleasant aspects of care. This type of relationship would occur in the majority of cases in palliative care.

- **An over-involved relationship** occurs when the patient has needs that are out of the ordinary and the nurse chooses to meet those needs. The nurse is committed to the patient as a person, which overrides her commitment to the patient's treatment regimen, the medical staff, the institution and her nursing responsibility to other patients. The relationship here goes beyond a professional relationship to a close personal relationship and is questionably therapeutic. The nurse, as a person, is overriding the nurse as a professional.

In a UK study, which examined the therapeutic potential of nurses' personal involvement with patients, Savage (1995) identified the relationship between nurse and patient as a crucial element in the effectiveness of nursing care. Savage referred, in particular, to the 'closeness' between nurse and patient, a concept she identified from the 'new nursing' literature. Pearson (1992), for instance, in his description of the work at Burford and Oxford Nursing Development Unit, stated that nurses achieve successful outcomes through the establishment of 'close relationships' with their patients and by using this closeness to therapeutic effect in a planned and systematic way. This 'closeness' can be seen as similar to the connected relationship described by Morse (1991). This closeness and connectedness is also explored in the work of Perry (1996), who examined the actions and beliefs of exemplary oncology nurses in Canada. She found that nurses used dialogue in silence, mutual touch and humour in the relationships they developed with cancer patients. Significantly in Savage's study, closeness is seen, in part, as developing from the performance of intimate activities, such as bathing a patient, in the context of a continuing relationship. Interestingly, these activities are largely undervalued by health care professionals.

Not surprisingly the nurses in Savage's study found the notion of 'closeness' difficult to explain but it often suggested to them proximity and occurred at a time when patients were more likely to open up. Likewise, nurses formed partnerships with patients in a mutually reciprocal role. Savage also found that close relationships were more likely to occur in an environment where nurses were well supported and satisfied with their work.

Practice of nursing

Another seminal research project, which has had an influence on the way that nursing is practised, managed and taught, is the work of an American nurse, Patricia Benner (1984). She identified five levels of competency in clinical nursing practice. These levels: novice, advanced beginner, competent, proficient and expert, were described in the words of nurses working in critical care units in the USA. Nurses were interviewed and observed, either individually or in small groups. Only patient care situations where the nurse made a positive difference were included.

Novice nurses were newly qualified nurses in a new clinical area, or student nurses. They were beginners who had little or no expertise of the situations in which they were expected to perform. They practised by rule-governed behaviour. The expert nurse, on the other hand, no longer relied on rules or guidelines to connect her understanding of the situation. They possessed an 'intuitive' grasp of each situation and 'zeroed in on the accurate region of the problem without wasteful consideration of a large range of unfruitful, alternative diagnoses and solutions' (Benner 1984, p. 32).

Additionally, in an Australian grounded theory study, Lawler (1991) explored the invisible aspects of nurses' work. She studied how the body is managed by nurses in their work and in particular what happens 'behind the screens'. She advocated that nursing involves not only doing things that are traditionally assigned to females in our society but also crossing 'social boundaries and breaking taboos and doing things for people which they would normally do for themselves in private if they were able' (Lawler 1991, p. 30).

She also stated that the relationship a nurse has with a hospitalised patient is context and situationally related. It is unlike a 'normal' social relationship as it occurs when the patient is experiencing one of the most stressful events that they will encounter. She proposed that nurses created an 'environment of permission' for the patient in which to reconcile what has happened to their bodies. She asserted that this is made possible by the construction of a particular kind of relationship and by the use of clinical strategies, which affect both the nurse and the patient.

She concluded that there was a widespread consensus that nursing is not a well-understood occupation in society generally and that a level of ignorance exists about the work of nurses. She advocated that people tend to focus on the aesthetically unpleasant or sexually related aspects of nursing practice. You only have to look at the current media portrayal of nurses to concur with this idea.

RESEARCH STUDIES ON THE ROLE OF THE NURSE IN PALLIATIVE CARE

It is apparent that nursing, as an occupation, is difficult to define. This may be in part to do with the fact that much of nursing is 'hidden'. In this respect an attempt will now be made to elicit what it is that palliative care nurses do.

Care of the dying patient and their family is primarily a nursing responsibility. As patients shift from the sick to the dying role it is principally the nurse who deals with the day-to-day task of supporting and helping them and their families to live with the psychological, social, physical and spiritual consequences of their illness.

■ REFLECTIVE PRACTICE 1.6   The dying patient

Think back to the first death you witnessed as a nurse.

- From that experience how would you prepare a student to deal with their first death in clinical practice?
- What do you consider are the most important aspects of the role of the nurse in palliative care and how would you explain this role to others?

Despite the fact that caring for the dying is and always has been a fundamental aspect of nursing, few researchers have examined this role and no research has examined patients' perceptions of this role and the effectiveness of palliative nursing. Much of the literature on the subject is anecdotal or descriptive. One of the difficulties in research of this nature is that few researchers have been able to articulate what it is that the experienced palliative care nurse does and how they influence patient and family outcomes.

Although research studies examining what nurses do are scant, the role of the nurse in palliative care has been defined in a variety of ways (see Box 1.2).

■ **BOX 1.2**

Definitions of the nurse in palliative care

Descriptor	*Author*
• Supportive	Davies & O'Berle 1990, 1992
	Heslin & Bramwell 1989
• Intensive caring, collaboration, continuous knowing and continuous giving	Dobratz 1990
• Fostering hope	Herth 1990
• Providing comfort	Degner et al 1991
• Providing an empathic relationship	Raudonis 1993
• Clinical, consultative with teaching, leadership and research functions	Webber 1993
• Being there and acting on the patient's behalf	Steeves et al 1994

ROLE OF THE PALLIATIVE CARE NURSE (GENERAL)

The few studies that have been carried out on the role of the nurse in palliative care are mainly North American.

Quint (1967) was the forerunner in this field. Her original research arose out of the grounded theory sociological study carried out in San Francisco, by Glaser & Strauss (1965, 1968) with Quint as a co-researcher in the team. Fieldwork from this study focused on what nurses do around dying patients in social relationships and work demands, in different ward settings. The nursing part of the investigation centred on what nursing students learn about death and *when* they learn. Quint's findings are still relevant today. Students are often inadequately prepared for dealing with death and dying and classroom teaching does not always match the reality of practice.

In a Canadian qualitative study, Degner et al (1991) identified seven critical nursing behaviours. Ten experienced palliative care nurses and 10 nurse educators were asked to describe situations in which student nurses or qualified nurses had displayed very positive or very negative attitudes towards care of the dying. The following seven critical behaviours were identified:

• Responding during the death scene
• Providing comfort
• Responding to anger
• Enhancing personal growth
• Responding to colleagues
• Enhancing the quality of life during dying
• Responding to the family

Using an extensive literature review the researchers compared theoretical findings with the results before returning to 15 of the respondents who identified that the descriptions accurately reflected their perceptions. Some of the language was, however, modified in accordance with their comments.

Interestingly, the authors have since used their results in their curricula content in Canada towards developing and testing a model of expert nursing practice in the care of the dying.

Williams (1982) in her American study examined the professional role in the care of the dying. Her subsequent conceptual framework for nurses engaged in the care of dying patients suggested that as the patient reaches a state of terminal illness they shift from the dependence of the sick role to a more independent and autonomous dying role. This role transition of the dying patient called for a complementary shift on the part of the doctor and nurse, the doctor's role essentially being that of curing and treatment orientation. Conversely, the nursing role was seen as caring and supportive, which became dominant when the patient was dying (Fig. 1.2).

These views could be viewed as somewhat simplistic and would not apply in specialist palliative care environments, such as hospices. They do, however, go some way to describe the fact that caring for the dying, particularly in the terminal phase of someone's illness, could be seen as fundamentally a nursing responsibility.

Brockopp et al (1991), in their North American study, examined the variables of anxiety, attitudes to death and perception of control in relation to the nurse's interaction with the dying patient. Data were collected, using questionnaires, from 105 palliative care, psychiatric and orthopaedic nurses in Canada. Significant differences were found in attitudes towards death and death anxiety between palliative care nurses and the non-palliative care nurses. The palliative care nurses who worked on a continuous basis with the dying had more positive attitudes about death than those who infrequently encountered death. In addition, palliative care nurses had less fear concerning their own mortality and the death of others. The results, however, do not explain how the palliative care nurses in the study developed their attitudes or their feelings regarding death. Neither do they substantiate the importance of such attitudes and feelings relative to patient care. Furthermore, the sample of palliative care nurses was an older and more experienced group of professionals. This factor may have had some bearing on their attitudes and feelings towards death.

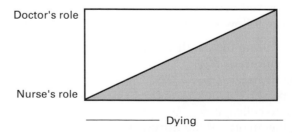

Fig. 1.2 Roles in the continuum of dying.

A FRAMEWORK FOR SPECIALIST PRACTICE IN PALLIATIVE NURSING CARE

Davies & O'Berle (1990, 1992) explored the dimensions of the palliative care nurse. The purpose of their study was to describe the clinical component of the nurse's role in palliative care. Data were collected, using a grounded theory approach, from in-depth retrospective descriptions of the care given by one clinical nurse specialist to 10 patients and their families. This included 25 hours of interviews.

Constant comparative analysis revealed that the nurse's role was a supportive one with multiple dimensions. From the findings, the researchers developed a model for palliative care nurses, which consists of six interwoven but discrete dimensions: valuing; connecting; empowering; doing for; finding meaning; and preserving integrity (see Fig. 1.3). Some of these dimensions are regarded as attitudinal, others are task-oriented, but all are regarded as playing a vital part in the support process (Davies & O'Berle 1990).

Valuing

There are two components to valuing: global and particular.

• **Global valuing** is having respect for the inherent worth of others. It involves being non-judgemental and having what Rogers (1967) would term 'unconditional positive regard'.

• **Particular valuing**, on the other hand, is about more individualised valuing and cannot occur until the nurse has developed a relationship with the individual.

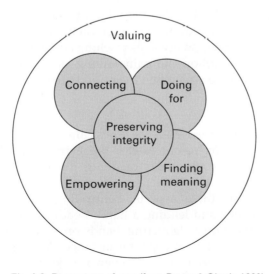

Fig. 1.3 Dimensions of care (from Davies & Oberle 1992).

Connecting

This refers to the nurse getting in touch with the patient and their family, entering their experience. There are three components of connection – making the connection; sustaining the connection; and breaking the connection.

Making the connection is about getting to know the patient in a deeper sense. It entails spending time with the patient or family, 'finding a common bond' and 'establishing rapport'. Central to making the connection is establishing trust: connection will not occur until trust has been established.

Sustaining the connection is about 'being available', 'spending time', 'sharing secrets' and 'giving of self'. Giving of self or self-awareness is central to the development of a trusting relationship.

Breaking the connection involves terminating the relationship. Although this often occurs with the patient's death, the nurse may continue to give bereavement support to the family after death.

Empowering

An important factor in nursing is enabling patients and families to care for themselves. It is 'strength giving' and 'invigorating'. There are five components to empowering: facilitating; encouraging; defusing; mending; and giving information.

Facilitating involves building on family and individual strengths by helping to plan strategies and make suggestions. The nurse recognises the patient's right to make decisions and gives the patient power to continue. Facilitating is also about recognising and accepting others' limitations and working with them towards a more positive outcome.

Encouraging acknowledges special abilities, gives approval, supports choices and encourages patient and family members to do what they want.

Defusing involves dealing with family members and patients' negative feelings and giving them the permission to have, express and deal with them.

Mending facilitates healing between family members by interpreting behaviours and enabling individuals to see each other's point of view.

Finally, giving information involves teaching and explaining about medication, changes in condition and pain. Giving factual information allows the patient and family to strengthen their ability to care for themselves.

Doing for

This is primarily concerned with the physical care of the patient. Doing for is about drawing on resources that are extrinsic to the patient and their family. The two components of doing for are: taking charge and team playing.

Taking charge has three aspects: controlling pain and symptoms; making arrangements; and lending a hand. Lending a hand is the aspect concerned with the nurse delivering hands-on care, usually when the family members can no longer cope; for instance, dealing with the patient after death. Hands-on care is not, however, a major remit of the specialist nurses' role.

Team playing involves negotiating the system on behalf of the patient, in other words acting as the patient's advocate. It involves sharing and consulting with other team members, working as part of a team, liaising with other members of the team, mediating on behalf of the patient and family and involving other members of the team. Much of this team work entails orchestrating the system for the benefit of the patient and their family.

Finding meaning

In palliative care the nurse helps the patient find meaning for their situation. It is empowering and strength giving and involves focusing on living and acknowledging death.

Focusing on living entails helping patients to make sense of their illness and prognosis. It involves helping them to live as fully as possible until they die. By acknowledging death, the nurse is able to talk openly about it when the patient and their family want to.

Acknowledging death requires the nurse not to run away from discussion of the subject. It involves giving or reiterating bad news and talking about death or the time left. The implication is that the nurse will enable patients and their families to come to terms with dying, by developing strategies to help them deal with the concept of dying and the actual process of dying.

Preserving integrity

The nurse in palliative care requires the ability to maintain feelings of self-worth and self-esteem. Maintaining energy levels is seen as integral to the effective functioning of the nurse. The nurse maintains energy levels and reduces stress by using particular strategies of distancing to regain self-control. For instance, she may use humour or hide personal feelings to protect herself.

The nurse maintains her self-esteem by: looking inward; valuing herself; and by acknowledging and questioning personal behaviour. Looking inward involves reflecting on the nurse's practice. This helps to reinforce the basic value of humanity and gives the strength to continue. The nurse may draw on her personal belief system or spirituality for this. Valuing self is of utmost importance in the preservation of integrity. Cues and reinforcements come from internal as well as external sources. Internal sources include reflecting on the nurse's practice; external sources include feedback from others. Finally, acknowledging one's own reactions involves continual self-assessment. The nurse must be satisfied that she is doing the right things for the right reasons. Identifying and recognising one's own feelings is important in maintaining perspective. Acknowledging and accepting one's own grief reaction is particularly important for integrated functioning. Recognising the need to set limits is also central to preserving one's own integrity. Only by preserving her own integrity is the nurse able to continue to find meaning in her work and to help patients and their families in their situations.

The key concepts here relate to the nurse as a person, as much as to being seen as central to the dimensions of nursing, thus implying that the nurse as a professional cannot be separated from the nurse as a person.

Despite the limitation in research design, i.e. using only one informant and relying on her reflections of her own practice, the findings of Davies and O'Berle's research have been widely adopted, including being the basis of the curriculum model for the palliative care courses.

ROLE OF THE NURSE IN HOSPICE

Surprisingly, there are no UK studies describing the role of the hospice nurse, despite the fact that the hospice movement was founded by Dame Cicely Saunders, herself a former nurse.

Dobratz (1990), an American nurse, examined the role of the hospice nurse in an extensive literature review. She identified four categories of nursing function in hospice care:

- Intensive caring, managing the physical, psychological, social and spiritual problems of dying persons and their families
- Collaborative sharing, the co-ordinated and collaborated efforts of the extended and expanded components of hospice care services
- Continuous knowing, the acquisition of the counselling, managing, instructing, caring and communicating skills/knowledge required for the specialty of hospice nursing
- Continuous giving, the balance of the hospice nurses' own self-care needs with the complexities and intensities of death and dying

This study goes some way to describing in detail what hospice nurses do. There is, however, a note of caution to be observed in generalising findings, with respect to the cultural context of the American health care system.

Raudonis' (1993) naturalistic field study explored patients' perspectives of the nature, meaning and impact of empathic relationships with hospice nurses. Data were collected through in-depth interviews with 14 terminally ill adults receiving home-based hospice care. The findings showed that an empathic relationship with the nurse developed through a process of reciprocal sharing in the context of caring and acceptance. This was based on being acknowledged as an individual, a person of value. The outcome of this empathic relationship between hospice nurses and their patients was maintenance or improvement of the patient's physical and emotional well-being. Understanding the patient as an autonomous person was seen as being critical for effective nursing intervention and a meaningful outcome.

This study is particularly important because the findings were elicited directly from patients. The most important aspect of the relationship for the patients was the acknowledgement of their individuality.

Hull (1991) also examined the caring behaviours of hospice nurses, as perceived by family caregivers in a hospice home care programme.

Semistructured interviews and participant observation were used to collect data from a sample of 10 families. Four areas of caring behaviours of hospice nurses were identified: 24-hour accessibility; effective communication; clinical competence; and non-judgemental attitudes.

It is evident from reviewing the literature, in relation to the role of the nurse in the hospice setting, that this area is under-researched.

CLINICAL NURSE SPECIALISTS IN PALLIATIVE CARE

Various authors in recent years have examined the role of the Macmillan Nurse (Cox, Bergen & Norman 1993, Bullen 1995, Graves & Nash 1992, M Kindlen, unpublished work 1987, Nash 1991, Sloan & Grant 1989, Webber 1993).

On the whole, the role of the Macmillan Nurse is perceived favourably by both practitioners and patients and their families. This role has provided a model for clinical nurse specialists in the UK. However, it should be taken into account that their perceived role is emotive to both professionals and lay people.

While existing research has advanced the body of knowledge regarding the role of the Macmillan Nurse, this has largely been from the practitioner's viewpoint. Attempts to elicit the views of patients and carers have been limited. This is partly due to ethical problems in facilitating such a study. The author conducted a major study using in-depth interviews and a repertory grid technique with patients and nurses to explore their perceptions of palliative nursing care. Findings demonstrated that there were marked differences between patients' and nurses' perceptions. For instance, all patients stated the importance of listening, the nurse being there and the nurse meeting their needs. On the other hand, the nurses stressed the importance of knowledge, experience and providing comfort (Johnston 1998).

■ REFLECTIVE PRACTICE 1.7   The role of the nurse

In Johnston's (1998) study there is a marked difference between nurses' and patients' perceptions about the nurses' role in palliative care.

• Do the nurses' views in this study reflect a patient-centred approach?
• What are the implications of this for palliative care nursing?

What then are the key characteristics of the role of the nurse in palliative care. This author would argue that in order to be an 'expert' nurse in palliative care, the nurse needs to have human qualities, such as compassion and empathy, combined with professional knowledge and experience of the specialty and effective communication skills.

WHERE DO WE GO FROM HERE?

What then is the future for palliative care and nursing? The future of nursing, despite recent reports that a generic health worker is the way forward, looks positive. With the implementation of the Calman and Hines report, numerous possibilities exist, particularly for those nurses working in cancer care (HMSO 1995, SHHD 1995). These reports have identified three contexts in which cancer palliative care will be delivered – the cancer centre, the cancer unit and the primary care setting – and makes a strong case for the establishment of key specialist nursing posts in each of these settings. In addition, the Royal College of Nursing Cancer Nursing Society has advocated the setting up of a structure which ensures that people affected by cancer will have access to expert nursing (RCN 1996).

Other initiatives that will serve to enhance the value of nursing in palliative care include nurse practitioner posts. Traditionally, nurse practitioner roles complement the role of the doctor. For example a nurse practitioner in an accident and emergency department would take on roles, such as treatment of minor injuries, without reference to a doctor, therefore allowing medical expertise to be applied where it is most needed (Scott 1995). In an innovative scheme in Hull, nurse practitioners were set up in a hospice. Their role incorporated: being consulted about pain and symptom control; being involved in research; taking on extra responsibilities clinically, including venepuncture and making decisions about readmission of patients; and being designated liaison contacts with outside agencies (Scott 1995).

With the development of an increasing number of specialist courses in palliative care at degree and postgraduate level, there will be more opportunities for developing specialist and advanced practitioners in palliative care.

SUMMARY

This chapter has emphasised the importance of the nursing role in palliative care and suggested ways in which that role might be enhanced in the future. It has explored the key characteristics of the role of the nurse in palliative care and explored the literature in this area. Finally, the words of Solzhenitsyn (1968) help to sum up the role of the nurse in palliative care:

> *How many adult human beings are there, now at this very minute, rushing about in mute panic wishing they could find a nurse, the kind of person to whom they can pour out the fears they have deeply concealed?*

REFERENCES

Addington-Hall J, McCarthy M 1995 Dying from cancer: results of a national population-based investigation. Palliative Medicine 9: 295–305

Ajemain I 1993 The interdisciplinary team. In: Doyle D, Hanks G W C, Macdonald N P (eds) Oxford textbook of palliative medicine. Oxford University Press, Oxford, pp 17–28

Anstey S 1993 Care in acute hospital units. Nursing Standard 7: 51

Bates T D, Hoy A M, Clarke D G, Laird P P 1981 The St Thomas' hospital terminal care support team – a new concept of hospice care. Lancet I: 1201–1203

Benner P 1984 From novice to expert. Addison Wesley Publishing Company, California

Brockopp D Y, King D B, Hamilton J E 1991 The dying patient: a comparative study of nurse care giver characteristics. Death Studies 15: 245–258

Buckman R 1993 Communication in palliative care: a practical guide. In: Doyle D, Hanks G W C, Macdonald N P (eds) Oxford textbook of palliative medicine. Oxford University Press, Oxford, 47–61

Bullen M 1995 The role of the specialist nurse in palliative care. Professional Nurse 10: 755–756

Campbell A 1984 Moderated love. SPCK, London

Cartwright A 1991 Balance of care for the dying between hospitals and the community. Perceptions of GPs; hospital consultants; community nurses and relatives. British Journal of General Practice 1: 10–14

Cox K, Bergen A, Norman I J 1993 Exploring consumer views of care provided by the Macmillan nurse using the critical incident techniques. Journal of Advanced Nursing 18: 408–415

Davies B, O'Berle K 1990 Dimensions of the supportive role of the nurse. in palliative care. Oncology Nurses Forum 17: 87–94

Davies B, O'Berle K 1992 Support and caring – exploring the concepts. Oncology Nurses Forum 19: 763–767

Degner L F, Gow C M, Thompson L A 1991 Critical nursing behaviours in care for the dying. Cancer Nursing 14: 246–253

Directory of Hospice Services 1998 Hospice Information Service, St Christopher's Hospice, London

Dobratz M C 1990 Hospice nursing: present perspectives and future directives. Cancer Nursing 13: 116–122

Douglas C 1992 For all the saints. British Medical Journal 304: 579

Doyle D 1992 The challenge of the disadvantaged dying in cancer nursing changing frontiers. Proceedings of the Weekend Symposium of the 7th International Cancer Conference, Vienna

Dunlop R J, Hockley J M 1990 Terminal care support teams. The Hospital–Hospice Interface. Oxford Medical Publications, Oxford

Dunn V 1992 Palliative care problems addressed and problems created in cancer nursing changing frontiers. Proceedings of the Weekend Symposium of the 7th International Cancer Conference, Vienna

Faulkner A 1993 Teaching interactive skills in health care. Chapman and Hall, London

Faulkner A, Maguire P 1994 Talking to cancer patients and their relatives. Oxford University Press, Oxford

Field D 1989 Nursing the dying. Tavistock/Routledge, London

Field D, James N 1993 Where and how people die? In: Clark D (ed) The future for palliative care. Open University Press, Bucks, 6–29

Glaser B G, Strauss A 1965 Awareness of dying. Aldine Publishing Company, New York

Glaser B G, Strauss A 1968 Time for dying. Aldine Publishing Company, New York

Gooch J 1988 Dying in the ward. Nursing Times 84: 38–39

Graves D, Nash A 1991 Macmillan nurse perceptions. Journal of District Nursing July: 4–6

Graves D, Nash A 1992 A friendship that inspires hope: a study of Macmillan nurses' working patterns. Professional Nurse April: 478–485

Griffin J 1991 Dying with dignity. Office of Health Economics, London

Harris L 1991 The disadvantaged dying. Nursing Times 86: 26–29

Heaven C M, Maguire P 1996 Training hospice nurses to elicit patient concerns. Journal of Advanced Nursing 23: 280–286

Herd E B 1990 Terminal care in a semi-rural area. British Journal of General Practice 40: 248–251

Herth K 1990 Fostering hope in terminally ill people. Journal of Advanced Nursing 15: 1250–1259

Heslin K, Bramwell L 1989 The supportive role of the staff nurse in the hospital palliative care situation. Journal of Palliative Care 5: 20–26

Higginson I, Wade A, McCarthy M 1990 Palliative care: views of patients and their families. British Medical Journal 301: 277–281

Hill D, Penso D 1995 Opening doors: improving access to hospice and palliative care services by members of the black and ethnic minority communities. National Council for Hospice and Specialist Palliative Care Services Occasional Paper, 7 Jan 1995

Hinton J 1979 Comparison of places and policies for terminal care. The Lancet i: 29–32

HMSO 1992 The provision of palliative care. Standing Nursing and Midwifery Advisory Committee and Standing Medical Advisory Committee. Her Majesty's Stationery Office, London

HMSO 1995 A policy framework for commissioning cancer services. A report by the expert advisory group on cancer to meet the chief medical officers of England and Wales. Her Majesty's Stationery Office, London

Hockley J M 1989 Caring for the dying in acute hospitals. Nursing Times Occasional Paper 55: 47–50

Hockley J M, Dunlop R, Davies R J 1988 Survey of distressing symptoms in dying patients and their families in hospital and the response to a symptom control team. British Medical Journal 296: 1715–1717

Hull M M 1991 Hospice nurses' caring support for caregiving families. Cancer Nursing 14(2): 63–70

Hull R, Ellis M, Sargent V 1989 Teamwork in palliative care. Radcliffe Medical Press, Oxford

Irvine B M 1993 Developments in palliative nursing in and out of the hospital setting. British Journal of Nursing 2: 218–224

Johnson I, Rogers C, Biswas B, Ahmedzai S 1990 What do hospices do? A survey of hospices in the United Kingdom and Republic of Ireland. British Medical Journal 300: 791–793

Johnston B 1998 A major study using indepth interviews and repertory grid technique to explore the perceptions of nurses and patients regarding palliative nursing care. In: RCN: the leading edge. International Nursing Research Conference, 3–5 April 1998, Edinburgh, UK

Lamerton R 1980 Care of the dying. Penguin Books Ltd, Harmondsworth

Lawler J 1991 Behind the screens: nursing, somology and the problem of the body. Churchill Livingstone, Edinburgh

Macleod Clark J 1983 Nurse–patient communication – an analysis of conversations from surgical wards. In: Wilson-Barnett J (ed) Nursing research: ten studies in patient care. John Wiley and Sons, Chichester, pp 25–26

Morse J 1991 Negotiating commitment and involvement in the nurse–patient relationship. Journal of Advanced Nursing 16: 455–468

Muetzel P 1988 Therapeutic nursing. In: Pearson A (ed) Primary nursing: nursing in the Burford and Oxford nursing development units. Croom Helm, London, pp 89–116

Murray Parkes C 1985 Terminal care: home, hospital or hospice. The Lancet 1: 155–157

NCHSPCS 1995 Specialist palliative care; a statement of definitions. National Council for Hospice and Specialist Palliative Care Services, London

Nightingale F 1980 Notes on nursing: what it is and what it is not. Churchill Livingstone, Edinburgh

Norum J 1995 Cancer patients dying at home: care providers' experience. Journal of Cancer Care 4: 157–160

Perry B 1996 Influence of nurse gender on the use of silence, touch and humour. International Journal of Palliative Nursing 21: 7–14

Quint J C 1967 The nurse and the dying patient. Macmillan, New York

Quint Benoliel J C 1988 Symposium on palliative care review lecture. In: Pritchard A P (ed) Proceedings of the 5th International Conference on Cancer Care. Cancer Nursing. A Revolution in Care. Macmillan Press Ltd, London, pp 178–181

Raudonis B M 1993 The meaning and impact of empathic relationships in hospice nursing. Cancer Nursing 16: 304–309

Reisetter K, Thomas B 1986 Nursing care of the dying: its relationship to selected nurse characteristics. International Journal of Nursing Studies 23: 39–50

Royal College of Nursing Cancer Nursing Society 1996 A structure for cancer nursing services. RCN, London

Saunders C 1991/2 The evolution of the hospices. Free Inquiry 12: 19–23

Saunders C 1993 Introduction – history and challenge. In: Saunders C, Sykes N (eds) The management of terminal malignant disease. Edward Arnold, London, pp 1–14

Savage J 1995 Nursing intimacy: an ethnographic approach to nurse–patient interaction. Scutari Press, London

Scott G 1995 Challenging conventional roles. Palliative Care Nursing Times 91: 38–39

Seale C F 1991 A comparison of hospice and conventional care. Social Science and Medicine 32: 147–152

Seale C F 1992 Community nurses and care of the dying. Social Science and Medicine 34: 375–382

SHHD 1995 Scottish Cancer Co-Ordinating and Advisory Committee; Commission Cancer Services Committee. Interim Report to the Chief Medical Officer, December 1995. Scottish Office, Edinburgh

Sloan D, Grant M 1989 Evaluating a Macmillan nursing service. Senior Nurse 9: 20–21

Solzhenitsyn A 1968 Cancer ward. Penguin Books, Harmondsworth

Spiller J A, Alexander D A 1993 Domiciliary care: a comparison of the views of terminally patients and their family caregivers. Palliative Medicine 7: 109–115

Stedeford A 1994 Facing death; patients, families and professionals, 2nd edn. Sobell Publications, Oxford

Steeves R, Cohen M Z, Wise C T 1994 An analysis of critical incidents describing the essence of oncology nursing. Oncology Nursing Forum Supplement 218: 19–25

Thorpe G 1993 Enabling more people to die at home. British Medical Journal 307: 915–918

Townsend J, Frank A O, Fermont D, Dyer S, Karran O, Walgrove A, Piper M 1990 Terminal cancer care and patients' preference for place of death: a prospective study. British Medical Journal 301: 415–417

Vachon M L S 1987 Occupational stress in the care of the critically ill, the dying and bereaved. Hemisphere Publishing Company, Washington

Walsh M, Ford P 1989 Nursing rituals: research and rational actions. Butterworth–Heinemann Ltd, Oxford

Watson J 1988 Nursing: human science and human care: a theory of nursing. National League for Nursing, New York

Webber J 1993 The evolving role of the Macmillan nurse. Unpublished Paper, Cancer Relief Macmillan Fund

WHO 1990 Cancer pain relief and palliative care. Technical Report Series 804. World Health Organization, Geneva

Williams C A 1982 Role considerations in care of the dying patient. Image 14: 8–11

Wilkinson S 1991 Factors which influence how nurses communicate with cancer patients. Journal of Advanced Nursing 16: 677–688

Non-specialist nurse education in palliative care

2

Margaret Kindlen   Sheena Walker

THE NON-SPECIALIST NURSE IN PALLIATIVE CARE

In this chapter we will focus on the registered nurse in the adult branch of nursing. We will examine how non-specialist palliative care nurses can develop knowledge, skills and attitudes to deliver, and to demonstrate to others, the highest possible quality of palliative care to their client group. In the context of education, we will encourage you to build your professional profile in palliative care through reflective practice. We hope to provide a stimulus for the reader to operate as a facilitator for student nurses, care assistants and others who have first-line contact with patients, thereby providing the opportunity for the principles of palliative care to be as widely available as possible.

LEARNING OUTCOMES

This chapter addresses the PREP categories of care enhancement and educational development. Having read this chapter you should be:

- Familiar with the principles of palliative care
- Aware of the different strategies appropriate to acquisition of competencies in palliative care
- Confident about how professional profiling can help you to develop competencies in palliative care

BACKGROUND OF PALLIATIVE CARE

Palliative care is the active, total care of patients whose disease is not responsive to curative treatment. Control of pain, of other symptoms and of psychological, social and spiritual problems is paramount. The goal of palliative care is achievement of the best possible quality of life for patients and their families. Many aspects of palliative care are also applicable earlier in the course of the illness in conjunction with anti-cancer treatment [WHO 1990].

Palliative care is not new. Its establishment as a medical and nursing specialty in the late 1980s raised its profile. Palliative care has been strongly influenced by the voluntary hospice movement and today this is reflected in the voice of the National Council for Hospice and Specialist Palliative Care Services (NCHSPCS). This organisation was established in 1991 as a co-ordinating and representative body for the hospice movement in England, Wales and Northern Ireland. Scotland has its equivalent organisation in the Scottish Partnership Agency for Palliative and Cancer Care. Both organisations have dialogue with the NHS, Government, politicians and other health care providers on policies and standards in palliative care. A major influence of the NCHSPCS has been its wide range of publications that provide guidelines for good practice in specialist and non-specialist palliative care. The integration of specialist palliative care into mainstream health care, as recommended by Wilkes (1980), has recently gathered momentum.

It has been long recognised that the experience gained from palliative care in cancer ought to be extended to the care of people with other chronic, diseases. This view is echoed in the 'Barcelona declaration on palliative care' (EAPC 1995) which states that 'Palliative Care must be included as part of governmental health policy as recommended by the World Health Organization'. It goes on to say that every individual has the right to pain relief and that 'Palliative Care must be provided according to the principle of equity, irrespective of race, gender, ethnicity, social status, national origin and the ability to pay for services'.

Various agencies and people have identified a need to consider palliative care in specialist and general practice (Finlay & Jones 1995, NHCSPCS 1995, SPAPCC 1996). The following definitions have emerged.

- **A palliative care approach** involves core skills for every clinician in health care. It aims to promote the principles of palliative care to all patients, whatever the illness, its stage or the context of the care setting. It emphasises the importance of considering psychological and spiritual, as well as the physical, aspects of illness and incorporates consideration of family and domestic carers.

- **Palliative interventions** include a number of non-curative treatments that are used by specialists in disciplines other than palliative care. The aim is to improve quality of life by managing symptoms. Examples of palliative interventions include surgical procedure, radiotherapy, chemotherapy and anaesthetic techniques used in pain relief.

- **Specialist palliative care** is delivered by a multiprofessional team, the members of which have specialist accredited training. Specialist palliative care is provided directly in a variety of settings, including in-patient, day care and home care, and indirectly through advice to other professionals, patients and carers. Specialist palliative care practitioners have a responsibility for research and effective education to widely disseminate the lessons learned. They must also be available to provide support to those giving care with a palliative approach.

Palliative care in context

Despite growth of palliative care services in the community, it is still the trend, in the UK, for the majority of deaths to occur in institutional settings. Although approximately one in 10 deaths worldwide are from cancer, many more are from other life-threatening conditions, i.e. those of cardiac, respiratory or neurological origin, or from AIDS and diseases of the elderly (EAPC 1995). This would suggest that all nurses working in hospital, the community, nursing homes and in specialist services need to be competent in their practice of palliative care. However, according to the WHO definition, 'many aspects of palliative care are also applicable earlier in the course of the illness in conjunction with anti-cancer treatment'. It is therefore possible that nurses in occupational health settings, health visitors, practice nurses and those working in custodial institutions will, from time to time, require to draw on the principles of palliative care nursing in order to meet the needs of their client group.

SPECIALIST PALLIATIVE CARE NURSES AND NURSING IN PALLIATIVE CARE

The specialist palliative care definition is mirrored in Webber's (1993) description of the evolving role of the clinical nurse specialist in palliative care. She noted that the primary concern of the clinical nurse specialist is to bring the highest standards of clinical care to the patient. There are two key principles involved. The first is that the clinical nurse specialist is not the primary carer and the second is the importance of research-driven practice feeding a role in the leadership and education of others. The Webber model (1993) presents three levels of expertise and specialist activity required for different palliative care situations (Table 2.1).

According to definitions, Level 1 of Webber's (1993) model represents a palliative care approach and the level of competencies identified should be expected of any registered nurse. Level 2 competencies would be expected of nurses who have had formal education in palliative care or who have acquired them through experience. Level 3 competencies are advanced and should be expected of nurses experienced in palliative care who have undertaken advanced educational programmes.

Webber's (1993) model underpins the RCN Cancer Nursing Society's statement, which differentiates between a nurse working within a specialty

Table 2.1 Levels of expertise and specialist activity required for different palliative care (after Webber 1993)

Level	Competencies required to assess and plan care	Specialist activity
Level 1 **Competencies expected of all registered nurses**	• Establish empathy • Listen • Elicit information • Give information • Assess needs, symptoms, psychosocial distress and the impact of these upon the patient and family • Recognise situations where referral is required • Represent patient and family needs to others	Indirect services • Formal and informal teaching • Consultancy • Support primary carers in the development and auditing of clinical standards • Ensure that policies are developed and monitored for use in the clinical environment • Disseminate research results and promote valid research findings as the basis for practice • Contribute to the creation of a working climate in which staff feel valued and supported Direct service There may be many clinical areas where Level 1 competencies have not been developed. In such cases the specialist may need to offer limited direct services until the foundation level of expertise has been reached
Level 2 **Competencies expected of nurses working within the specialty of palliative care**	• Assess patients and families presenting with clearly identified and treatable physical and/or psychological problems and needs • Implement protocols and monitor their effect • When appropriate assist clients to express and explore emotionally distressing feelings • Utilise interventions to prevent physical and psychological problems developing or escalating • Recognise situations and problems requiring referral	Indirect services • Consultancy • Formal and informal teaching • Develop and evaluate interventions and protocols to be used by primary nurses • Provide support for staff in stressful situations Direct service • Undertake joint assessments with primary nurses • Assist primary nurses to plan and implement care • Modelling good practice • Accept referrals

Table 2.1 Levels of expertise and specialist activity required for different palliative care (contd)

Level	Competencies required to assess and plan care	Specialist activity
Level 3 **Competencies expected** **of advanced** **practitioner**	• Assess, plan and implement interventions for patients experiencing complex or intractable physical symptoms • Assess, plan and implement care for those with multifaceted complex psychosocial problems • Provide psychological support using a recognised therapeutic framework or model • Seek personal supervision when required • Recognise situations requiring referral	Indirect services • Assist with problem definition • Explore approaches to complex problem management • Provide supervision for nurses offering short-term psychological care of patients and families • Provide information about resources available to achieve objectives • Research and refine interventions • Support staff in stressful situations Direct services • Accept referrals • Assess degree of complexity of need and problems • Provide ongoing care and support for those with intractable/multifaceted physical and psychosocial problems

and a specialist nurse. The nurse working within a specialty provides the day-to-day care for patients in units specialising in, for example, palliative care. The specialist nurse is someone who has studied to a higher and advanced degree and has in-depth and specific knowledge and skills in palliative care. In contrast, there is also the registered nurse, who requires a knowledge of the principles of palliative care in order to apply these to patients nursed in more general and other specialist contexts, e.g. general medical, surgical or care of the elderly (RCN 1996). Using Webber's model, Level 1 and 2 competencies could be expected of non-specialist palliative care nurses and nurses working within the specialty of palliative care. Nurses working in specialist palliative care positions, offering consultancy to others, would be expected to have achieved Level 3 competencies.

■ REFLECTIVE PRACTICE 2.1   Profile in palliative care: registered nurses' experience in palliative care

At any one time the population of practising nurses will include those who have qualified over a period of 40 years. Inevitably there are changes in health care policy, professional practice and education philosophy and many of these occur during the working life of a nurse. The PREP requirements are the first statutory requirement for nurses to show that they are credible in their particular field of practice.

With specific reference to the group of nurses that you currently work with, do you recognise Level 1 competencies as identified in the Webber (1993) model (Table 2.1)?

Ask each of the nurses with whom you work if:

- The preregistration education they received effectively prepared them to care for chronically ill and dying patients
- They think they are competent and confident with this group of patients. To what do they attribute this confidence?

Finlay & Jones (1995) stress that recognition of the difference between general and specialist palliative care may serve to reduce confusion about the 'legitimate province' of palliative care. They illustrate this in the example of a patient with advanced cardiac disease requiring palliative intervention from a cardiologist. A specialist in palliative medicine may become involved to advise on opiates and sedation for chest pain or intractable dyspnoea and may provide additional help in supporting psychological distress in both the patient and family.

Finlay & Jones (1995) further state that in the business culture of health care provision, it is important for those purchasing and providing palliative care services to ensure that palliative care, according to the three definitions cited on page 28, is identified and integrated to the maximum for the benefit of patients, carers and professionals. The implication is for all nurses, regardless of their clinical setting, to adopt the principles of palliative care.

PRINCIPLES OF PALLIATIVE CARE

What are the principles of palliative care? The modern hospice movement was founded on the premise that there were large deficits in the care for people approaching death. The goal of the pioneers in hospice care was to remedy that situation: to build a philosophy and body of knowledge that would permeate the entire spectrum of health care, in the belief that every human being and those who matter to that person would receive compassionate care at the end of life. To deliver this type of care the professional requires the skills to 'be with' a person in suffering, whether the source of distress be physical, emotional, spiritual or social. These were the elements of total pain that Saunders (1978) posited in her early philosophy and around which a multidisciplinary approach to care was developed. To 'be with' someone in suffering requires the ability to:

- Respect the identity and integrity of other human beings
- Be sensitive and non-judgemental
- Know when to listen and when to speak
- Have the knowledge and skills to intervene in a way that promotes the best possible quality of life as perceived by the patient

One might argue that these qualities cannot be taught but are learned through life experiences. The counter argument is for a model of education to promote value and respect for students during the formative years of preparation for their chosen career and for organisations to continue to respect and value members of staff, the principle being that to deliver 'whole person care' the professional needs to feel a 'whole person' (Doyle 1996, Sheldon 1996). In this chapter we are concerned with palliative care in the context of ongoing professional education and how that education can be acquired.

POSTREGISTRATION EDUCATION FOR PRACTICE (PREP)

In the UKCC (1992a) document 'The scope of professional practice', nurses are reminded that they are personally accountable for their practice and, in the exercise of professional accountability, each nurse must:

- Maintain and improve his professional knowledge and competence
- Acknowledge any limitations in his knowledge and competence
- Decline any duties or responsibilities unless able to perform them in a safe and skilled manner

In its position statement, the UKCC also states that postregistration education equips practitioners with additional and more specialist skills that are necessary to meet the special needs of patients and clients. There is a broad range of postregistration provision and the UKCC regards adequate and effective provision of quality education as a prerequisite of quality care.

The education structure for nurses has changed. There is now emphasis on preparation to diploma and degree level with further opportunities for advanced study at postgraduate diploma, master and doctorate levels. Such academic preparation encourages evidence-based reflective and questioning practice. Nurses have sufficient insight to identify deficits in their own knowledge, skills and attitudes, which can be addressed through professional development.

PREP requires:

- Nurses to maintain and enhance standards of care in order to meet the needs of patients, clients and health services
- That newly registered nurses are supported in their practice
- Professional development for the nurse and achievement of advanced practitioner status

There is a statutory requirement for every nurse, during the 3 years leading to periodic registration, to provide evidence of appropriate learning by completing a minimum of 5 days of study (UKCC 1990).

PROFESSIONAL PORTFOLIO AND PROFILES

The UKCC requires nurses to build an individual portfolio. Within this, there is scope for a profile on palliative care. In the RCN Nursing Update programme, Kelly (1995) defined portfolio and profile.

A portfolio is a personal collection of evidence, private to the owner, which demonstrates the continuing acquisition of skills, knowledge, attitudes, understanding and achievement. It deals with the past, present and future and should cover both professional and personal life

A profile is a selection of evidence extracted from your portfolio when you have a specific need. It will be shown to others to fulfil a specific function.

In this chapter our concern is about how the non-specialist nurse can develop competencies in palliative care. We have chosen to do this by encouraging the development of a palliative care profile.

The ENB guidelines (1995) on profiling recommend its use to:

- Record evidence of professional experience, thus meeting the requirements for PREP
- Support a job application
- Facilitate reflective practice
- Feed individual performance reviews by helping employee and employer identify and plan how an employee's personal goals within an organisation can be achieved
- Focus on organising personal learning
- Support learning from practice and clinical supervision
- Demonstrate evidence of learning
- Assist towards assessment for an education award
- Provide evidence to support a claim for accreditation of prior learning

We have discussed PREP, and our intention throughout this chapter is to demonstrate reflective practice as a fundamental skill in the learning process. In the context of job application it is sufficient to say that a well-maintained professional portfolio will feed a CV document. Here we are more concerned about building a profile in palliative care and will deal with this below the headings of Continuing professional education, Individual personal review (IPR), Personal learning and Organising a profile.

Continuing professional education

Our code of professional conduct requires every nurse 'to maintain and improve his professional knowledge and competence' (UKCC 1992b). We have already stated that a palliative care approach should be within the repertoire of every registered practitioner. So how can non-specialist nurses develop this approach within their continuing professional education?

Webber (1993) suggested levels of competencies expected of every registered nurse and those which ought to be acquired alongside growing participation in palliative care interventions and specialist care. How these are achieved is dependent on the overall philosophy that exists in organisations towards continuing professional education of nurses. Maggs (1996) places continuing professional education in the context of career development. He describes continuing professional education as a 'partnership involving the individual practitioner, the profession and the employer'. This supports Roache & Baldwin's (1995) conceptual model that practice and education are an equal partnership involving personal professional and political influences.

Individual performance review

As an employee you are subject to periodic individual performance reviews (IPR). This process involves both retrospective and prospective reviews of one's own performance, together with an agreement, drawn up between employee and an employer, that is representative of the employee's future performance objectives over a stated period, usually 1 year. Your portfolio has a major contribution in this process. Evidence can be produced of achievements and non-achievements of previously planned objectives. The prospective element of the review provides an opportunity for development of a plan of personal goals identified to the benefit of employee, employer and the client group. The third stage of the IPR process is an agreement with the employer, which is representative of what is achievable through personal effort (independent of employer support) and what resources can realistically be offered through employment support to facilitate achievement of the employee's professional development.

With regard to formal education, there may be agreed arrangements with identified education institutions, thus giving practitioners formal study time. Alternatively, many education agencies now provide flexible open and distance-learning programmes for practitioners to choose from without having to negotiate study leave.

Personal learning

IPR is one way of identifying personal learning needs. Organisation of these can be difficult without the focus of a formal programme of study.

It is worth pausing to consider what learning is. We all know colleagues who, until PREP's statutory requirements, claimed not to have continued their education beyond their professional qualification. Yet, many of these nurses are skilled and informed in their practice. The explanation for this lies in an individual's perception of education and failure to value private reading, consultation with colleagues and specialists, together with personal professional experience, as education. Your portfolio is a way of 'formalising' this 'informal' education.

Adult education recognises the wealth of experience that people accumulate and that meaningful learning is guaranteed when its relevance is seen in practice. Kolb's (1984) learning cycle explains the connection between experience and learning (Fig. 2.1). Learning often begins with a concrete experience. You then make observations, reflect and decide on what new knowledge or skill you need to become more effective in your professional practice. With help from a variety of resources, you generate and refine new ideas. Finally, you test out and obtain feedback on these ideas.

As you proceed further through this chapter we hope to provide you with opportunities to examine ways in which reflection on practice can help you to develop your practice in palliative care.

Reflective practice

Schon (1983) described two aspects of reflective practice: 'reflection on action' and 'reflection in action'. Reflection on action is a retrospective review of a situation. This increases self-awareness and provides an opportunity to refer to theory and to better understand actions and decisions that were taken. In contrast, reflection in action involves the application of learning base on theory, from a previous experience into a current situation. Both activities feed a systematic approach to personal, professional development.

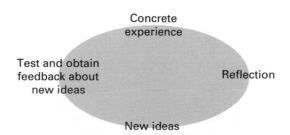

Fig. 2.1 The Kolb learning cycle (adapted).

■ REFLECTIVE PRACTICE 2.2   Portfolio in palliative care: acquiring competencies

Earlier in this chapter we identified from Webber's (1993) work competencies what every registered nurse should possess to deliver palliative care. Take a moment to think about your current clinical practice and how often a specialist palliative care nurse is requested to deliver *directly* the skills listed below.

• Establish empathy
• Listen
• Elicit information
• Give information
• Assess needs, symptoms, psychosocial distress and the impact of these upon the patient and family
• Recognise situations where referral is required
• Represent patient and family needs to others

If you are not confident with your level of the above competencies, or if it is usual practice to invite a specialist palliative care nurse to 'take over' the care of a patient, then you should formulate some personal learning objectives around each of the above competencies. For each, consider the knowledge, skill and attitude component. Each will require a different strategy for achievement.

Your aim should be to use the specialist palliative care nurse as a consultant, a source of support and an information resource as you develop the above competencies.

If, on the other hand, you are confident with these Level 1 competencies and are satisfied that specialist palliative care nurses are appropriately consulted, review the Level 2 competencies in Table 2.1 and work through the above process.

ORGANISING A PROFILE

Hull & Redfern (1996) promote profiling as a major activity in professional development, which encourages practitioners to consider their preferred style of learning, to identify what prevents their learning and how to overcome such difficulties. It also requires reflection upon past experience and working out how best to learn. They further recommend that you use your profile to:

• Collect relevant articles and references
• Write notes on a regular basis about what you have learned and what you need to find out more about
• Record the outcomes of any self or peer assessment and the necessary action that you subsequently need to take

■ REFLECTIVE PRACTICE 2.3   Portfolio in palliative care: resources

What are the different resources that you can use for your personal learning in palliative care?

Resources

On a personal basis, keeping up to date with principles and practices in palliative care requires you to regularly scan your library catalogues for journal articles and textbooks in all health care disciplines.

There is a range of multiprofessional journals in palliative care now available, in addition to the non-specialist publications, which do publish research in palliative care articles. To help you find these, the British Library publishes 'Palliative care index' (an abstract index) every month as does the Leeds Medical Information bimonthly ('Progress in palliative care'). Hospices and palliative care units invariably have education resources, such as journals, textbooks, videos and self-directed learning packages, which you may be able to negotiate the use of. If you have access to the internet, there is a growing number of website addresses with palliative care information.

Information on study days and conferences is available from the Hospice Information Service, through various newsletters and journals from palliative care specialist organisations. The RCN update series has included palliative care and this can be viewed on the television 'learning zone programme' in the UK. Finally, there are a growing number of specialist palliative services in hospitals and the community. All such specialists are involved in education through local, and often national, education initiatives and have consultancy and support of primary carers as part of their professional role.

Stating competencies

Recording development in competencies requires practitioners to be acquainted with the knowledge, skills and attitude components of learning and to be aware that different levels of learning are reflected in their clinical practice. Using the management of pain as our example, Table 2.2 maps out competencies, i.e. how a practitioner demonstrates understanding of knowledge in clinical practice. According to this table application, analysis, synthesis and decision-making, based on understanding of knowledge of pain management, can be demonstrated in a practitioner's clinical performance. In Table 2.2 this is stated as competencies or may also be described as learning outcomes. If Table 2.2 is viewed alongside Table 2.1, which depicts Webber's model, it would be fair to suggest that the non-specialist nurse, i.e. Level 1 and 2 in Webber's framework, could be expected to develop competencies that demonstrate application of understanding of knowledge of pain management.

Evidence of learning

When taking responsibility for your own professional education it is important to be able to supply evidence that learning has occurred. When, for example, you attend a lecture, study day or short course you may be provided with a certificate of attendance to present in evidence of your professional development. A well-documented record of evidence of meaningful learning can be submitted in application, for consideration of prior learning, towards formal academic accreditation. Such evidence can be demonstrated through an account of your reflective observation on practice. The following sections might be used:

- Brief details of the event
- Significant learning points from the content
- Personal learning outcomes
- Action plan
- Evidence of integration of new learning into practice, e.g. by providing narratives examining application of new learning in your clinical experience
- A record of new or improved level of competence

Feedback on learning can be obtained both formally and informally. Your professional colleagues are perhaps the most frequent source for you to check out your competencies. We have already discussed how feedback on clinical performance can be obtained in a formal way through IPR. Clinical supervision and formal education experience are other ways of validating the evidence that can be produced through your profile.

Clinical supervision

The aim of clinical supervision is to promote good clinical standards and innovative practice. Fowler (1996) states that the purpose of supervision must be clearly understood and followed by both supervisor and the practitioners being supervised. One criterion that he identifies for supervision combines professional development, pastoral care and assessment. This is echoed by Darley (1996) who describes clinical supervision as:

> ... a medium for encouraging practitioners or a group of practitioners to work with a supervisor to reflect on practice.

The supervisor uses her skills to enable practitioners to problem solve and to consider new ways to think about their practice. Accordingly, lecturer practitioners and clinical nurse specialists in palliative care may well be called upon to act as supervisors for non-specialist nurses who are developing their competencies in palliative care.

Formal education

Evidence of learning can, of course, be demonstrated by accreditation through formal education. The principle of self-directed education being followed through this chapter is intended to enable practitioners to select out formal education appropriate to their learning outcomes. It must be recognised that the importance of 'time out' of clinical areas to study and practice skill development in a formal educational setting is not being dismissed by the authors of this chapter. We are, however, recommending that the correct balance for individual practitioners is reached.

Formal education in institutional settings have financial, time and resource implications for the consumers. Directly, this means the practitioner who is undertaking the course. You might, however, consider employers and patients as indirect consumers of the education being undertaken. Bearing

Table 2.2 Competencies in pain management

	Factual knowledge	Understanding factual knowledge	Application of the understanding of knowledge	Analysis of the application of knowledge	Synthesis of knowledge	Decision-making
Level of learning	**Know** • Concept of total pain • Typology of physical pain • Definition of different types of pain • Pain is managed according to its source • A systematic approach to pain management	**Understand** • The concept of total pain • How personal and professional attitudes can influence and exacerbate pain • The definitions of the different pain types • Pathophysiology of pain • Different modalities for pain management • How to assess and plan management for effective pain relief	→	→	→	→
Competencies or learning outcomes	**Recall** • Describe the elements of total pain • The different types of pain • Definition of the different types of pain • Principles of managing the different types of pain	**Explain** • The significance of the different elements of total pain • How personal and professional attitudes can affect the experience and effectiveness of pain management	**In clinical situations** • Elicit psychological, social, spiritual and physical factors that influence pain with different patients • Be effective in listening and responding to patients' concerns	**Examine** • Data generated in assessment of pain • Listening and responding skills of self and others • Attitudes displayed by patients,	**Initiate and implement** • Protocols and policies in pain management • Teaching of the principles of pain management to others	**Take responsibility for** • Transferring knowledge of the principles of pain management to different disease processes • Evaluation of

Table 2.2 Competencies in pain management (contd)

Competencies or learning outcomes (contd)			
• The stages of the problem-solving cycle	• The different pain types • The pathophysiology of pain • The different modalities and their effectiveness in pain management • A systematic approach to pain management	• Be aware of personal and professional attitudes towards the experience and management of different elements of pain • Identify different types of physical pain • Discuss management of specific types of pain with colleagues, patients and others • Explain the effectiveness of different pain modalities for specific types of pain • Assess, plan and evaluate specific types of pain and its management	professionals and the public towards the experience and management of pain • Symptoms of the different pain types • Pharmacological and non-pharmacological techniques of pain management • Protocols for pain management	• Structures of emotional support for client and professional groups	protocols and policies in pain management • Ensuring that a positive attitude towards pain management prevails amongst a staff group • Ensuring that education in all aspects of pain management is available to a staff group • Actions taken in specific circumstances • Conduct scientific enquiry about pain and its management

in mind the latter points, if funding is being sought for a course of study, the choice of a course needs to be justified alongside the practitioner's desired competencies to meet his own learning needs, the needs of patients and the clinical area in which employed. It would therefore seem reasonable to develop a checklist for examining whether certain programme-driven courses meet the stated criteria. Such a list might include:

• The aims and content of the course
• The stated learning outcomes of the course
• The method of teaching/learning employed, i.e. how the stated learning outcomes will be enabled
• The credibility of staff directing and delivering the curriculum
• The accreditation awarded

WHAT IS PALLIATIVE CARE EDUCATION?

The multiprofessional approach in palliative care is central to providing whole-person care. The professionals involved require to work in partnership with the patient and family members in order to understand and address the physical, psychological, social and spiritual aspects of dying, death and bereavement. The National Council for Hospice and Specialist Palliative Care Services recommends five principles, based on the hospice philosophy, that must feature in any palliative care education programme whatever topic is under consideration and in all disciplines (NCHSPCS 1996a). These are:

• Promotion of as high a quality of life as possible
• Assurance of whole-person care
• Inclusion of the dying person and those who matter to her
• Respect for patient autonomy and choice
• Openness and sensitivity in all communication

Nurse education in palliative care

Corner's (1993) review of nursing education in palliative care revealed a disappointing picture reflected in nursing practice. Nurses in Birch's (1993) study reported dissatisfaction with the preregistration education preparation they received to care for dying patients and their families. Birch noted that it was largely the behavioural aspects of care that the nursing curriculum failed to adequately address. Field & Kitson (1986) reported, from 192 schools of nursing in the UK, that the average number of hours of formal teaching on death and dying was 10 and this was largely delivered in a didactic mode. In Hockley's (1989) study, first-year students were reported to find it difficult to cope with their emotions in clinical practice. This was reflected in Hurtig & Stewins' work (1990), which identified a theory practice gap; in the clinical environment the primary focus on work tended to be task driven rather than on developing relationships with dying patients and their families. They recommended experiential methods as the most effective way of teaching about death and dying.

Research studies carried out in the 1980s unveiled very similar findings to those of 20 years previously. When exposed to the complex situations in clinical practice, the old adage that attitudes are caught and not taught rang true. Nurses learned about coping with death and dying by working along-side other members of staff. Defence systems against anxiety, such as dis-tancing, busyness and giving routinised care, as described by Menzies (1960) in her study of student nurses, were still evident in the research findings of Mills et al (1994). Dying patients were left alone for lengthy periods and, overall, received much less attention from nurses and doctors than did other patients. There is evidence of failure of nurses to recognise the need for ongoing and symptom management. Corner (1993) concluded that although there are now a greater number of education programmes available, these will be of little benefit unless education targets nurses of all levels.

PROFESSIONAL ISSUES IN PALLIATIVE CARE EDUCATION

Having dealt with technicalities of profiling in palliative care, we will now turn our attention to a range of professional issues in palliative care that are transferable between nursing contexts of care. We will examine quality of care, quality of life, teamwork and communication. In each we will highlight the educational issues that require non-specialist nurses in palliative care to develop their competencies to a level which demonstrates effective applica-tion of understanding of the principles of palliative care (Tables 2.1 & 2.2).

Quality of care

The political and economical climates within which health care services operate have seen radical change over the last decade. A market economy is now well established in the NHS where purchasers are seeking the most realistic or lowest price for a service, whilst obtaining competitive quality purchaser/provider relationships. The client also has a right to receive the care and services that they require and expect (HMSO 1990). How does this relate to palliative care?

The Calman and Hines report (1995) on the future of cancer services proposed a range of services for cancer patients from the first point of contact in primary care to the specialist cancer hospital. Underpinning this plan is the integration of specialist palliative care services in hospital and community to provide seamless care at the point of delivery. Earlier in this chapter we referred to definitions for palliative care and established that the palliative care approach ought to be an integral component of all clinical practice. These principles must now be addressed at an organisational level (NCHSPCS 1996b). For the non-specialist palliative care nurse this means that health authorities have a responsibility to purchase or to provide a specialist service to back up those providing a palliative care approach, whether or not the patient has cancer. In their executive summary the NCHSPCS (1996b) state that:

> Trusts should ensure that appropriate educational programmes, policies and standards are in place to promote this aim throughout the hospital. Evaluation and audit of palliative care should be promoted.

When speaking of audit, the term 'quality of care' springs to mind. Quality, according to the current Oxford English Dictionary, 'is a degree of goodness or excellence'. It follows that quality of care is the degree to which good standards are maintained in clinical practice.

Standards of care

Standards of care are fundamental to quality assurance, which is characterised by a flexibility that encourages innovation and creativity. Donabedian (1989) described quality as:

- Goodness of technical care
- Goodness of interpersonal relationships among all concerned with care, with special attention to the relationship between the patient and the health care practitioner
- Goodness of the amenities of care

In the context of palliative care, quality (as described above) can be clearly identified in Table 2.3, which presents both the Donabedian definition of quality and the WHO statement about palliative care.

A standard is an agreed level of performance which is achievable, observable, desirable and measurable [Kitson 1988].

The Donabedian (1966) model of structure process and outcome has provided the framework for standard setting amongst health care professionals. Briefly described:

- **Structure** – combines human, physical and financial resources necessary to provide health care
- **Process** is the use of resources, including measures of throughput, which assess whether patients are cared for according to agreed criteria
- **Outcome** is the result of an intervention and relates to whether any change in a patient's health status or psychosocial well-being can be attributed to the health care provided

Table 2.3 Defining quality: a comparison of definitions (after Donabedian 1989, WHO 1990)

Quality of care (Donabedian 1989)	Palliative care (WHO 1990)
Goodness of technical care	Provides relief from pain and other distressing symptoms
Goodness of interpersonal relationships among all concerned with care, with special attention to the relationship between the patient and the health care practitioner	Affirms life and regards dying as a normal process and neither hastens nor postpones death
	Integrates the psychological and spiritual aspects of patient care
Goodness of the amenities of care	Offers a support system to help patients live as actively as possible until death
	Offers a support system to help the family cope during the patient's illness and their own bereavement

Standards can be defined at personal, clinical and organisational level. At all three levels standards refer to the intended goals for patient care set in relation to what an individual professional, a team or the organisation can expect to provide. Standards set at an individual, team and organisational level are interdependent. In setting and using standards, nurses can empower themselves and patients. Added to this is a feel-good factor of ownership, which helps nurses to feel valued as members of a multiprofessional team.

The level of standard will, however, ultimately depend on resources such as skill-mix of staff, finance, education, equipment, drugs and availability of specialist support services within the organisation. Copp (1993) identified the frustration of health professionals at not being able to provide the standard of care felt to be appropriate. It is unlikely that standards will be realistic or achievable without full consideration of what the organisation can provide.

Standards on their own can only provide an operational framework. When included in an audit cycle, Fig. 2.2, measuring current standards, provides evidence to justify a request to the organisation for improved resources.

■ **REFLECTIVE PRACTICE 2.4   Portfolio in palliative care**

Non-specialist palliative care can be involved in three types of audit. Take a few minutes to review what you believe to be the standard of palliative care that you personally deliver and that which is offered by your team and by the organisation for which you work.

Kitson (1988) strongly advises that nursing standards be realistic, understandable, measurable, believable and achievable. She recommends that the following questions are asked when reflecting on present practice and as a way towards setting standards for good practice:

- Do all members of your multiprofessional team agree that there is a need for improvement in practice?
- Are goals that you wish to set achievable?
- Do other team members agree with your goals?
- Do you have the necessary authority to tackle the problem?
- Do all the team agree that setting standards is important and which standards require to be set?

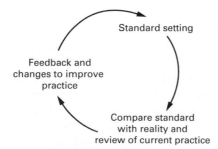

Fig. 2.2 The audit cycle.

Clinical standards in palliative care

There are a number of factors that need special consideration when setting standards in palliative care. The definitions given on page 29 for palliative care approach, palliative interventions and specialist palliative care, together with the levels of competencies defined by Webber (1993) (Table 2.1), are important in relation to making the clinical standards set in a non-specialist palliative care context understandable, realistic, believable and achievable. Standards are essential for monitoring patient care.

Hinton (1980) said 'If we believe that the recognition of a patient's awareness of dying affects our approach to his care, it is pertinent to discover, to what extent people recognise that they are dying, whom they are likely to tell and why'. These words suggest that palliative care demands certain skills. For the non-specialist nurse wishing to review the standard of palliative care which he delivers, competencies should be developed to a higher level in:

- Relieving symptoms that impair quality of life
- Encouraging and maintaining a patient's independence within ever-changing and deteriorating physical and, perhaps, psychological state of health
- Promoting and providing open and honest dialogue
- Facilitating support for patients, relatives, carers and colleagues
- Liaison with other professionals, services and agencies when appropriate
- Empowering patients
- Improving interpersonal communication

Quality of life

Quality of life is a central consideration in palliative care. It is a personal construct, but one in which many people become involved in making judgements, often based on personal attitudes towards life and death issues. Such attitudes are influenced by personal experience, society and, to some extent, politics. In clinical practice, nurses have to come to terms with their own attitudes towards physical, emotional, social and spiritual suffering. Decisions about care are often a compromise, influenced by patient choice, professional judgement and the resources available. Such decisions may not always be 'balanced' or judged to be fair by all the professionals involved. We invite you to consider quality of life in palliative care. What does it mean to you? How do you relate that to patient care?

Quality and value of life are sometimes used synonymously. Quality of life in health care has come to mean a measure which assesses quality of care given by professionals. The perception of value of life, on the other hand, is individual and rests with the person whose life it is. Value, for some, is in the exchange of a balance of simple human interaction, such as facial expressions, touch, close body proximity. For others, value of life will equate with the highest possible degree of perfection according to health, ability, intellect, power and strength. Many more will place value for life somewhere between the two. It is from this notion of value, combined with the sanctity of human life, that the will to live, die, to accept, demand or reject treatment, to engage in suicide and choose euthanasia, arise. Both quality and value of life issues constantly raise ethical considerations, problems and dilemmas in palliative care. These are issues that professionals are not always adequately prepared to deal with.

■ REFLECTIVE PRACTICE 2.5 Portfolio in palliative care: quality of life

The clause on personal responsibility within the UKCC (1992b) code of professional conduct requires you to ensure that no action or omission on your part or within your sphere of influence is detrimental to the condition or safety of patients.

Think of a situation where, in your opinion, a decision was made about a patient's future without full consideration of her perception of value or quality of life.

• What was the subsequent effect on that patient in terms of her physical, psychological, social and spiritual well-being?
• What input did you have in the decision and would you now act differently?
• This activity combines reflection on action and reflection in action.

In their document 'Education in palliative care' members of the working party for the NCHSPCS (1996a) stated their concerns about the neglect of education for health care professionals in ethics. Although the curricula for 'Project 2000' students in nursing and for 'Tomorrow's Doctors' have attempted to redress this, there are many nurses and doctors in clinical practice who have not benefited from ethics and ethical theory being taught within the context of clinical practice (GMC 1994, MCCC 1992, UKCC 1986). Although ethical considerations and decisions, and how they are dealt with in clinical situations, are reflected in the overall approach and interprofessional relationships across the whole spectrum of health care, they are brought into sharper focus in palliative care. (MCCC 1992, Randall & Downie 1996).

Sellman (1996) examined the rationale for teaching ethics to nurses in the preregistration context. Much of his discussion is applicable to the postregistered nurse. Nurses need to be prepared for the types of ethical difficulties that they will encounter in the palliative care context. They may be involved in quality and value of life decisions: whether treatment should be commenced, continued or withdrawn. Furthermore, patients may express views to nurses that suggest a desire for ending their life. Also, there are the ethical considerations that accompany all aspects of nurse–patient communication: dealing with fears, with information needs and sometimes interpreting the effects of poorly communicated information, such as bad news. Because nurses are involved in ethical decision-making they, at least, need a knowledge and understanding of ethical language. With the right vocabulary, nurses will be more able to justify their contribution towards decisions. It will also enable them to question, rather than be persuaded to be involved in, activities that cause them concern. Teaching ethics to nurses, or at least exposing them to ethical arguments in health care, strengthens their position within the multiprofessional team and provides them with the confidence to act as an advocate, when appropriate, on behalf of patients. These points are discussed in more detail in Chapter 10.

Jeffrey (1993) proposes an ethical model for palliative care that combines respect for autonomy with a caring ethos within a professional/patient partnership. His model promotes the value of teamwork. A team approach, he argues, allows health care professionals to share problems and co-ordinate different skills for the benefit of the patient. Not all teams, however, share Jeffrey's philosophy. In contrast is a paternalistic approach when patients are faced with an unequal partnership. Professionals are 'the experts', with knowledge and skills not accessible to patients. Patients cannot make informed decisions in circumstances where professionals seek to protect patients at all costs. Another danger is the assumption about a shared system of values amongst team members. Each professional will have their own system of value, based on their individual circumstances.

Jeffrey's (1993) definition of quality of life challenges us to include a balance between the impact of a treatment and its side-effects: to recognise and respect the patient in body, mind and spirit in the context of social relationships with family and friends. This is reflected in his model of autonomy, which combines the concepts of freedom of choice, dignity, individuality, independence, responsibility, rationality and critical reflection. When a person is ill it is important for the health care professionals involved in providing care to consider the patient's right to information and the subsequent choices made in relation to sustaining dignity, individuality, independence and responsibilities. This inevitably has implications for how you work within your team.

Teamwork

Leathard (1994) describes hospice teams as the exemplars in interprofessional teamwork. Vachon (1996), however, writes:

> ... from the early days of the palliative care movement, it was identified that, to function effectively, a palliative care team needed to clearly recognise its members' expertise and value. Yet, from early on, it was also recognised that – much like a family – the hospice/palliative care team could simultaneously be the source of much strength and satisfaction, and the root of much conflict and distress.

Broadly speaking, there are two elements in teamwork – people working together and a task to be achieved. A closer examination of both will enable us to select the educational issues for the non-specialist nurse in palliative care.

According to Vachon (1996) there are four specific characteristics that distinguish a team from a group. These are:

- A reason for working together
- The recognition of the value of each member's experience and ability
- Effective decision-making
- Accountability in an organisational context

Ovretveit (1996) refers to the confusion which arises in the different inter-pretations that are made of teams involving different professionals working together. He points out that many problems in teamwork 'arise out of poor management and "perverse incentives" rather than from the more popular explanation of "personality conflicts".' (Ovretveit 1993, p. 3).

Understanding the management of and the task of the team is paramount to its functioning. The five ways in which he describes multiprofessional teamwork include and expand on the characteristics identified by Vachon (1996). Ovretveit (1996) talks about the:

- Degree of integration between professionals
- Extent of collective responsibility
- Membership
- Client pathway
- Management structures

Degree of integration

On a continuum of loose/close integration, the specialist palliative care team might be described as a closely integrated team. Workload and clinical decisions are governed by multiprofessional protocols in manage-ment. There is a single entry point for the patient and the team have an agreed policy for designating patient care to a particular team member.

Multiprofessional teams, in hospital and community, by Ovretveit's (1996) description are network groups. Practitioners belong to a team because of their involvement with a specific client group. Each practitioner is, however, accountable to his respective professional manager for the service provided. Also, each team member works closely with colleagues within their own professional domain and keeps the multiprofessional team informed about the patient's progress, e.g. a district nursing sister may consult a specialist palliative care nurse about a nursing matter with-out necessarily having to first consult the full team. The network meeting of professionals thus provides an opportunity for the update and exchange of ideas. This leads to a common purpose and shared goals for client care. The team meeting enables cross-referring, enables co-ordination of care for patients and avoidance of unnecessary overlap of professional roles. It is the latter that might infringe the privacy of the patient or cause role dysfunction and conflict amongst professionals. Attendance at network meetings may vary, depending on the priorities and accountability of individual professionals to their respective professional manager and wider workload, e.g. the social worker might have an 'emergency on-call' commitment within the wider social work service.

Extent of collective responsibility

Specialist palliative care teams in hospital and community, managed and financed as a single entity, have collective responsibility for the service that they provide. In such teams all members are accountable for pooling and using their collective resources to meet the priority and special needs of patients who require palliative care. The notion of collective responsibility has management implications in deciding if, for example, specialist palliative care teams have responsibility for all patients requiring palliative care or, according to the definition on page 29, only those with specialist palliative care needs.

Ovretveit (1993) stresses that if, in the organisational context, the client population is not defined for the team there is a risk of work overload and inappropriate use of resources. From the example above where the specialist palliative care team have a defined responsibility for those patients with complex and specialist palliative care needs, the non-specialist practitioner is presented with the challenge of developing competencies to deliver a palliative care approach and networking with the specialist practitioners to complement their team resources. In their discussion of interdisciplinary teamwork, Randall & Downie (1996) advise that team decisions have ethical and legal implications and professionals entering into collective decisions must be prepared to take responsibility, both professionally and legally, for the consequences of such decisions.

Membership

Membership of a team is an important issue. Network membership is fluid and the loyalties that individual practitioners have outside the team may be considered a priority within the more closely integrated team. Team membership may be core or extended. This distinction may help to see how decisions about palliative care can be reached in the non-specialist palliative care setting. Ajemain (1993) points out that it is not necessary for all members of a team to be consulted each time a decision is made. Some decisions are made by individuals and others within a core membership of a team, which might include two or three professionals. Other decisions require the combined expertise of the whole team and sometimes an extended team, which involves additional members who have intermittent contact with the team. This might mean the primary health care team calling on a hospice consultant to assist them to formulate a protocol for the management of pain within the practice. It may be that in the experience of most nurses, team meetings involve only core members. In this case it is vitally important, for the overall healthy functioning of the full team, to keep all members informed about decisions made. When arranging meetings, Ajemain (1993) encourages us to consider:

- Who has the information necessary to make decisions
- Who needs to be consulted
- Who needs to be informed once a decision has been made

Team membership, of course, must take account of personalities and abilities. No single practitioner has the ability to provide holistic care for patients. Such care requires the ability to recognise, understand and value the experience and competencies of other practitioners from similar and different professional backgrounds. This involves the recognition that there may be overlap of roles, and individual team members require the skills of advocacy, assertiveness and the quality of humility in order to deal with potential conflict arising from these grey areas of practice. Teamwork depends on good professional relationships founded on effective communication skills. Membership of teams who are involved with patients with serious and life-threatening illnesses, requires a combined subjective and objective perspective on human relationships to provide support. Vachon (1996) talks about sharing sorrow and joy and advocates remembering that in any team, whatever their specialist focus, there will be a degree of grief work to attend to.

Client pathway

Ovretveit (1996) describes routes or pathways that patients follow with different teams. He refers to different processes in which teams engage, for example: initial contact or reception, short-term response, referral, assessment, intervention, review, discharge and follow-up. The hospital team is likely to have a well-defined pathway for patients, including reception, assessment, planning, intervention, review, discharge and follow-up. The primary health care team, on the other hand, may operate multiple pathways, depending on patient needs. Different professionals might follow their own care plans with patients and at team meetings update or refer a patient onto another professional. Ovretveit calls this phenomenon 'parallel pathways'. Another team function is when the specialist community palliative care team receives a referral from hospital. Following assessment, the patient might be referred to the primary care team for ongoing care with the palliative care team being further involved in reviewing the patient's progress. This is called 'reception assessment and allocation pathway'. In other situations, referred to as 'hybrid parallel pathway', two teams may work together – the primary care team may seek admission of a patient to a specialist palliative care unit for assessment and symptom management. Subsequently, both teams will remain involved in the patient's care.

Ovretveit (1996) suggests that mapping patient pathways through a team helps to clarify professional/patient relationships, increases patient participation, enables teams to evaluate their decision-making and utilises their resources for the optimum benefit of all concerned. The spin-off benefit for practitioners is a strengthening of their professional autonomy.

Management structure

The fifth way of describing a team is in terms of leadership. Decision-making within a team is integral to the beliefs about leadership and the model of practice followed. In any interdisciplinary team, doctors and nurses will have a strong presence and it is on their approaches to care that we need to focus.

The nursing reforms in the 1970s forced nurses to look at their practice: at the relationships between themselves and patients and between themselves and other health care professionals, particularly doctors. From this emerged a proliferation of models of care with the common denominator of partnership with patients, and a deliberate move away from the disease-orientated model.

Combined with this we need to look at models of medicine to understand some of the leadership difficulties within health care teams. Veatch (1972) described four models:

- Engineering
- Priestly
- Collegial
- Contractual

• **The engineering model** emphasises a heavily dominated scientific approach to medicine with the temptation to focus on data rather than the individual circumstances of patients.

• **The priestly model** attributes an expertise in life issues to the doctor as part of his medical responsibilities. It upholds the principles of providing care that produces the greatest benefit for the patient, without causing undue harm, with paternalism as the modus operandi.

• **The collegial model** promotes a partnership between the patient and doctor based on trust and confidence in a developing relationship.

• **The contractual model** is akin to a business relationship with negotiations being entered into according to the circumstances and the resources for any given encounter between doctor and patient.

In his attempt to place patient autonomy at the heart of team decisions, Jeffrey (1993) describes a broad approach and a narrow approach to team decision-making in palliative care.

• **The broad approach** includes taking account of the patient's informed decisions. This involves a certain amount of risk taking and the possibility for patients of 'getting it wrong'. Such an approach acknowledges patients' total circumstances, their feelings and values, and it is cautious with professional interventions that will prolong life.

• **The narrow approach** excludes patients from decisions. It is strongly paternalistic, seeking to protect the patient's well-being and to prolong life at all costs. Decisions are greatly influenced by scientific data and professional interventions are high on the team agenda.

In summary, teamwork presents a complex network of working patterns and professional relationships, all of which affect the quality of care for patients. The educational issues emerging from this discussion about teamwork focus first on a clear understanding of the exact function of the teams to which you provide professional expertise and, second, an examination of your professional and personal relationships that contribute to the dynamics of the different teams. Self-awareness and confidence in professional and personal values, knowledge, experience and skills should form the basis of reflection when considering education for professional development.

■ REFLECTIVE PRACTICE 2.6   Portfolio in palliative care: teamwork

Many of us work in a variety of teams: some uniprofessional, others multipro-fessional.

Ovretveit's five ways of describing the multiprofessional team is relevant also to the uniprofessional team. Using these descriptors think about the different teams that you are directly involved with. How would you describe each in terms of:

- Degree of integration between professionals
- The extent of collective responsibility
- Membership
- Client pathway
- Management structure

Following this 'reflection on action' return to the previous reflective practice and, in relation to the personal responsibility clause of the UKCC (1992b) code of professional conduct, consider what personal professional development you need to think about to improve your own performance within the different teams to which you belong.

Communication

Effective communication has been described as the essence of effective health care. Fielding (1995, p. 2) defines effective care as 'a crucial higher-level communication skill dependent on more specific skills like question style and eye contact'. Heaven & Maguire (1996) write that 'good com-munication is one of the most important aspects of care, since it pervades every part of the nurse–patient relationship, from before diagnosis to death or cure'. The study of nurses' communication skills has escalated since the late 1970s. The use of blocking tactics by nurses is consistently reported. This observation dates back to Menzies' (1960) work when she observed the behaviour of student nurses during training in the late 1950s and again in Webster's (1981) study. Using field observation, Webster conducted her research in four different hospitals and involved 53 learner nurses, each over a 4-hour period. Data were also collected about other members of staff who were involved with the learner during the observation period, from ward sisters, staff nurses, enrolled nurses and nurse tutors. Webster reported that both the trained nurses and the learners involved in the study had difficulties in communicating with dying patients. The most frequent tactics used were:

- Denial of the seriousness of the patient's condition
- Abrupt change of the subject of conversation
- Behaving as though the patient had not spoken at all
- Intense concentration on the physical task in hand
- Pursuing the least-threatening aspect of conversation
- Introducing a joking atmosphere
- Disappearing from a stressful situation

In Webster's study, nurses were aware of using blocking tactics, both in protecting themselves and patients from being upset. She concluded that the need for increased teaching on communication skills was not the only problem. Ward orientation, the amount and quality of information passed on to learners from trained nursing staff and medical staff, together with society's attitudes towards death and dying, all play a role in influencing the learners' attitude and ability in communicating with dying patients. The findings in Webster's research reappear as themes of self-awareness, and predictor variables for facilitating verbal behaviours in studies conducted through the 1980s and 1990s.

Self-awareness

Morrison & Burnard (1989) described the views of nurses about the level of their own interpersonal skills. They used Heron's six-category intervention analysis (Table 2.4) with groups of student nurses (84 in all) selected at different stages in training. The nurses were introduced to and allowed to familiarise with Heron's categories before being asked to rank their perception of the level of their own intervention skills. The findings of this study were compared with an earlier investigation (using the same inventory) where 93 trained nurses from different backgrounds were asked to rank their self-perception of the level of their own interpersonal skills. A pattern emerged with both student and trained nurses rating themselves as most skilled in prescriptive, informative and supportive elements of intervention and least skilled in confronting, cathartic and catalytic skills. It is worth noting at this stage in the discussion that Heron (1986) subdivided the six categories into authoritative skills (which allows the practitioner to stay in control of the relationship) and facilitative skills (when control lies with the patient). Heron placed no greater emphasis on any of the intervention skills but argued that skilled communicators would move in a balanced way between the authoritative and facilitative groups of interventions.

Table 2.4 Heron's six-category inventory (after Morrison & Burnard 1989)

Category	Intervention
Authoritative	
Prescriptive	To offer advice or make suggestions
Informative	To give information, knowledge or instructions
Confronting	To challenge verbal or non-verbal behaviour
Facilitative	
Cathartic	To facilitate the release of emotion through tears or other emotional response
Catalytic	To enable reflection through use of questions or review of circumstances
Supportive	To confirm self-esteem by validating thoughts, feelings, behaviours, etc.

Predictor variables for facilitating verbal behaviours

Wilkinson's (1991) study identified factors that influenced the quality of nurse/patient verbal interaction. She involved a group of 54 trained nurses (registered and enrolled from two hospitals, one of which was specialist). The nurses were selected from three wards in each hospital. Each was asked to conduct three audiotaped histories: one with a patient with a new diagnosis of cancer, one with a patient with a recurrence of tumour, and the third with a patient receiving palliative care. In addition, the nurses completed a self-administered questionnaire and a semistructured interview. Wilkinson (1991) explored:

- The extent to which nurses use facilitative or blocking behaviours when communicating with cancer patients
- If nurses are aware that the verbal behaviours used are blocking or facilitative
- The relationship between nurse verbal behaviours and levels of anxiety, social support, work support and attitude towards death
- Nurses' feelings about caring for cancer patients

Wilkinson's study (1991) supports the findings of Webster (1981). Although blocking behaviours were generally prominent in the interviews, the researcher identified four groups of communicators – facilitators, ignorers, informers and mixers. The latter were found to be more aware of using blocking techniques than any of the others. An interesting observation from the informer group was that one nurse consistently gave inappropriate advice. This could be worrying in light of Morrison & Burnard's (1989) work wherein both trained and student nurses ranked prescriptive and informative interventions as their better skills. It has implications for the trust that is generated from the accuracy of advice and information given to patients. Overall assessments of patients in Wilkinson's (1991) study were poorly rated in the analysis of the tape-recorded data. The physical assessment was deemed to be superficial and the psychological element was rated low in comparison with the physical component. Verbal behaviours were analysed in respect of ward environment, nurses' religion and their own anxiety about death. In her conclusions, Wilkinson (1991) suggests that the way in which nurses communicate may be affected by the environment created by the ward sister, the nurse's religious belief and society's attitudes towards death, rather than by their education in communication skills. Interestingly, Heron (1986) noted that in respect of his intervention categories, the cathartic category is most likely to be avoided and that such skills may not be highly developed in a society where expression of strong emotion is discouraged. The research findings discussed here have bearing on observations of practice when it has been noted that nurses more readily become involved in the physical care of patients.

Based on the premise that 'patient assessment underpins every aspect of nursing care and the evidence that many nurses lack the skills necessary to communicate effectively with patients', Heaven & Maguire (1996) examined the outcomes of training hospice nurses to elicit patient concerns.

In their review of literature on the effectiveness of training in communication skills, they divided studies into those which focused on the structure and process of interaction and those which concentrated on outcome. They concluded that no study had attempted to examine both the acquisition of skills and the subsequent impact on nurses' ability to assess patient needs. Their study sought to determine the outcome of assessment skills training by examining nurses' ability to elicit patients' concerns in a ward situation where all staff had been trained together. Forty-four nurses and 87 patients from two hospitals were involved in the study. A pretest/post-test design was used. This incorporated a 10-week teaching programme and a 9-month follow-up to ascertain if skills were retained over time. The test involved conducting an audiotaped assessment interview followed by writing out a list of the concerns elicited. The patient was then interviewed by a trained research worker using a validated anxiety and depression questionnaire and a concerns checklist. Overall, the research demonstrated an improvement in skills from pretest to post-test and follow-up, particularly in the number of open questions. In contrast, however, training did not influence the nurse's ability to identify the patient's concerns. Heaven & Maguire (1996) comment that although the incidence of blocking techniques rose in the post-test and subsequent interviews, the incidence was not as frequent as Wilkinson (1991) found in her data. It appeared that patients were prepared to disclose their problems as they got to know their nurses but there was no corresponding willingness on the part of nurses to listen. This echoes the suggestion from Heron's (1986) work about a society that does not encourage the expression of strong feelings.

There is much here to reflect upon in educational issues. Heaven and Maguire (1996), with different colleagues, have demonstrated that training using video demonstration and audio feedback improves skill in the short term but the improvement is not always sustained over time. In the study discussed here the researchers trained a full staff group together and offer this as a possible explanation for the retention of skill. To some extent this again agrees with Wilkinson's (1991) suggestion that the ward environment, and particularly the ward sister, was a variable that affected the communication skills of nurses. By training a full staff group, an environment of mutual support and understanding was created.

To conclude this section we will reflect upon the findings discussed above and consider what might happen in practice. Imagine or reflect upon a real incident where you are with a patient who asks 'Nurse, am I going to die soon?'. In the research reviewed, competencies have been identified for effective communication between nurse and patient. Equally important factors in facilitating effective communication are environment and attitudes.

The situation identified demands insight into the nature of the situation, a level of self-awareness that enables honesty and the ability to make an 'on-the-spot' decision in the patient's interest. To deal effectively, the nurse requires competencies in:

- Empathy
- Trust building
- Negotiating time and boundaries

- Eliciting information
- Listening, exploring and responding to patient needs
- Self-awareness of strengths, limitations and vulnerability
- Making decisions
- Advocating for the needs of a patient
- Assertiveness in justifying action and decisions taken

SUMMARY

The considerations in this chapter fuel an argument for palliative care to be within the repertoire of all health care professionals. Doyle (1996) reminds us that palliative care is an unusual specialty. It emerged because of identified deficiencies in caring for a group of patients with a diagnosis of incurable disease. The knowledge, skills and attitudes that underpin palliative care are required by all professionals but inevitably there will be those patients with complex needs who require attention from a group of specialists. Our aim throughout this chapter has been to enable the non-specialist nurse to access the education required to develop the competencies to deliver the optimum standard of palliative care in different care settings.

We have attempted to demonstrate that the principles of palliative care are core skills and we suggest that they are recognised as such through preregistration courses. The challenge, however, goes beyond the formal setting of pre- and postregistration courses. Ongoing professional education includes taking responsibility for one's own learning, a process that we have endeavoured to encourage through creating a profile in palliative care.

REFERENCES

Ajemain I 1993 Interdisciplinary teamwork. In: Doyle D, Hanks G, Macdonald N (eds) Oxford textbook of palliative medicine. Oxford Medical Publications, Oxford, pp 17–27

Birch J A 1983 Anxiety and conflict in nurse education. In: Davis B (ed) Research into nurse education. Croom Helm, London, pp 11–25

Calman K, Hine D 1995 A policy framework for commissioning cancer services, DOH, London

Copp G 1993 Frequency and difficult problems perceived by nurses caring for the dying in community hospice and acute settings. Palliative Medicine 7: 19–25

Corner J 1993 Education and training in palliative care: the nursing perspective. In: Doyle D, Hanks G, Macdonald N (eds) Oxford textbook of palliative medicine. Oxford Medical Publications, Oxford, pp 781–790

Darley M 1996 UKCC guidance on clinical supervision. Macmillan Nurse Newsletter 2: 4–5

Donabedian A 1966 Evaluating the quality of medical care. Millbank Memorial Fund Quarterly 44: 166–206

Donabedian A 1989 Institutional and professional responsibilities in quality assurance. Quality Assurance in Health Care 1: 3–11

Doyle D 1996 Education in palliative care. Palliative Medicine 10: 91–92

EAPC 1996 The Barcelona declaration on palliative care. Progress in Palliative Care 4: 113

ENB 1995 Using your portfolio. A resource for practitioners. English National Board Publications, London

Field D, Kitson C 1986 Formal teaching about death and dying in UK schools of nursing. Nurse Education Today 6: 270–276

Fielding R 1995 Clinical communication skills. Hong Kong University Press, Hong Kong

Finlay I G, Jones R V H 1995 Outreach palliative care services: definitions in palliative care. British Medical Journal 311: 754

Fowler J 1996 How to use models of clinical supervision in practice. Nursing Standard 10: 42–47

GMC 1993 Tomorrow's doctors: recommendations on undergraduate medical education. General Medical Council, London

Heaven C, Maguire P 1996 Training hospice nurses to elicit patient concerns. Journal of Advanced Nursing 23: 280–286

Heron J 1986 Six category intervention analysis, 2nd edn. Human potential research project. University of Surrey, Guildford

Hinton J 1980 Whom do dying patients tell? British Medical Journal 281: 1328–1330

HMSO 1990 Working for Patients. Her Majesty's Stationery Office, London

Hockley J 1989 Care for the dying in acute hospitals. Nursing Times 85: 47–50

Hull C, Redfern L 1996 Profiles and portfolios: a guide for nurses and midwives. Macmillan, London

Hurtig W, Stewin L 1990 The effect of death education and experience on nursing students' attitude towards death. Journal of Advanced Nursing 15: 29–34

Jeffrey D 1993 There is nothing more I can do: an introduction to the ethics of palliative care. Paten Press in association with Lisa Sainsbury Foundation, Cornwall

Kelly J 1995 RCN nursing update series: the really useful guide to portfolios and profiles. Nursing Standard 9: 32

Kitson A 1988 Steps to setting achievable nursing standards. RCN Standards of Care Project, London

Kolb D 1984 Experiential learning: experience as a source of learning and development. Prentice Hall, New Jersey

Leathard A 1994 Going interprofessional. Routledge, London

Maggs C 1996 Towards a philosophy for continuing professional education in nursing midwifery and health visiting. Nurse Education Today 16: 98–102

MCCC 1992 Teaching ethics: an initiative in cancer and palliative care education department of education. Marie Curie Cancer Care, London

Menzies I 1960 A case study in the functioning of social systems as a defence against anxiety. Tavistock, London

Mills M, Davies H T O, Macrae W A 1994 Care of dying patients in hospital. British Medical Journal 309: 583–585

Morrison P, Burnard P 1989 Students' and trained nurses' perceptions of their own interpersonal skills: a report and comparison. Journal of Advanced Nursing 14: 321–329

NCHSPCS 1995 A statement of definitions. National Council for Hospice and Specialist Palliative Care Services, London, Occasional paper 8

NCHSPCS 1996a Education in palliative care. National Council for Hospice and Specialist Palliative Care Services, London, Occasional paper 9

NCHSPCS 1996b Palliative care in the hospital setting. National Council for Hospice and Specialist Palliative Care Services, London, Occasional paper 10: 3

Ovretveit J 1993 Co-ordinating community care: multidisciplinary teams and care management. Open University, Milton Keynes

Ovretveit J 1996 Five ways to describe a multidisciplinary team. Journal of Inter-professional Care 10: 163–171

Randall F, Downie R S 1996 Palliative care ethics: a good companion. Oxford Medical Press, Oxford

RCN 1990 Quality patient care. The dynamic standard setting service: Royal College of Nursing standards of care project. Scutari, Harrow

RCN 1996 A structure for cancer nursing services. Royal College of Nursing, London

Roache J, Baldwin M A 1995 Quality through partnership. International Journal of Palliative Nursing Care 1: 96–100

Saunders C 1978 The management of terminal illness. Arnold, London

Schon D 1983 The reflective practitioner. Basic Books, New York

Sellman D 1996 Why teach ethics to nurses? Nurse Education Today 16: 44–48

Sheldon F 1996 Life so short, the craft hard to learn: a model for post basic education in palliative care. Palliative Medicine 10: 99–104

SPAPCC 1996 Palliative cancer care: the integration of palliative care with cancer services. Scottish Partnership Agency for Palliative and Cancer Care, Edinburgh

UKCC 1986 Project 2000: a preparation for practice. United Kingdom Central Council for Nursing Midwifery and Health Visiting, London

UKCC 1990 Report on post registration education and practice project. United Kingdom Central Council for Nursing Midwifery and Health Visiting, London

UKCC 1992a The scope of professional practice. United Kingdom Central Council for Nursing Midwifery and Health Visiting, London

UKCC 1992b Code of professional conduct. United Kingdom Central Council for Nursing Midwifery and Health Visiting, London

Vachon M 1996 What makes a team? Palliative Care Today 5: 34–35

Veaton R 1972 Cross-cultural perspectives in medical ethics. Jones and Barnett, Boston

Webber J 1993 The evolving role of the Macmillan nurse. Cancer Relief Macmillan Fund, London

Webster M 1981 Communicating with dying patients. Nursing Times June 4: 999–1000

WHO 1990 Cancer pain relief and palliative care. Report of a World Health Organization Expert Committee, Technical Report Series 804

Wilkes E 1980 Terminal care: report of a working party standing advisory committee. HMSO, London

Wilkinson S 1991 Factors which influence how nurses communicate with cancer patients. Journal of Advanced Nursing 16: 677–688

Holistic assessment of patients' and relatives' needs

3

Christine Pearce   Jean Lugton

Palliative care is patient centred, tailored to meet the patient's and relatives' constantly changing and complex needs wherever the patient is, whether at home, in residential care or nursing home or in hospital. Because needs change, a range of skills, expertise and facilities is necessary, starting with the palliative care approach. [National Council for Hospice and Specialist Palliative Care Services 1995]

ASSESSMENT

Assessment of needs is not new but the Department of Health's NHS and Community Care Act (1990) makes it a legal requirement for health authorities and health boards to assess the needs of their populations for services. It is now expected that needs assessment will have a growing input by users of health services and their carers. This challenges us to make proper assessment of our patients' needs, and good case management the cornerstone of our care. There are various definitions of need. A classification of need by Bradshaw (1972) included:

• Felt need – the subjective views of service users
• Expressed need – the demand placed on services
• Normative need – assessment of need in a particular society often made by professionals and politicians

- Comparative need – a comparison between two groups in similar circumstances

Assessment of need not only involves a systematic approach to identification of problems and sources of distress but also the forming of clinical judgements on the basis of which nursing care can be planned and tailored to preserve the autonomy and dignity of the individual concerned.

LEARNING OUTCOMES

This chapter stems from the authors' interest in the assessment of need from personal, clinical, and teaching and research experience in palliative care. It will fulfil the requirements for PREP in the categories of: reducing risk – health problem identification, protection of individuals, risk reduction; care enhancement – developments in clinical practice and treatment, new techniques and approaches to care, and empowering consumers.

By the end of this chapter, the reader will have:

- Increased awareness of factors influencing expressions and responses to need
- Explored the concept and principles of assessment
- Reviewed a broad range of research and literature on assessment
- Identified important factors in making assessment of needs
- Considered frameworks for use in holistic need assessment
- Considered the stages of assessment
- Examined attitudes, knowledge and skills used in assessment

FACTORS INFLUENCING EXPRESSION AND RESPONSES TO NEED

Sheldon (1993) noted that whether individuals can express needs often depends on factors, such as their expectations, and their confidence that they can contact someone who will help them meet their needs.

Patients may find it more difficult to express certain needs because they are uncertain of how professionals will respond. Chapter 6 of this book describes a frequent lack of recognition by health care professionals of the sexual needs of patients with advanced disease and the effects that this may have on their ability to express their sexual needs.

■ REFLECTIVE PRACTICE 3.1   Assessment overview

- When making an assessment, do I tend to focus on areas of interest to me?
- If so, what are these areas?
- Are there other areas of assessment which I tend to spend less time assessing?
- What are these areas?
- Why do I sometimes neglect them?

Make some notes and review these when you have completed the chapter.

Sometimes, groups of people may be relatively disadvantaged in terms of needs assessment and the quality of palliative care they receive. Sheldon (1993) maintained that there is increasing recognition that specialist palliative care services have not been meeting the needs of people from some cultural groups in the UK. Rather than examining what difficulties people from ethnic minorities experience in using palliative care services, it has been implied that it was the users' fault if they did not come forward. A social bias, such as a negative attitude towards the homeless, could result in a less thorough assessment of the individual.

Palliative care of patients with cancer has greatly improved over the years. However, patients with serious illnesses (other than cancer) may be relatively disadvantaged in terms of accurate assessment of their needs and the quality of care they receive. In a review of needs assessment in palliative care, Clarke & Malson (1995) maintained that:

We must become clearer on how complex social, psychological and physical needs can be described and conceptualised, allowing unexpressed needs and the needs of disadvantaged groups to be more fully articulated.

Skilbeck et al (1997) used a holistic approach to assess the needs of patients (and their main carers) admitted to hospital with an exacerbation of their chronic obstructive airways disease and found that their quality of life scores were very low when compared with the quality of life scores of those dying from end-stage cancer (Osoba 1991). Skilbeck et al (1997) asked patients with chronic obstructive airways disease about the symptoms they were experiencing and the level of intensity. As expected, the most debilitating physical symptom was extreme breathlessness but the extent of other symptoms, such as thirst, pain and fatigue, was surprising to these authors. Patients were asked about how the illness was affecting their activities of daily living and it was found that their functioning was extremely limited. Most people felt that their social lives had been greatly affected by the illness. They also felt a sense of loss because they were unable to undertake roles that had once been an accepted part of their lives. This sense of loss produced anxiety and depression. These people whose lives were greatly affected by their illness knew very little about the details of it.

Assessing the needs of patients whose illnesses have progressed from the acute to the palliative stage can be difficult and may be neglected, especially if they continue to receive treatment in acute hospital wards. Writing from an Australian perspective, Prior & Poulton (1996) found that sometimes introducing the palliative care role to patients was difficult, especially when they had not fully accepted their prognosis. Palliative care staff had first to establish credibility with ward staff by explaining the potential of palliative care. One of the authors of this chapter (Lugton 1994) observed the difficulties faced by patients, with recurrent breast cancer, in accepting palliative care when other patients were receiving potentially curative treatment for their disease. There were problems for health care professionals in maintaining patients' hopes, despite a poor prognosis, and of controlling distressing symptoms.

■ REFLECTIVE PRACTICE 3.2 Palliative care needs

How knowledgeable am I about the palliative care needs of:

a) people from ethnic groups other than my own?
b) people with serious illnesses other than cancer?

   Choose an example from a) and b). Are there any needs about which I know little? Are there needs to which I would find it difficult to respond? What knowledge, skills and attitudes must I acquire to improve my ability to help these people?

ASSESSMENT RATIONALE

Carpentino (1995) has defined assessment as the systematic collection of data to indicate a person's current and past health status and functional status and to evaluate present and past coping patterns. The importance of structure and system in assessment is also stressed by the WHO (1987, p. 173) in its study of nursing care needs of two groups of people in the European region. It concludes:

> Through the use of a structured health assessment protocol, needs other than physical can be identified.

PRINCIPLES OF ASSESSMENT

The following factors will be important in any assessment of the needs of sick people:

- Establishing relationships of trust with the patient and relatives
- Identifying and classifying the patient's and relatives' needs
- Prioritising the patient's and relatives' problems
- Developing a multiprofessional approach to needs assessment
- Making a diagnosis of nursing needs

Establishing relationships of trust with the patient and relatives

To establish trust, when making an assessment, it is important to believe what the patient says. However, studies have indicated that nurses' beliefs about patients' suffering are largely based on their own culture, socioeconomic level and ethnic background (Davitz 1981, Davitz & Pendleton 1969, Davitz et al 1976). For example, research has suggested that one of the most important factors in effective treatment for patients with chronic pain is to be believed about its nature (McCaffery 1980, Seers & Friedli 1996). An effective nursing assessment contains two-way communication whereby patients can receive new information or clarification about their expectations, the practical aspects of their care and a forum to express fears and hopes. When this happens, the patient's experience of care in whatever setting, home, hospital, or hospice, will be a positive one. It is important to explore the patient's expectations of health care providers. This information assists in planning goals of nursing care as well as determining whether the patient's expectations are realistic.

Identifying and classification of the patient's and relatives' problems

The main purpose of any assessment is the identification of problems and sources of distress and generation of possible solutions to these. Ill individuals, whether in their own homes, hospital, hospice or nursing home, will inevitably report a number of symptoms. However, it is important not only to identify symptoms but also to assess symptom distress. This means noting the intensity and frequency of symptoms and establishing which of them troubles the patient most. Warden et al (1998) noted that it is important to recognise that pain and suffering are two distinct concepts, even though pain is often accompanied by suffering. Copp (1974) defined suffering as a state of anguish of one who bears pain, injury or loss.

Prioritising the patient's and relatives' problems

When making an assessment, the nursing diagnosis should take account of both the clinical and the patient's priorities. The nurse must know what essential information it is necessary to collect immediately and what can be collected over a period of time. Clearly, the reversal of a life-threatening situation, such as haemorrhage or airways obstruction, will require immediate action based on only the most specific and rapid physical assessment. On the other hand, if a patient is admitted for a review of current medication for symptom relief, the assessment should be more detailed. The nurse will spend time explaining what will happen and gaining the co-operation of the patient in the associated activities. Unless there is clearly a priority, such as pain relief, Lyke (1992) suggested a sequence for assessing patients' needs that is based on Maslow' (1970) hierarchy of human needs.

- Oxygenation
- Physical safety
- Comfort
- Hydration
- Nutrition
- Bowel elimination
- Urinary elimination
- Hygiene and skin/tissue integrity
- Activity/mobility
- Rest and sleep
- Psychosocial needs
- Emotional security
- Communication and cognitive needs
- Need for love and belonging
- Self-esteem and self-actualisation

Developing a multiprofessional approach to needs assessment

In palliative care, assessment of needs is often complex as patients may have a wide range of problems. A holistic approach is therefore required and this implies multiprofessional involvement in assessment and care planning. With so much information to collect, the risk of duplication is great and can cause unnecessary stress to the patient. For this reason, good documentation and communication with other members of the multiprofessional team is very important. Prompt verbal reporting of the assessment findings to relevant team members should be followed by a written report, which is factually correct, concise but sufficiently detailed to communicate a holistic picture of the individual. The use of the patient's own words in report writing is helpful.

Having written up her assessment report, the nurse should also read what others may have written and listen to what others have said. Pooling of information gives all concerned the opportunity to share knowledge and skill and enhances care.

Making a diagnosis of nursing needs

While recognising the importance of co-operation with other professionals in care planning, a detailed assessment of patients' *nursing* needs is essential if nurses' clinical decision-making is to be accurate and appropriate nursing care is to be given. One way of achieving this is through making a nursing diagnosis. Lyke (1992) noted that:

> Today's nurse can no longer afford to rely on what happens to attract his or her attention while caring for the patient or that might be reported by another staff nurse or health care professional. The information required for nursing diagnosis must be systematically investigated.

Because the patient's situation may be changing continually, nursing assessment is also a continual process and nurses have to make judgements about the frequency of reassessment.

FRAMEWORKS FOR NEED ASSESSMENT

While there are a variety of nursing models, all require similar assessment data. Having a clear idea about what to include in an assessment is vital if some aspects important to patients are not to be omitted. Organisational traditions, such as the way in which documentation is formatted, may lead to weakness or errors in data collection.

The person is viewed by Rogers (1970) as a unified being. Maslow (1970) maintained that the person is engaged in a lifelong attempt to maximise his potential with a range of needs extending from basic physiological needs to needs for self-actualisation. Assessment of patients' needs include:

- Physical needs
- Psychological needs
- Social needs
- Spiritual needs

A holistic approach

A holistic approach requires the fostering of hope, choice and autonomy, which help people to adapt to illness more effectively (Rideout & Montemuro 1986). There are now several frameworks for assessment that adopt a holistic approach. Many nursing models adopt a holistic approach to assessment and care planning. For example, Roper et al (1980) viewed patients' needs in terms of the activities of living. These authors identified need for assessment of physical, psychological, social and spiritual problems associated with dying, and the inclusion of needs of the family in the assessment process. Holistic nursing involves sharing information with the patient and relatives who are then involved in setting goals and making decisions. Gordon (1994) proposed a Functional Health Patterns assessment framework.

The functional health patterns model of assessment: an example of holistic assessment (Gordon 1994)

The 11 aspects of this framework are as follows:

- Health perception/health management pattern
- Nutritional/metabolic pattern
- Cognitive perceptual pattern
- Assessment of pain
- Self-perception pattern
- Role–relationship pattern
- Elimination pattern
- Activity/exercise pattern
- Sleep/rest pattern
- Coping/stress tolerance
- Value/belief pattern

During her research into the support of patients with breast cancer by health visitors, one of the authors of this chapter (Lugton) found that a Domiciliary Assessment Form adapted from a form devised by Tait et al (1982) helped to ensure that health visitors made a holistic assessment of patients' needs. Health visitors reported it to be a valuable tool. The form included general observations about the patient, her physical adjustment to breast disease, effects of the disease on her key relationships, her interactions with the health care team since leaving hospital, social adjustment and psychological adjustment. The assessment of psychological adjustment included guidelines on the recognition of clinical depression and anxiety state. In the final section of the form, key problems were identified and the actions taken or pending were described.

■ REFLECTIVE PRACTICE 3.3   Frameworks for need assessment

- Do you and your colleagues use a framework to help you to assess your patients' and relatives' palliative care needs?
- Does the framework enable you to make **holistic** assessments?
- Are there any changes you and your colleagues would like to make to the framework for more effective identification of needs?

  Discuss with your colleagues and note any agreed changes.

The use of assessment tools

A number of tools have been designed and validated for use in assessing the problems and in evaluating the quality of life of people receiving palliative care. The appropriateness of these tools and the areas measured are discussed in Chapter 11 of this book. The use of assessment tools such as pain scales or mood measures can significantly add to the quality of an assessment. Formal assessment tools can promote effective communication and reduce the chance of error. Simple 0–10 rating scales are helpful in establishing the intensity of pain. A number of quality of life instruments have been validated in cancer care, and palliative care audit tools such as STAS (Higginson 1993) are being developed. When the use of a tool is being considered, the following factors should be taken into account:

• For which group of patients was the tool designed?
• Was the tool designed to be completed by patients, relatives or professional carers?
• Does length makes it inappropriate for the very ill?
• Is it simple enough to be understood by very ill patients?
• Is the tool equally useful in any setting (home, hospital)?

While the use of tools may be helpful during initial assessments, their continuous use may cause the patient to focus too much on a particular symptom to the detriment of quality of life.

Assessment of the needs of patients' relatives

As stated above, holistic assessment involves considering the family as a unit. Worden (1994) maintained that attention should be given to family dynamics and the position of the person receiving care within the family. Neale (1991) pointed out that a patient's carers often experience physical, emotional, social and economic burdens as a result of the illness and that too often professionals have accepted these as inevitable. Children should be included in any assessment of relatives' needs because they suffer when a loved parent or relative is ill and can often be excluded from the support that professionals give to adult family members. Chapter 8 of this book describes the stress which patients' relatives often experience, arising from the patient's illness, from within themselves and from the hospital environment. Sheldon (1993) singles out three areas where carers' needs are great and are not always met. First, they need good communication and attention to their emotional strain. Second, they need well-co-ordinated domiciliary support. Third, they need advice on financial problems, which they may experience as a result of caring for a sick person. An assessment of their needs is therefore vital in order that their support is planned and not left to chance encounters with different health care professionals.

Aspects of holistic assessment

Aspects of holistic assessment will now be considered in more detail.

Assessment of physical needs

While all needs are important, none can be dealt with until physical/functional (symptom) problems are addressed. In addition to exploring the severity of patients' symptoms with them it is important to ask questions about how they are experiencing their symptoms. In relation to pain, Carr (1997) recommends asking:

- What makes the pain better (what strategies are currently being used)?
- What makes the pain worse?
- What is the patient's desired goal for pain relief?
- What does this pain mean to the patient?

Some areas of physical assessment are neglected. For example, weakness and fatigue are common complaints in patients with advanced disease and have a variety of causes: drugs, metabolic disturbances, electrolyte disturbances, tumour load, infections. Co-existing symptoms, such as pain, nausea, vomiting and dyspnoea, aggravate tiredness and require treatment.

Assessment of psychological needs

In a study evaluating nurses' communication skills, before and after a 26-hour training course, Wilkinson et al (1998) found that prior to the course, nurses' scores were low in every key area of assessment, particularly in areas of psychological assessment: assessing how patients were feeling; introducing themselves and stating the purpose of the assessment, and ascertaining patients' understanding of their admission. Wilkinson et al (1998) noted that:

> Overall the assessments were physically oriented and superficial. There was little structure to most of the assessments. This resulted in an enormous amount of repetition.

All nurses benefited from the training and this benefit was transferred into their working environments. Nurses needed most help with emotionally loaded areas, such as patients' awareness of their diagnosis and prognosis, handling difficult questions, psychological assessments, and dealing with patients' and families' emotions, such as anger and denial. Reid-Ponte (1992) noted that primary nurses who showed empathy towards their patients had an ability to explore patients' feelings, to express sympathetic understanding and to act in a caring way. There was a significant relationship between the empathy skills of the nurse and relief of the patient's distress.

Taking account of the person's need for self-esteem and self-actualisation (Maslow 1970), nursing assessment should include data related to the patient's self-concept. How does the patient describe himself and how do his descriptions link in with his behaviour? In Chapter 4 of this book, the effects of advanced disease on patients' identities is discussed and the role of nursing support in maintaining patients' identities and helping them to adapt to change is described.

Facing a diagnosis of serious illness and an uncertain future can provoke great anxiety. Maguire et al (1995, p. 74) noted that such anxiety could reduce the threshold of physical suffering and hinder the disclosure of important practical and emotional concerns. These authors stressed the importance of:

- Offering supportive communication
- Offering information (if the patient wishes this)
- Encouraging the patient to disclose concerns and associated feelings
- Looking for links between thoughts and feelings

- Exploring possible solutions with the patient
- Reviewing any procedures causing anxiety

Maguire et al (1995) stressed the importance of differentiating between moderate anxiety, which is a natural reaction to the individual's serious illness, and an anxiety state, the relief of which may need drug therapy. In a clinical anxiety state, the person has felt apprehensive for longer than 2 weeks and evidence of mood disturbance has been present for at least 50% of the time.

Another emotion that is difficult for nurses to assess and cope with is patients' and relatives' anger. Anger can be expressed in words, tone of voice, facial expressions and non-verbal behaviour. Faulkner et al (1995) noted that anger can result from unrealised ambitions, feelings of loss of control, feelings of hopelessness and from spiritual causes. They maintain that it is important to acknowledge the anger and, when appropriate, its legitimacy. This gives individuals permission to express their feelings. Ideally, anger should be explored in private and without interruption. Assessment should be made of whether the anger is normal for that individual, whether it is rational or irrational, and of the causes of the anger.

■ REFLECTIVE PRACTICE 3.4   Psychological needs

Are there any aspects of assessment of patients' psychological needs which I find difficult? Why is this so?

Discuss with your colleagues how you could improve your assessments of patients' psychological needs.

Assessment of social needs

Assessment of social needs is important as problems in this area can severely impact on people's quality of life. Social need can be related to the following factors:

- Altered relationships/social isolation
- Ill health/disability of another family member
- Loss of work/role
- Financial problems

The aim of care for the patient and family is maintenance of the integrity of the family unit and the well-being of each family member during that process. The illness of one family member profoundly influences the physical and psychological well-being of the others. Normally, families can provide for the needs of their members. However, in times of crisis, they may need us to help them do this. We should ask patients about the reactions of family and close friends to their illness and enquire about the kinds of support they may or may not have received from them. It is important to assess whether the patient and family are experiencing any difficulties in their relationships or communications. Glaser & Strauss (1965) noted that 'open awareness' and discussion of the terminal illness eased communication for staff while 'closed awareness' increased their difficulties. In a study of the needs of relatives of hospice patients, one of the authors (Lugton 1989) found that communication was good in 34 of the 50 families who participated. There were problems in seven families because the patient was confused and, in nine families, communication was poor for other reasons. Difficulties in family relationships may be intractable and longstanding or may have arisen more recently as a consequence of the patient's illness. Where the difficulties in relationships appear to have arisen during the patient's illness, there may be instances where the nurse could talk to the person concerned and encourage him to be more supportive to the patient. Sometimes, children become very anxious about a parent's or grandparent's illness and this may manifest itself in 'difficult' behaviour, for example, becoming upset at school or being apparently unable to cope with school work. The nurse may be able to speak to the child concerned about his anxieties or encourage the patient to be more open with the child about his illness.

Any assessment should include questions about the health of other family members. Such illnesses obviously cause anxiety to patients while they are coping with their own treatment or may mean that care at home is impractical.

Some patients may have become unemployed as a consequence of their illness. Not only may they be on a low income but they may also be missing the status and social side of being at work.

Financial problems may have arisen because of the patient's low income or unemployment. Low income may mean that there is no money for extras that would have made a difference to quality of life, for example, new clothes for themselves or their children, or a holiday. The nurse or social worker may be able to help with some of these problems, for example, finding funding for holidays or helping patients to claim benefits.

■ **CASE HISTORY 3.1   Susan: an assessment of social needs**

Susan, who had advanced breast cancer, was living in a small room within a hotel which was overcrowded and which had totally inadequate bathroom facilities. As a consequence of assessing her social needs, her health visitor made application for rehousing her and she moved into a flat in the same area. The health visitor also applied for financial assistance on her behalf for flat furnishings, an attendance allowance, mobility allowance and money for clothes. All of this considerably improved her quality of life.

Assessment of spiritual needs

Some needs, for example spiritual needs, may be less easily articulated by the patient and therefore more difficult to assess. Renetzky's (1979) definition of the spiritual dimension summarises many attempts to define this concept. He defined spirituality in three parts:

- The need to find meaning, purpose and fulfilment in life, suffering and death
- The need for hope/will to live
- The need for belief and faith in self, others and a power beyond self/God as defined by the individual

Cohen et al (1996) have argued that existential concerns need to be included in any health-related quality of life assessment. Using a quality of life instrument to explore quality of life of cancer patients and their spouses receiving palliative home care, Axelsson & Sjoden (1998) found that the items that received the lowest scores throughout were: ability to do what one wants, physical strength, global quality of life, meaningfulness, and ability to feel joy. They stressed the importance of assessing such items because their findings indicated that when the patient's condition deteriorates:

> Existential issues gain in importance as determinants of global quality of life. We suggest that it will be difficult to substantially improve the overall quality of life of these patients if the existential domain is not considered.

Meaningfulness was also the item that correlated most strongly with global quality of life of patients' spouses. In an unpublished paper, Whyte (1995) acknowledges that suffering is part of the human condition and that it may be more helpful for nurses to work on alleviating suffering and helping the individual to find meaning in suffering than to insist on healing as a goal. Ross (1994a) conducted a survey of nurses' perceptions of spiritual need and spiritual care. Her respondents were 685 staff nurses and charge nurses on 'care of the elderly' wards in Scottish NHS hospitals. She presented spiritual care as part of the nurse's role and stressed the importance of identifying patients' spiritual needs through conducting a spiritual assessment, implementing appropriate interventions to meet needs and evaluating the extent to which interventions had been successful. She maintained that in order to conduct an assessment of spiritual needs nurses would need to know:

- What spiritual needs are
- How they can be recognised (i.e. indicators of spiritual distress)

The highest proportion of nurses defined spiritual need in terms of the need for belief and faith. It appeared that there was a tendency for nurses to view spiritual needs in religious terms. Nurses used a variety of indicators to identify patients' spiritual needs. It emerged that in 70% of cases, spiritual needs were recognised through non-verbal communication. Ross noted:

> This finding suggests that spiritual needs are perhaps more subtle and more difficult to identify than some other needs and that whether or not they are identified may depend on the sensitivity of the nurse.

Ross conducted semistructured interviews with 12 nurses to gain insight into possible factors influencing the spiritual care given. Four main factors emerged. These related to the patient, other professionals, the environment and the nurse. Factors that interfered with nurse–patient communication, such as deafness and dementia, made it more difficult for nurses to identify spiritual needs. Spiritual care was sometimes hindered if there was lack of communication between nurses and the clergy. Nurses reported that a lack of time, coupled with a lack of peace, quiet and privacy, interfered with the giving of spiritual care. Finally, nurses who gave spiritual care at a deep level were aware of the spiritual dimension in their own lives, had experienced personal crises that seemed to act as growth points, perceived spiritual care as part of their role and appeared to be particularly sensitive, perceptive people. Ross (1994b) postulated that it might be possible to maximise nurses' awareness of patients' spiritual needs and confidence in giving spiritual care through self-awareness/sensitivity teaching. It would also be important to encourage nurses to recognise their own limitations in this area and to know when and how to refer to someone else (Ross 1996). She recommended adapting admission sheets to include a spiritual assessment, communicating more with clergy and including clergy in patient profile discussions. Where the patients have difficulties in communicating, collaboration with families and friends may be needed to ascertain what gave these people meaning and hope in their lives prior to the deterioration in their condition.

STAGES OF ASSESSMENT

Assessment of each need is divided into three stages (Lyke 1992).

- A review of the database
- A screening assessment
- A focused assessment

Review of the database

This involves collecting, from charts or case notes, data that have been documented by others. This information is concerned with who this person is, reasons for his admission, the provisional diagnosis and how he is progressing. Much is to be gained by reading any existing medical or nursing notes concerning the patient as it may be possible to see changes in his attitude and medical condition over a period of time. This may have implications for the way in which he is likely to respond to current treatment and nursing care.

Screening assessment: eliciting the current problems

This comprises a brief patient interview with concurrent observation followed by a short examination. It can be used as an initial assessment of a newly referred patient to identify unmet needs. Seeing the person alone is preferable. Maguire et al (1995) maintain that people often deliberately withhold important information if they are first seen with a partner, relative or friend. Lyke (1992) noted that this initial nursing assessment should be confined to:

> The key factors essential to detecting whether a possible, potential or actual problem exists. It is intended only for ruling out or identifying problem areas, not for making a definitive diagnosis.

When we first meet a patient, we will notice a number of things about that person, the way he moves, for example, or facial expressions and demeanour. The behaviour of those accompanying that individual may also be of importance. We can use senses, such as touch and smell, to help us build a picture of what may be happening. A handshake when introducing oneself to a patient will provide us with information about the patient's skin condition. It may be cool and damp or dry and warm. Try to establish which problem the person most wants help with, its nature and severity and how the person feels about that problem. Taking notes avoids forgetting important cues about problem areas. Sharing information with the team is important.

■ **CASE HISTORY 3.2   Anthony, part 1: review of database and screening for problems**

Anthony was a 43-year-old gentleman with a rapidly progressing lymphoma diagnosed 10 months earlier.

Review of database
Anthony had managed well on his own for 5 months but had become debilitated and anxious. He agreed to come for an out-patient appointment at the hospice and it was suggested that a 1-week admission for assessment and symptom relief would be appropriate.

Screening assessment: eliciting the current problems
The hospice used a multidisciplinary approach to assessment of patients' needs. The initial assessment was carried out, with Anthony's agreement, by the doctor and nurse together. This practice was developed in order to minimise repeated questioning and allows the nurse to build on information shared at that time, clarify issues discussed and confirm the plan of care. Only essential information is sought at this initial assessment. Anthony was asked what was troubling him most and what he had been able to do to help the problems. He was an articulate and open individual and this made it easier to assess and meet his needs.

Assessment of physical needs
At the point of Anthony's first admission to the hospice, he was reporting the following symptoms:

- Anxiety
- Sleep loss
- Poor appetite
- Constipation

Anthony spoke openly about his difficulties and saw his sleep loss and poor appetite as the two most distressing symptoms.

At this stage, Anthony's lymphoma, although sizable, was causing him little concern and no pain. Anthony had much faith in complementary therapies, including relaxation and meditation techniques, and was reassured to hear that the hospice would facilitate his continuing those practices whilst an in-patient. The hospice would be able to offer him aromatherapy and massage if he wished. Anthony was independent for much of his needs but needed some help with bathing and shaving.

Assessment of psychological needs

In the hospice, involvement of patients in treatment decision-making is a high priority and need for negotiation, concerning care, is recognised and acted upon. At the initial assessment, we explored what Anthony understood about his illness and what his expectations were for this admission. Anthony was keen to feel a little better but was fully aware and open about his prognosis, which at the time of his admission was thought to be a matter of a few months only. Anthony stated that although he was told by family and friends that he 'looked fine' and was 'doing well', he knew that he was becoming weaker and was beginning to worry a great deal about how his death would occur, what he should expect and what there was to help him through what he had to face, given that he was not willing to take orthodox medicines.

Assessment of social needs

Both Anthony and his family were involved in assessment of his needs to ensure that any information given was the same for all parties. We learned that Anthony was divorced from his wife but had remained friends with her and regularly saw his two sons. However, Anthony's mother had been his main carer since his illness and planned to care for him at home for as long as possible. On admission, Anthony was offered a single room so that he could spend time with his children and family if he wished.

Focused assessment

A focused assessment is much more comprehensive and is indicated whenever the screening assessment indicates a possible problem. This assessment involves a thorough investigation of a specific need and provides substantial evidence to support or rule out such a need.

For example, the comfort of the patient is obviously a priority when curative treatment is no longer possible. However, Lyke (1992) noted that many patients are reluctant to directly verbalise discomfort. Patients' spontaneous descriptions of pain may not be adequate. In most instances, thoughtful and compassionate interviewing is necessary to obtain the information needed for its successful control. Lyke (1992) recommended that the patient should be asked to describe his discomfort or pain and the following information sought:

- Location and radiation
- Character, intensity (a visual analogue scale may be used)
- Duration and constancy
- Precipitating factors
- Alleviating factors and usual length of time to relieve
- Related symptoms (nausea, sweating, anxiety, depression)

Lyke also recommended close observation of the patient during the interview to observe the patient's use of hands to describe or locate the pain, any associated behaviour, such as moaning, crying or pacing, and any changes in thought processes, such as irritability, inappropriate responses or confusion. If the area of discomfort is accessible, the nurse could lightly palpate the area and examine it for redness, swelling or distention.

Another area for focused assessment might be sleep. The quality of sleep that a person has can provide a respite from the pain, worry and hardship that can be associated with terminal illness. The inability to get adequate sleep may compromise the quality of life in the terminally ill person, resulting in fatigue, depression and increased pain. If a patient who is being cared for at home is not sleeping well, the relatives may also become exhausted, thus precipitating the patient's admission into hospital. This fact is well recognised by the Marie Curie Foundation in the UK who provide a night sitter service to both care for the patient and to give respite to tired relatives. Sateia & Silberfarb (1996) estimated that insomnia may affect as many as 50% or more patients with advanced cancer. They noted that depression and anxiety are common in terminally ill patients and can cause insomnia. They recommended that a brief review of current sleeping patterns should be part of the information obtained from all patients receiving palliative care. Assessment should include inquiry about the quantity and quality of sleep at night, any unusual or worrying nocturnal events and the degree of alertness during daytime. The first priority should be to establish the nature of the complaint:

- Trouble getting to sleep
- Frequent awakenings
- Inability to return to sleep
- Unrefreshed sleep
- Not enough sleep

Sateia & Silberfarb advocate that efforts should be made to identify any factors causing insomnia, such as pain, worry or dyspnoea, and to assess the patient's emotional reaction to the sleep disturbance. A review should be made of the 24-hour sleep–wake schedule, including napping, to determine the role that circadian rhythm disturbances play in the presenting complaint. The evaluation of an insomnia complaint should also include a review of the patient's current physical disorders and current medication. Some medications, such as corticosteroids, may contribute to insomnia.

■ CASE HISTORY 3.2   Anthony, part 2: focused assessment

During the initial assessment Anthony became quite tired and the assessment interview was stopped. It was considered important to spend time sharing necessary information at a pace set by the patient. The nurse and doctor arranged to go back to Anthony after he had rested for an hour. On their return, they asked Anthony what he wanted to talk about most. Anthony stated that he needed to know more about what to expect over the next month or so.

Progress of the disease and future care
The doctor explained that he would expect Anthony to gradually become weaker and less able to care for his own needs. The nurse and doctor discussed

with Anthony the options for minimising the distress this might cause him and the help that community and Hospice services could offer. These included:

- Carers to help his mother
- Practical modifications to his home
- The loan of specialised equipment, if necessary

Needs for symptom control

As Anthony had complained about a poor appetite, a dietitian visited to assess his nutritional needs.

It was decided to administer an oral senna preparation for the relief of Anthony's constipation. Anthony was happy with this treatment because of the natural origin of this substance.

Anthony asked if he should expect much pain, which had not been a feature of his illness so far. It was explained that he might experience some pain at a later stage. Treatment options were described briefly. These ranged from simple measures, such as massage, to appropriate analgesia. Anthony restated his desire to avoid orthodox medicines but suggested that perhaps he needed to know more about them before he could be sure. The nurse arranged to spend whatever time he needed with him to discuss various drugs used in treatment of pain and how they could be administered. Anthony wanted to know about both desirable and side-effects of the drugs. The nurse showed Anthony a video that had been produced to help patients to learn about morphine. The use of morphine in treatment of pain had been a particular concern of Anthony's. The information was shared with Anthony over a 4-day period.

Other fears that Anthony expressed were that he might bleed to death or suffocate. These possibilities were discussed with him and the actions that would be taken, should they occur, described.

Psychological and spiritual needs

Anthony said that it was largely fears about how his death would occur and what help he would receive which were causing his sleepless nights. He felt unable to stop these thoughts and had not been able to talk to his family about them for fear of upsetting them. He had visited his GP but felt that the time he needed to discuss his problems was taking other patients' time so he did not make a second appointment. Anthony agreed to receive aromatherapy and massage to help him relax. He continued with his meditation exercises. Soon Anthony was reporting better sleep and said that he was beginning to regain a sense of control. Even though he knew that this would not last he could use this time to plan things the way he wanted them.

Social needs

Anthony said that he wanted to die in the hospice and not at home. A meeting was arranged for Anthony, his mother and the hospice staff to discuss the practicalities of implementing this wish. At the close of the meeting, Anthony's mother confided in the nurse that she was relieved that Anthony had taken this decision. Anthony's mother had always been really fearful of what to expect and did not think she could have coped. She had not felt able to suggest an alternative to home.

CONTINUOUS ASSESSMENT

The assessment of patients' and relatives' needs requires great sensitivity and skill from nurses, not only at the time of diagnosis, but in the following weeks or months of the terminal illness. If we have the opportunity to get to know a patient and his family over several weeks, our assessment of their needs should become increasingly expert because our judgement is informed by our knowledge of them as individuals.

Knowing the patient

Benner et al (1996) noted that a central aspect of clinical judgement of expert nurses was 'knowing the patient'. This meant knowing the patient's typical pattern of responses and knowing the patient as a person. This was especially difficult if the patient was unable to communicate normally. Describing such a case, Benner et al (1996, p. 21) maintained that as we get to know a patient and what is important to him, it sets up the possibility to:

> ... see him in new ways, to challenge the prevailing view of his quality of life, to notice indications of what life meant to him. This was particularly noteworthy in a situation where possibilities for verbal communication were virtually non-existent so other ways of knowing and understanding the person must be relied on. Through narrative accounts of his life, the nurse came to understand who he was as a person, what was important to him and what his concerns might be.

Through these these accounts, nurses come to know the patient in a way that is essential for planning and conducting his care. It was noted earlier that when people are critically ill, their identities are threatened. As nurses, we must find ways to preserve our patients' personhood. In the course of continuous assessment, we can develop detailed knowledge about an individual's pattern of responses, how he moves, what positions are comfortable, what timing of care works best. Benner et al (1996, p. 22) noted several particular aspects of 'knowing the patient':

- Responses to therapeutic measures
- Routines and habits
- Coping resources
- Physical capacities and endurance
- Body topology and characteristics

For example, the frequency of assessments for the patient with pain should be determined by the nature of the pain, the expected duration of effect of analgesics and on whether the patient tends to report or conceal discomfort. Benner et al (1996) claimed that 'knowing the patient' goes beyond formal assessments in several ways. As the nurse is familiar with the typical patterns of responses of a patient, certain aspects of the situation become salient while others recede in importance. This allows for particularising his care from prescriptions and abstract principles. The case history of the patient, Anthony, illustrates how the familiarity of Hospice staff with his attitudes to the use of morphine in pain control, to use of complementary therapies for relaxation and to diet, helped them to create a care plan that was tailored to his expressed needs.

■ **CASE HISTORY 3.2   Anthony, part 3: continuous assessment**

At the end of a week Anthony was able to return home. His sleep pattern was much improved and he was eating and drinking more. He attended the hospice at intervals for out-patient visits to see the doctor and to have aromatherapy and massage. Two more Hospice admissions were necessary over the next 2 months for symptom control. On the second of these, pain had become a problem.

Needs for symptom control

Anthony agreed to try one dose of morphine, which relieved his pain but made him feel sleepy. The nurse spent time explaining to Anthony that drowsiness is common at first but reminded him of the video that he had watched during his first admission. This video had explained that drowsiness resulting from the administration of morphine usually lifts after about 48 hours. Anthony agreed to 'stick it out' and was pleased to find that the drowsiness had gone after only four more doses. As Anthony's condition deteriorated, he experienced difficulties with swallowing and it was agreed that the route of administration of his analgesia should be changed from oral to a syringe driver.

As the lymphoma had increased markedly in size at this point, Anthony was experiencing some difficulties in swallowing solid food. The hospice catering staff modified Anthony's meals, making purees and reconstituting them with a thickener, refashioning the puree in moulds into the shape of the original food, for example, carrot, fish. As Anthony said that he had been a vegetarian for many years his meals included pulses and soya protein, which blended well and reformed convincingly.

Stridor became a feature when Anthony was lying in bed so it was assessed that he needed careful positioning and administration of a nebuliser to give some relief.

Psychological needs

Anthony wanted to take an active part in the decisions about his care and this was encouraged throughout his contact with the hospice. He found this greatly comforting.

Outcome

Anthony died peacefully on the first night of his last admission. The hospice staff had been alongside Anthony throughout his illness. None of the fears concerning the manner of his dying had become realities. Anthony's mother had been with him at his death and found the dignity with which the death occurred of great comfort.

■ **REFLECTIVE PRACTICE 3.5 Knowing the patient**

Benner et al (1996) indicated particular aspects of 'knowing the patient':

• Responses to therapeutic measures
• Routines and habits
• Coping resources
• Physical capacities and endurance
• Body characteristics

Think of a patient receiving palliative care whom you had come to know well. How did this 'knowledge of the patient' help you to meet his needs? Are there any aspects of knowing the patient that you would like to add to Benner's list?

ATTITUDES, KNOWLEDGE AND SKILLS IN ASSESSMENT

Attitudes

As indicated above, nurses' attitudes will influence how assessments are conducted, what is considered important to include in assessments and whether patients are considered partners in their assessment. For example, it has been well documented that nurses do not manage patients' pain effectively and several factors have been identified that contribute to this outcome. In an American study, Warden et al (1998) conducted a survey of graduate nurses' beliefs about suffering as a potential barrier to pain management. Results indicated that nurses held a neutral view of suffering and ineffectively managed hypothetical pain scenarios. Warden et al (1998) postulated that nurses were socialised into viewing situations objectively, to prevent their personal beliefs from influencing patient care. It is only more recently that the importance of subjective pain ratings from patients have been emphasised in nursing curricula.

Knowledge and evidence-based palliative care

To be a skilled assessor, a sound knowledge base of both health and illness is necessary and experience essential. Nurses rarely work entirely alone but are part of a team with access to other nurses and health professionals who have experience and knowledge to share. One of the most recent paradigm shifts in nursing and medicine has been the 'evidence-based care' movement. To be evidence based, the assessment and management of symptoms should rely on existing knowledge from research or respected authorities, based on clinical evidence. In an American study concerned with improvement of care towards the end of life, Field et al (1997) reported that too many people suffered from pain and other distress that could have been relieved or prevented, using existing knowledge. Dunne et al (1997) stressed the need to validate assessment data through published work and with family members so that correct inferences are made. For example, if the cue is a complaint of insomnia and pain from the patient, supporting evidence is that pain is a common cause of insomnia in the terminally ill (Kaye 1992).

Assessment skills

The assessment of patients' and their relatives' needs represents a significant time commitment in any nurse's working day but how accurately do we assess and how well do we communicate our findings to members of the multiprofessional team? Research suggests that nurses are not always effective in their assessment activities, so how can we improve our assessment abilities? When observing colleagues' interaction with patients, we can see the most effective and successful approaches used. When time allows, efforts should be made to discuss the methods employed and to reflect on how we can incorporate such skills into our own practice. The WHO report (1987: p. 183) on Europeans' needs for nursing care, described assessment as follows:

> *Assessment is defined as the first step in the nursing process. Assessment consists of receiving and gathering data about the needs of persons for nursing care. This means perceiving incoming data as well as systematic seeking out of data. It involves the use of skills of observation, communication, analysis and interpretation. It documents data as the interaction with the person proceeds as recorded on the health assessment form or nursing care plan.*

Looking more closely at this, we can see that for a nurse to collect data systematically, knowledge and a certain set of skills are required:

- Holistic observation
- Communication: verbal and written
- Discrimination, analysis and interpretation
- Decision-making

Holistic observation

We need to be sensitive to signs or cues that patients give as to what is troubling them. It does take time and commitment to gain such skills but a great deal can be learned in the workplace itself. Lyke (1992) maintained that accurate assessment involves critical thinking. She claimed that nurses must observe carefully and thoughtfully and learn to describe their observations precisely.

Communication skills

With the perceived increase in the pace of nursing activities and demands made on nursing time, it becomes even more important to make the best use of the time there is. Maguire et al (1995) stressed that assessment of a patient or relative should be conducted in a way that:

> *... maximises the opportunity of the individual disclosing all their main problems, whether physical, social or psychological in nature.*

Communication skills are obviously important in achieving this objective and various aspects of these skills will now be considered:

- Introductions/greetings
- Setting the scene

- Timing
- Eliciting problems
- Note taking/documentation

Introductions/greetings Irrespective of whether you are going into the patient's home or the patient is entering hospital or visiting a surgery, the manner in which the individual is greeted will have a significant and lasting effect on him. On meeting patients for the first time, a welcoming handshake, a smile and the appropriate use of the patient's name will provide a good foundation on which to build a therapeutic relationship. Good practice dictates that if you do not know the name of the patient in advance, then establish what he would like to be called. The use of nicknames or preferred names can be comforting to the individual who is under stress. Similarly, some people prefer to be addressed formally by strangers, a wish that must be respected.

Setting the scene Where possible, see the patient alone to carry out the assessment interview. In this way, you will be truly assessing the patient and not the family or carers. This can be done separately. There are, of course, situations that call for you to interview the patient and family together but this normally occurs in response to the initial assessment carried out with the patient. It will have a specific purpose, for example, to discover how the family views the situation at home or the patient's progress. When interviewing a patient, ensure that he is comfortable and that you are not interrupted. If circumstances do not allow you to interview the patient in a quiet area, then try to minimise the noise by informing staff who are working close by.

Timing A number of points need to be considered here, the most important of which is the negotiation of time. Good assessment takes time but the patient may not be able to tolerate a lengthy interview.

Before the assessment begins, the patient should be informed about how long the interview might take and given permission to stop if he wishes. If the nurse knows that time is limited, then the patient should be told what time is available. In this way the patient has the option to prioritise the information given to the nurse. There is a secondary benefit in this situation. It affords the patient a degree of control at a time when control is being lost in other ways.

If the patient does not communicate problems in terms of priority, then it is for the nurse to ask what troubles the patient most. Assessment can take a day or two to complete in full, which will allow the patient and nurse to develop a relaxed relationship where necessary information can be collected in the least obtrusive way.

Eliciting problems A good assessment strategy contains a sequence of events leading to disclosure of information. It is necessary to plan the assessment process so that it is ordered and clear. Maguire et al (1995) offer the following strategy:

- Elicit the current problems
- Clarify the general nature of the main problems

- Summarise and screen any other problems
- Prioritise and explain
- Summarise and agree on the list of problems
- If the patient becomes distressed always ask, 'Are you able to talk about this?'

When a patient has a cognitive impairment or cannot respond verbally, assessment of needs is more difficult and relatives should be involved.

Questioning A good questioning technique is of paramount importance if the nurse is to assess effectively and within a realistic timescale. It is important to use open, as well as closed, questions.

For factual information, such as that relating to mobility, the nurse may begin with broad, open questions such as:

How much can you do for yourself?

The answer to this question may be:

Hardly anything now. My family have to care for me all the time.

The nurse will need to know what effect that is having on the patient emotionally. She can ask another open question:

How does this make you feel?

This gives the person an opportunity to express their concerns in his own way. Having reached this point, it should be possible to find out exactly what care the patient thinks he will need and how it may be offered so as to minimise associated distress. If something is too painful to discuss then you risk harm to insist that the person continues talking.

Active listening An active listener is someone who listens not only to what is being said but observes what is not being said. An active listener hears the tone of the voice being used (inflections), notices body language and picks up cues to investigate what may be behind them. The response to our original question 'How much can you do for yourself?' was 'Hardly anything now'. This presents the assessing nurse with two options. The first is to assume that the patient is dependent on someone else for all his needs. The second and correct option is to ask more questions. What does the patient mean by 'Hardly anything?' If the patient has lost function, what function is lost and over what timeframe have these changes occurred? When nurses' time is perceived to be in short supply, it is only too tempting to make assumptions and to fill in the gaps of information with guesswork. Assumptions are not only misleading, they can be dangerous if they lead to a series of erroneous decisions about care.

Note taking/documentation In order that important information is not forgotten, the assessing nurse must take notes during an assessment. The notes will include facts but also cues that the patient may give, in the form of statements or behaviour, which may be necessary to follow-up as the assessment proceeds. Whenever taking notes, however, it is essential to tell the patient that you will need to do so before you begin. This will ensure that disclosure is not hindered in any way.

We must also remember that the way in which we document assessment findings must be non-judgemental. If we accept the patient's subjective reports of what he thinks is happening, then we will have the basis of good care already underway.

Accurate and sensitive documentation of nursing assessment is fundamental in initiating an appropriate and effective care plan. In view of the amount of information that can be collected about a patient, it is essential to document only such data that is relevant to the patient's current situation and is necessary to know. Documentation tools are available to guide assessment.

Confidentiality must be maintained at all times if the patient's trust is not to be abused and the potential for a therapeutic relationship lost. A good assessor, therefore, is one who sits beside or shares another's position as well as a collector of data.

As indicated above, sharing of information about the patient and relatives among health care professionals is important, except in instances where one professional has been the recipient of confidential information given in trust by a patient or relatives. Of course, patients are partners in their own care and have access to their notes should they wish to read them. The hospice movement has had, for some years now, an established tradition of shared documentation. All the health care professionals write in the same set of notes. This allows the person reading them to get a clear picture of everyone's view about the person's ability, emotional status and progress. In particular, hospice documentation contains some considerable detail about how the patient and the relative/carer feels about what is happening. This document, sometimes known as the 'Significant Communication Sheet', is where the nurse, social worker, doctor and physiotherapist will record patients' emotions relating to their adjustment to dying and any wishes they have in the way they want to be cared for. Any concerns or difficulties of relatives and carers are also included, as they will clearly have implications either for the future care of the patient or for their own health in bereavement.

Decision-making

Effective nursing assessment necessarily involves the patient in a great deal of disclosure in response to questions asked. Some of the information gained may be relatively superficial but much could be of a highly personal and sensitive nature and will require equally sensitive handling by the nurse. The assessing nurse must make a number of decisions during assessment. These decisions fall into four categories:

- How much of the disclosed information is relevant to the patient's current situation?
- What is the priority order of the information disclosed, as the patient and the nurse perceive it?
- How is the assessment information to be communicated within the multidisciplinary team?
- What are the implications for planning care?

SUMMARY

As indicated above, when considering these factors, we must be aware of the role of any personal and social biases and organisational traditions that may affect the assessment outcome. In an exploratory study of general nurses' perceptions of palliative care, Holmes et al (1997) found that:

This sample of nurses focused primarily on the disease and that which the patient had 'lost', regarding him not as a living person but as a dying patient. The nurses' role is seen to be that of 'taking over' all activities for the patient so as to reduce suffering.

If made in partnership with the patient (and relatives), assessment is not only an important basis for effective, individualised nursing care, it can be an invaluable support to the patient in appraising his own situation, the adequacy of his coping resources and in indicating the professional support which is available to him.

Assessment is the foundation upon which effective, person-centred nursing care rests. It is vital therefore, that no important elements are neglected or overlooked so that nursing care is a true response to our patients' needs.

REFERENCES

Axelsson P, Sjoden P O 1998 Quality of life of cancer patients and their spouses in palliative home care. Palliative Medicine 12: 29–39

Benner P, Tanner C A, Chesla C A 1996 Expertise in nursing practice: caring, clinical judgement and ethics. Springer Publishing, New York

Bradshaw J 1972 A taxonomy of social need. In: McLachlan G (ed) Problems and progress in medical care. Oxford University Press, London

Carpentino L J 1995 Nursing diagnosis: application to clinical practice. J B Lippincott, Philadelphia

Carr E 1997 Assessing pain: a vital part of nursing care. Nursing Times 93: 46–48

Clarke D, Malson H 1995 Key issues in needs assessment. Progress in Palliative Care: an International Journal 3: 53–55

Cohen S R, Mount B M, Thomas J J, Mount L F 1996 Existential well being is an important determinant of quality of life: evidence from the McGill Quality of Life Questionnaire. Cancer 77: 576–586

Copp L A 1974 The spectrum of suffering. American Journal of Nursing 74: 491–495

Davitz A J 1981 Compassion, suffering, morality: ethical dilemmas in caring. Nursing Law and Ethics 2, 1, 2, 6

Davitz J R, Pendleton S H 1969 Nurses inferences of suffering: cultural differences. Nursing Research 18: 100–103

Davitz L J, Sameshima Y, Davitz J R 1976 Suffering as viewed in six different cultures. American Journal of Nursing 76: 1296–1297

Department of Health 1990 NHS and Community Care Act. Her Majesty's Stationery Office, London

Dunne K, Coates V, Morgan A 1997 Functional health patterns applied to palliative care: a case study. International Journal of Palliative Nursing 3: 324–329

Faulkner A, Maguire P, Regnard C 1995 The angry person. In: Regnard C, Hockley J (eds) Flow diagrams in advanced cancer and other diseases. Edward Arnold, London

Field M J C 1997 In: Field M J, Cassel C K (eds) Approaching death: improving care at the end of life. National Academy Press, Washington DC, pp 1–12

Glaser B G, Strauss A L 1965 Awareness of dying. Aldine Publishing, Chicago

Gordon M 1994 Nursing diagnosis: process and application. Mosby, St Louis

Higginson I (ed) 1993 Clinical audit in palliative care. Radcliffe Medical Press, Oxford

Holmes S, Pope S, Lamond D 1997 General nurses' perceptions of palliative care. International Journal of Palliative Nursing 3: 92–99

Kaye P 1992 A–Z of hospice and palliative medicine. EPL Publications, Northampton

Lugton J 1989 Relatives: making plans. Nursing Times 85: 44–45

Lyke E M 1992 Assessing for nursing diagnosis. J B Lippincott, Philadelphia

McCaffery M 1980 Nursing management of the patient with pain, 2nd edn. J B Lippincott, Philadelphia

Maguire P, Faulkner A, Regnard C 1995 Eliciting the current problems. In: Regnard C, Hockley J (eds) Flow diagrams in advanced cancer and other diseases. Edward Arnold, London

Maguire P, Faulkner A, Regnard C 1995 The anxious patient. In: Regnard C, Hockley J (eds) Flow diagrams in advanced cancer and other diseases. Edward Arnold, London

Maslow A 1970 Motivation and personality, 2nd edn. Harper Row, New York

NCHSPCS 1995 Specialist palliative care: a statement of definitions. National Council for Hospice and Specialist Palliative Care Services, London, Occasional Paper 8

Neale B 1991 Informal palliative care: a review of research on needs standards and service evaluation. Trent Palliative Care Service, Occasional Paper 3, Sheffield

Osoba D 1991 Effect of cancer on quality of life. CRC Press, Boca Raton, Florida

Prior D, Poulton V 1996 Palliative care nursing in a curative environment: an Australian perspective. International Journal of Palliative Nursing 2: 84–90

Reid-Ponte P 1992 Distress in cancer patients and primary nurses' empathy skills. Cancer Nursing 15: 283–292

Renetzky L 1979 The fourth dimension: applications to the social services. In: Moberg D O (ed) Spiritual well-being: sociological perspectives. University Press of America, Washington

Rideout E, Montemuro R N 1986 Hope, morale and adaption in patients with chronic heart failure. Journal of Advanced Nursing 11: 429–438

Rogers M E 1970 An introduction to the theoretical basis of nursing. Davis, Philadelphia

Roper N, Logan W W, Tierney A J 1980 The elements of nursing. Churchill Livingstone, Edinburgh

Ross L A 1994a Spiritual aspects of nursing. Journal of Advanced Nursing 19: 439–447

Ross L A 1994b Spiritual care: the nurse's role. Nursing Standard 8: 33–37

Sateia M J, Silberfarb P M 1996 Sleep disorders in patients with advanced cancer. Progress in Palliative Care 4: 120–125

Seers K, Friedli K 1996 Patients' experiences of their chronic non malignant pain. Journal of Advanced Nursing 24: 1160–1168

Sheldon F 1993 The needs to be met. In: Robbins (ed) Needs assessment for hospice and specialist palliative care services: from philosophy to contracts. National Council for Hospice and Specialist Palliative Care Services, London, Occasional Paper 4

Skilbeck J, Mott L, Smith D, Page H, Clark D 1997 Nursing care for people dying of chronic obstructive airways disease. International Journal of Palliative Nursing 3: 100–106

Tait A, Maguire P, Faulkner A, Brooke M, Wilkinson S, Thomson L, Sellwood R 1982 Improving communication skills. Nursing Times 78: 2181–2184

Warden S, Carpenter J S, Brockopp D Y 1998 Nurses' beliefs about suffering and their management of pain. International Journal of Palliative Nursing 4: 21–25

WHO 1987 People's needs for nursing care: a European study: a study of nursing care needs and of the planning, implementation and evaluation of care provided by nurses in two selected groups of people in the European region. World Health Organization Regional Office for Europe

Wilkinson S, Roberts A, Aldridge J 1998 Nurse–patient communication in palliative care: an evaluation of a communication skills programme. Palliative Medicine 12: 13–22

Worden W 1994 Grief counselling and grief therapy. Routledge, London

FURTHER READING

Benner P, Tanner C A, Chesla C A 1996 Expertise in nursing practice: caring, clinical judgement and ethics. Springer Publishing Company, New York

Regnard C, Hockley J 1995 Flow diagrams in advanced cancer and other diseases. Edward Arnold, London

Support processes in palliative care

Jean Lugton

4

INTRODUCTION

The purpose of this chapter is to unravel something of the meaning of the concept of support, a term in everyday use in nursing but not often clearly defined. The chapter will address the question, 'What do nurses need to do to give support to patients who are receiving palliative care?'. Various theories and aspects of support will be explored, giving readers an opportunity to reflect both on the meaning of this important concept and on the implications for their practice. Illustrations of the meaning of social support, as perceived by women with breast cancer and their health visitors, are taken from my own research, which explored the links between support and social identity (Lugton 1994). The importance of the concept of identity in nursing will, therefore, also be examined.

LEARNING OUTCOMES

This chapter addresses the PREP 'categories' of care enhancement, and patient, client and colleague support. It also encourages the growth of reflective practice.
  After you have read this chapter, you should be able to:

• Identify relevant dimensions of social support (verbal, non-verbal, actions)
• Be aware of the effects of social support in maintaining or changing aspects of individual identities

- Recognise ways in which the identities of dying people and their relatives are threatened by the illness
- Plan nursing interventions to care for people whose identities are threatened by serious illness and provide support for their significant others
- Recognise sources of material to assist in developing your support skills

DIMENSIONS OF SUPPORT

Let us not diminish the power of waiting by saying that a life saving relationship cannot develop in an hour. One eye movement or a handshake can replace years of friendship when a man is in agony. Love not only lasts for ever, it needs only a second to come about. [Nouwen 1979]

At all phases of life-threatening illness, the aim of professional carers should be to maintain and promote the realistic hopes of patients and their significant others and to preserve the best possible quality of life for both.

We communicate our support to others, both verbally and non-verbally, and there must be consistency between these two forms of communication if we are to be perceived as genuine. We should therefore try to relate to dying people on a personal, as well as a professional, level. Benjamin (1981) emphasised the necessity of congruence between verbal and non-verbal communication in effective counselling and the importance of increasing our awareness of our non-verbal communications. Speaking about the insights gained through the use of video during counselling training sessions he noted that:

We can judge for ourselves to what extent our words match our actions ...
We can see ourselves as the interviewee may see us ... Most of all, do we only sound genuine or do we look genuine as well? [Benjamin 1981, p. 67]

Although effective verbal communication is an important channel of support, there are other powerful, but less-recognised, dimensions. It has been estimated that non-verbal communication carries four times the weight of verbal communication (Henley 1973). For example, three major themes emerged from Perry's (1996) study of exemplary oncology nurses. Two of these concerned the importance of non-verbal communications in providing support, that is 'dialogue in silence' and 'mutual touch'. Silence emerged repeatedly as an approach that was used by exemplary nurses in the study.

Most of these silences were rich in non-verbal communication. Messages that were difficult or even impossible to speak were sent from nurse to patient and from patient to nurse in silence.

Silence was important for listening and hearing the message and Perry recommends listening with openness. Sometimes, silent messages were 'encoded in actions' of the nurses. Small details like 'folding their pyjamas', 'warming up their milk if they like it that way' seemed trivial but transmitted powerful messages to patients. The second non-verbal theme identified by Perry was mutual touch. Sometimes this was 'non-physical' as when nurses were skilled at 'encircling' a patient by having an arm just behind the patient's back or around the patient's shoulders. Sometimes, eye contact was combined with touch to provide a potent communication medium. Perry's third theme encompassing non-verbal and verbal behaviour was the use of humour. This was described as a light-hearted attitude, common among the skilled nurses in the study. These nurses deliberately chose, most of the time, to see the positive and humourous side of situations for the benefit of both themselves and their patients. Benjamin (1981) also advocates the use of humour as a means of support. He is careful to point out that he does not mean sarcasm, ridicule or cynicism, but a light touch of humour which stems from empathic listening and which reflects a positive outlook on life.

> *It may well consist of no more than a raised eyebrow, a smile, a gesture. When it breaks through, it brings the two partners in the interviewing process closer together by establishing an additional bond. For want of a better term, I can only call this bond genuine caring for each other and confidence of the helping nature of human rapport. [Benjamin 1981, p. 159]*

■ REFLECTIVE PRACTICE 4.1   Dimensions of support

Please take a few moments to recall the last time you nursed a dying patient. Note down the following points:

- To what extent did you use non-verbal support?
- What kinds of non-verbal support did you use?
- What was the patient's response?
- Do you think that this kind of support helped? In what ways?
- Are there any forms of non-verbal support that you do not use? Why is this?

Once you have read this chapter and the chapter on complementary therapies, reflect on how you could improve your non-verbal support to your patients.

SUPPORT AND IDENTITY IN HEALTH

The greater part of identity or sense of 'self' is developed and maintained through interaction with others. Everyday interactions among family members have profound effects upon the development of the self. Mead (1934) argued that the individual develops a self-concept through role taking. In the first stage of this process, children play roles other than their own and become aware of the differences between themselves and the roles they play. In the second stage, children come to see themselves from others' perspectives as participants in the game. Mead's theories have been developed by other sociologists who recognised that individuals incorporated only the norms of the groups in a society that had become significant to them but of which they might not yet be members (e.g. Sherif 1953). These reference groups influenced attitudes and behaviour and moulded identity. Hirsh (1981) maintained that people's social networks can both support and assist in redefinitions of their identities. However, these social networks also reflect people's values and choices. The process of maintaining social identities is thus interactive between people and their significant others. Of a number of social identities, a few can be described as core identities because they form the basis of the individual's perceived self, being those self-perceptions that seem most important to the person. Examples of core identities for most people are their body image and sexuality. People's significant others, such as their partners, parents, siblings and children, are likely to be included in their self-concepts. The attitudes and behaviour of people in these close relationships are important to individuals' self-esteem and security. Combs & Snygg (1959) claimed that in their interactions with others, people seek to maintain and enhance their identities.

SUPPORT AND IDENTITY IN ILLNESS

The self-concept represents the person's fundamental frame of reference and is usually very stable and resistant to change. In a crisis, such as illness, when a redefinition of self may become necessary, much encouragement may be needed to make this shift possible. Social interactions can undermine people's identities if they negatively label or stigmatise them. Labelled people are grouped into 'types' of person and certain kinds of behaviour are expected of them. In a study of patients' experiences in self-management of diabetes mellitus, Nyhlin (1990, p. 64) found that diabetics worked hard at creating an appearance of normality.

The diabetic person would rather be shown consideration primarily as the person he is instead of having to show that he is diabetic.

The literature suggests that the majority of female patients with cancer continue to be sustained by most of their close relationships as they adjust. However, isolated instances of rejection are relatively common (Bard & Sutherland 1955, Dunkel-Schetter 1984).

■ REFLECTIVE PRACTICE 4.2   Identity

Reflect on the subject of core identities and consider the core aspects of your own identity: your sexuality, important relationships, beliefs, values, skills, strengths and weaknesses. How might these core identities be affected by illness and how would you feel if they were so affected? Discuss with a friend. For example:

- What are your most important beliefs and values?
- How important to you is your sexuality, aspects of your physical appearance?
- What personal qualities do you most value in yourself, for example, your independence, your cheerfulness?
- How important is it to you to develop and use your skills and talents, for example, professional skills, being musical, being artistic?
- Which are your most important roles, for example, at home, at work, in organisations to which you belong?
- Which relationships, are most important to you, for example, with family, friends, work colleagues?

Effects of support in maintaining and changing aspects of identity

Support is integral to effective palliative nursing. Much has been written about nurses' responsibility to communicate both with people who are approaching death and with their distressed friends and relatives. However, support is still a concept that we use frequently, but loosely, without really examining what we mean. How does our support promote a sense of well-being in others? My own research into the experiences of women with breast cancer indicated that the underlying 'essence' of social support is the way it maintains individuals' identities, their sense of 'self', both in every-day life and in crisis situations such as illness (Lugton 1994). In some circumstances, support also helps people to make necessary changes in their self-concepts by adapting their self-perceptions to their changed circumstances.

Effects of advanced illness on identity

Research has shown that it is often difficult for people to maintain adequate concepts of self when undergoing changes caused by serious illness, which can spoil aspects of their established identities (for example, Anderson 1986, 1988, Kelly 1991, 1992, Tait 1988). The degree to which an illness affects the individual's core identities varies from person to person. People who are terminally ill are likely to face several identity crises. They have to move through these crises towards a more peaceful acceptance of their situation. Failure to do so means that identities remain under threat and the crises are unresolved. Although most women with breast cancer were beginning to get back to normal living a year after treatment, aspects of their identities remained under threat (Lugton 1994). Many patients still spoke of fears of recurrence, dissatisfaction or lack of confidence in their body image and sexuality. One woman was still very preoccupied with the effects of mastectomy on her body image and sexuality 3 years later, to the extent that it severely limited her social life.

THE NURSE–PATIENT RELATIONSHIP

We need to think about our patients' identities much more and, in some cases, help patients make changes to their identities as they struggle to cope with the effects of illness. Proctor (1996) pointed out that nursing is about relationships and interactions, not, as some nursing models imply, about what the nurse does to the patient. It is about continuity of relationships to maintain growth. Proctor notes:

> This implies a high degree of autonomy on the part of the nurse and the patient but this is often not allowed by the system.

Nurse–patient relationships are, to an extent, invisible, and therapeutic relationships may not be so highly valued by health care organisations as more obvious measures of effective nursing care. Indeed, much of the information required by management as an indication of the effectiveness of nursing services seems to be quantitative. Morse et al (1992) claimed that the heart of effective nursing support was the nurse's ability to identify with patients' experiences.

> *The caregiver must be emotionally involved or able to identify with the sufferer. The caregiver must be willing and able to experience or share with the others suffering and to respond meaningfully and appropriately to the sufferer ... The essence of the nurse–patient relationship is the engagement, the identification of the nurse with the patient. [Morse 1992, p. 811]*

However, emotional involvement with patients can leave aspects of nurses' identities exposed and vulnerable. Morse et al (1992) recognised that it was not desirable for caregivers to be constantly engaged in relationships. Other responses were often appropriate to protect the caregiver or were needed by the patient. Health visitors sometimes found their involvement with patients with breast cancer stressful (Lugton 1994). Anna had advanced breast cancer and her health visitor had this experience:

> *It's quite involving. You tend to think about it as you come away as well. The visits can take quite some time. In fact Anna has almost gone through a grief type reaction. I see a big need there. Mind you it would be very draining.*

There are compensations for making an emotional commitment to the patient. The caregiver often receives reciprocal support. However, it is important that professionals support each other in these situations. Nurses working in the community can be particularly vulnerable if there are fewer opportunities for sharing their feelings with colleagues.

Johns (1996) noted that the advent of the reflective practitioner will shift reliance on prescriptive models of nursing towards reflective practice, which is grounded in reflective cues that tune the practitioner into the human encounter.

> *It always involves a process of grasping and interpreting the moment (assessment) in the light of past experience (evaluation) and responding with appropriate intervention in light of envisaged outcomes (planning) ... Transcending the nursing process, reflective models utilise a narrative mode of writing, responsive to the unfolding relationships between the person receiving care and the caregivers.*

This reflection on experience develops the quality of interventions. Professional relationships with patients can often be supportive because they are not embedded in any past or future roles and do not carry expectations of reciprocity, as do relationships with kin and friends. During illness, many patients feel obliged to protect their network members by hiding their true feelings. Women with breast cancer commented on the supportiveness of confiding in someone 'outside' their social circles (Lugton 1994). For example, Carol, who had advanced disease, reported that her family was unwilling to talk about her illness because they could not cope. Being separated from her husband, she wanted to share her worries about herself and her sons' future. She was unable to do this.

My mother, sisters and brother don't seem to have much time for me. I don't think they can actually cope with it. They just don't talk about it.

She felt she could confide in her health visitor.

It's nice to have someone who knows what I'm talking about but is sort of an outsider. It helps because I'm beginning to see it from her point of view as well as my own. The family is hopeless about this.

We should be aware that patients' protective attitudes can sometimes extend to professional helpers as well (Lugton 1994). Patients may protect their doctors from their anxieties, putting up with discomforts without complaint, presenting a bright face. A health visitor attending the hospital out-patients' breast cancer clinic noted:

The thing that struck me about those clinic sessions was what a false impression the doctors might get about the patients. The patients on the whole were quite bright and positive with the doctors and joked with them. At some of the clinics, the patients would stay in the rooms and get undressed. I would stay with the patients and they would say, 'This is a nightmare' or something totally opposite to how it sounded to the doctor.

Patients' coping ability is increased by the availability of nurses who are perceived as accessible and approachable and able to provide personalised support. This support can be in the background, available if needed. In this respect nurses can be like the 'attachment figures' described by Bowlby (1975, p. 234):

Presence of an attachment figure is to be understood as implying ready accessibility rather than actual or immediate presence and absence implies inaccessibility. Not only must an attachment figure be accessible but he/she must be willing to respond in an appropriate way to someone who is afraid.

This perceived availability in relation to health visitors was described by several patients with breast cancer (Lugton 1994). Anna commented on her relationship with her health visitor:

She's my lifeline. I know she's there. I suppose it's a bit like a kid with a night light. You know it's there if you want it. She's really made a tremendous difference.

We have to be able to convey to patients, verbally and non-verbally, that we can both understand and cope with their distress. Power plays a more obvious role in professional than in informal relationships. Professionals who control their relationships with patients by dominating interactions and controlling accessibility are seen as unsupportive. By contrast, those who are openly available to see patients and to discuss anxieties are perceived to be very supportive. Adverse effects of power on effective support are evident when professional agendas dominate their interactions with clients. Thus, professionals can use their expertise to exercise power over patients or to empower them. For example, Ina, who had been receiving treatment for breast cancer, was worried about a lumpy breast following radiotherapy. She unsuccessfully sought professional reassurance (Lugton 1994):

The radiotherapists didn't notice. It's just their own wee bit they are interested in. Then the doctor says, 'Take your things off'. Then he just goes, 'Oh yes'. I mean it's ridiculous. Why do we bother because they don't look at the thing. I never felt he asked me anything. I thought, 'I'm going away'. I can't get out quickly enough.

ASSESSMENT

The process of protecting and building identities starts with careful assessment of the person. Important questions are:

- How is this person feeling?
- What important aspects of this person's identity (including significant relationships, future plans, important roles) are threatened in the present situation?
- What professional and informal support does this person have?

How is this person feeling?

It is important to assess how sick people are feeling. Expressing these feelings is vital in enabling them to come to terms with their situations, to cope, and for nurses to respond with sensitivity. Awareness of serious illness does not always mean acceptance of its implications. Denial may be the way in which some people cope with their illness. Janet, who had advanced breast cancer, was not ready to see herself as 'dying' and was frightened by her GP's apparently pessimistic view of her future and his inability to see that denial was helping her to cope.

I feel that he [GP] takes a more pessimistic view of my illness. I always get the impression when he speaks to me that he's surprised that I'm as well as I am. He seems to think it was much worse than I thought.

Having a debilitating illness may sometimes cause people to review their lives and may enhance any existing feelings of failure. Anna had periods of depression and had once attempted suicide. Her health visitor empathised with her feelings and this helped Anna to cope:

She sees her life as being a failure because there's two marriages that have broken down. To us it seems that she's been terribly, terribly hard done by. Why should she have this as well? She's had a miserable upbringing. She remains very depressed. She confided to me that she felt life was not worth living and had attempted to commit suicide by trying to overdose with tablets. As time goes by she won't be nearly so well. I don't feel I could drop off from seeing her.

What important aspects of this person's identity are theatened in this present situation?

A person with advanced disease is likely to pass through several identity crises, described here as threats.

The threat of illness to life and future plans

In health, most individuals are able to plan for the future with some confidence because they do not imagine they will become ill and be unable to do the things they presently take for granted. Ideas about personal invulnerability and immortality begin in early childhood. Young children, for example, are often unable to understand the permanence of death, thinking that a relative who has died will return. Teenagers and young adults tend to see themselves as relatively indestructible with an unlimited future. Many apparently healthy, middle-aged people have an expectation of living to an old age. Often, people do not think much about their deaths when they are in apparent good health. If they become aware that they have a potentially fatal disease, they are stopped in their tracks. It is a threat to the very core of the self and can undermine their sense of security and ability to plan for the future. Women with breast cancer had to cope with their fears of dying of the disease (Lugton 1994). For example, if there was a history of breast cancer in a patient's family, this increased her worries about her own prognosis. Phyllis coped by perceiving herself as indispensable to her family.

> You've got to die of something in the end. My mother died of lung cancer.
> She had secondaries before they discovered it had come from the breast. I'm not
> planning on doing that just now! I've got far too many responsibilities.
> I'm far too busy.

Another woman, Susan, had been afraid of dying from cancer since her youth. She confronted her fears by remembering that she was only 46, strong enough to fight the disease.

> I suppose when I was younger I thought 'What if I die of cancer?' That's
> everybody's fear, to die of cancer. I never thought at 46 I would have cancer. Folk
> will say to you, 'You'll get on all right. You are strong enough. You're okay.'

Eleanor felt that she needed to face up to her mortality before she could move on.

> I did go through a week like that, thinking negatively, but you have got to go
> forward. Some people suppress their thoughts. Some people suffer from
> depression because they can't express themselves.

These examples show various ways in which one group of women with breast cancer coped with the threat to their survival. To be effective, palliative support should begin early, rather than in the latter stages of the disease process. Dixon et al (1996) noted the importance of including patients' fears of recurrence as an integral part of the nursing assessment of cancer patients because such patients worry about: how their families would cope if they should die; how they would be treated and by whom; whether they would be allowed to stay at home or be admitted to a hospital or a hospice; whether medical staff would say that there was nothing more that could be done, leading to a sense of abandonment and a feeling that no-one cared; and how they would die and if they would be in pain or experience severe symptoms.

The threat of illness to physical and psychosocial independence

In health, most people regard themselves as competent and independent people. Disease often makes them feel temporarily or permanently uncertain of their physical and psychological coping abilities. Erikson (1965) maintained that gaining autonomy is an important part of development of the self. Loss of independence can be shattering to self-esteem. Johnson (1991) found that the process of regaining control after a heart attack involved three dimensions: an ability to predict outcomes, make informed decisions and act on decisions. Heart attack victims had a sense of uncertainty, which diminished predictability. They also lacked understanding of their bodies, undermining their sense of power and control. No longer able to trust their abilities, and relying on others' support, undermined their independence.

The ability to make decisions is an important aspect of this autonomy. Maier & Seligman (1976) proposed a 'learned helplessness' theory of depression, suggesting that a stressful situation could lead to depression if the individual believed it was impossible to control the situation.

The threat to body image and sexuality

The threat of advanced disease to the sexual identities of sufferers is discussed in depth in Chapter 6 of this book and is only briefly mentioned here. The threat to life posed by the illness does not always override anxieties about sexual identity, which is so much a part of personhood. For example, in my own research (Lugton 1994), Carol, who had advanced breast cancer, disliked her appearance because she had a fungating tumour. She always took a foam bath to avoid looking at herself, saying that she felt dirty because of her cancer. Even patients in longstanding, apparently good relationships, were anxious about the possible effects of cancer on their sexual relationships. Retaining her femininity, despite having a double mastectomy and hair loss, was important to Margaret.

> It's very important to have a good wig. To be caught without it can be really shattering. You think, 'I can't look so terribly different with no hair,' but oh my goodness you do. Your head looks so wee. It's as if half your personality had been whipped off as well. But wanting to wear a wig and having to are two different things. It's nice to have your own hair. It's part of being feminine isn't it?

Edith, whose cancer had caused her to lose a lot of weight, often felt depressed about her physical appearance. Her husband was supportive.

> It's all my false bits. Once you take them off you think, 'Oh dear.' Then I lost an awful lot of weight. Then I swelled up in the tummy. I looked like one of those poor little mites you see on TV with the thin arms and thin legs and pot tummy. I don't have a light on to go to bed. My husband and I had our first little barney for a long time. It sparked off over a dress he wanted me to get. I said, 'Oh what's the point? I've got that much in my wardrobe that I can't wear because I'm going up and down in size.' I've always put on this brave face. Just now and again you can't. It's only you and your husband that has to accept it and mine never showed any repugnance.

Janet was also cachectic and depressed about her appearance.

I don't look at my mastectomy very much. If I have a bath and I look up I think, 'Oh my goodness, you do look awful!' I'm so thin and scraggy looking. My husband has been very kindly and gentle with me. We've come to terms with it. We're a bit past a sex life. He's not got the energy you know. He says, 'If you had seen yourself when you were really ill, you're a miracle now.'

The threat to social roles and status

With progression of disease, people are likely to feel less confident in their roles as partners, parents, friends and workers. Some roles may have to be given up. Lynam's (1990) research into the support of young adults with lymphoma and sarcoma emphasised the importance, to identity, of their ability to fulfil social roles. All her respondents defined themselves in terms of their social roles and relationships and the feelings derived from them. Women with breast cancer (Lugton 1994) also worried about their competence to carry out their normal social and work roles. Many found themselves temporarily unable to do so and a few were permanently unable to cope. Serious illness, and its treatment, imposes physical limitations. These are often temporary and are cast aside on the road to recovery. However, in advanced disease, physical dependence often increases as the disease progresses.

Physical limitations mean that sufferers are unable to carry out their normal social and work roles; this has implications for self-esteem. Northouse & Swain (1987) found that the greatest concern of many hospital patients recovering from surgery for breast cancer was whether they would be able to return to their previous lifestyle. Women with small children said that family concerns were their primary worry. They reported vocational, domestic and social problems. Vocational difficulties centred on taking time off work. Domestic difficulties resulted from limited arm movement interfering with housework, and social difficulties resulting from tiredness. The domestic problems echo research by Oakley (1974), which drew attention to how female identities could be moulded around the housewife image. Many women are anxious to resume their normal household tasks in spite of feeling tired and debilitated as a result of illness. They are often encouraged to do so by other family members. Maintaining their employment was important to many patients with breast cancer (Lugton 1994). Carol, who had advanced breast cancer, had prided herself on taking little sick leave from work, until she had to take time off for hospital treatment. Her disease and treatment made her feel tired. However, her work was important to her identity. She wanted to continue full time for as long as possible.

There are a lot of girls in the work who take one day here and two days there. I'm not that sort of person. Before all this happened I was never off you know. I find that if I'm working I feel that much better. I think it gives you a purpose. It takes your mind off the problems. I do feel I need to work.

Anna, who had advanced cancer, wanted to work but was unsure of her ability to cope.

Being at home and not being able to do anything, it's driving me mad. I don't know if I could cope with work. I think fear is a big part of it.

She later had a course of chemotherapy but this made her feel tired and old. Her illness and its treatment had undermined her self-esteem.

The chemotherapy is working but I keep asking myself, 'Is it worth it to be like someone in their dotage?' It took me an hour last night to wash up dishes.
I'm going in to work today. God knows how I'm going to do it. I'll have to try. I shouldn't be feeling sick like this. There's so many things I want to do and I just can't do them. You just can't help doubting yourself.

The threat to relationships

In health, many people feel secure in their important relationships. Close relationships form part of a person's identity and give feelings of security and competence. As the seriousness of their illness becomes manifest, people often go through a period of feeling less confident in their relationships. Indeed, they may experience negative reactions from some relatives and friends whose own security is threatened by the illness. My own research among 35 women with breast cancer (Lugton 1994), revealed that for 14, their social networks were predominantly supportive. Their relationships were good. Relatives and friends seemed able to cope with the patients' illness without perceiving it as in any way threatening to themselves. However, 20 networks offered women with breast cancer a mixture of support and strain. There were longstanding relationship difficulties between some women and their network members in this group. In a number of instances, a relative was ill or unable to cope with the woman's illness, regarding it as in some way threatening to herself. One woman had a predominantly stressful network owing to dysfunctional relationships within the family and a lack of friends. The strain existing in some social networks illustrates the potential for professional staff to both provide the missing support themselves and to facilitate improved relationships between patients and their significant others. Glaser & Strauss' (1965) research showed that communication within families could become closed when one member was seriously ill and others became anxious. Family members were aware of the situation but were unable to discuss their concerns. This is an area where nurses can be helpful in trying to open up communication.

Sick people may be unable to fulfil their normal roles and this may affect their relationships. Sometimes, relatives and friends do not want to recognise the seriousness of an illness because the patients' inability to fulfil their normal roles threatens their own accepted roles and identities. For example, Janice was very depressed after breast surgery and felt that her husband and children made light of her illness, not acknowledging her feelings.

When you are feeling low you need a bit of understanding, don't you? It was quite hard because it wasn't until I was really quite down that they sort of acknowledged that I was feeling low. I had to shout quite loudly about it.
In fact Ben [husband] has always been very busy and he was rushing around. He was perhaps the last one to notice.

Carol found her work tiring while having chemotherapy. Her work supervisors showed little understanding of her situation.

When I did get the letter the first time about the hours of work changing I said to my boss, 'Are we not supposed to be asked about this?' She said, 'Look if you go upstairs about it, you'll be out.' That's the way they work. If you don't like it you're out.

However, illness also offers opportunities for increased richness in relationships because of increased awareness of how much others care. Margaret had advanced cancer. Her husband, who was a doctor, decided to spend more time with her.

He decided he would retire early. He decided last year when I was getting chemotherapy and he was getting home late. It meant I had to wait sometimes the whole day till he was finished. We thought, 'This is silly. We should be spending more time together, not muddling on trying to get this one to pick me up and he having the stress of not being able to do this.'

The threat of stigma and isolation

In health, most people regard themselves as 'normal', integrated into their families and their communities. Serious illness can make them feel powerless and unsure of their status, especially if they are subjected to others' negative expectations and labelling. For example, anyone with cancer has to face society's fatalistic attitudes to malignant disease. The sufferer is often reduced in people's minds from being a whole and normal person to being a tainted, discounted one, a stigmatising experience shared by families of patients with cancer. Anna found her advanced breast cancer embarrassing because it was incurable and some people avoided her.

It's an embarrassing disease. At times I feel as if I've got a big sign up saying 'Beware cancer'. There are a lot of people who'll not come near you if they know you've got something like that. You feel as if you should be ringing a bell saying 'Unclean' or something. You tend to keep it to yourself. I mean it's not the sort of thing you go spreading around. Other people, you feel, are watching you, just waiting on you popping off.

A disease like cancer is a mystery to many people as its causes are unknown, adding to its aura of fatality.

The threat to faith and hope

A life-threatening illness may cause a person to grow spiritually or fall into doubt and despair. Sometimes patients speak of the need for spiritual support. For example, Sheila valued the spiritual support offered by her church friends.

There's a lot of prayers being said by a lot of people. I'm in their thoughts. You don't think it's doing anything but it does. It brings you through.

A person's spirituality is much broader than her religious beliefs or lack of them. It is an important part of identity. Chapter 5 explores ways in which spiritual distress can manifest itself during terminal illness and ways in which nurses can care for clients who have spiritual problems.

■ REFLECTIVE PRACTICE 4.3   Threatened identity

Think about some crisis in your own life that was difficult for you to cope with. What aspects of your identity came under threat? Make notes about the following:

• How did you feel?
• How did you cope?
• Did you emerge from the crisis as essentially the same person or were you changed in some ways by the crisis?
• In what ways, if any, were you changed?

What professional and informal support does this person have?

We should ask patients about the practical and emotional support that they are receiving from their key relationships. People with advanced disease can lose many social contacts owing to their own increasing incapacity (Lugton 1994). Edith suffered anxiety attacks since her recurrence. Tension and tiredness made it difficult for her to do the things she enjoyed.

> My friends say, 'Do you read? Do you sew?' Well, when you are ill you can't do these things. That's what makes the day so long. Sometimes my nerves are that bad that I can't thread a needle and I haven't got the concentration either. It makes you realise how basic life is.

Jane was typical in losing contact with her peers who were diagnosed with breast cancer at the same time.

> Gradually you lose touch a little bit because we've all gone different ways. They haven't required any further treatment as far as I know.

Rita did not want contact with other patients because she felt unable to cope if they became more ill.

> I haven't kept in contact with any other patients. I didn't really feel I could cope with that, it might be difficult if anyone was ill.

Sometimes, people with advanced illness experience rejection by others who in some way perceive the illness as threatening to themselves. Families may react negatively to disruptions in their routines and the threatened expectations that family members hold for one another as members of an interdependent system. Helen's son, aged 15, had to cope with both his mother's breast cancer diagnosis and his father's illness caused by a subarachnoid haemorrhage.

> He went away when I was in hospital to stay with my cousin, who he's very fond of, because he couldn't hack it anymore, he said. I know it's certainly affected his school work. He's lost a lot of self-confidence but the school is aware of why.

Mary's children, 4 and 3 years old, initially coped well with their mother's illness. However, the little boy's nursery school work was affected by his mother's illness. Lichtman et al (1985) also found that a minority (12%) of their respondents with breast cancer reported a deterioration in one or more of their relationships with their children. Patients may be unwilling to talk about their fears about their illness to friends and neighbours if any of these have reacted negatively. For example, Betty did not want to discuss her cancer recurrence with many people, remembering a neighbour's reaction when she was first diagnosed with breast cancer.

Last time after I got better, I was at the bus stop and there was a woman who kept looking at me as if she expected me to drop dead at any minute. I've always remembered that and this time I did want to keep it quiet.

Edith, who had developed ascites and had had a paracentesis performed, experienced rejection by patients who felt threatened by her illness.

In hospital I just went up to these two women. They hadn't long had their operations. I said 'How do you feel?' Then they said, 'Have you had an operation?' I said, 'No.' I had this bag of water I was carrying round (from paracentesis). I said 'Mine's a hiccup. I had mine 5 years ago.' This other one said, 'I don't want to hear any more about it.' She said, 'I've had enough of people talking about it.'

Despite their difficulties, some respondents managed to maintain their involvement in family, community and work life. This was mainly a result of personal determination.

Patients should be asked to indicate both positive and negative reactions of their relatives and friends to the illness (perhaps through a simple diagram). This will enable nurses to assess which aspects of support are not being provided informally. They are then in a position to ask, 'Can existing network members be assisted to provide the kind of support that is needed?' Serious illness poses a threat to the future of families, as well as of patients, yet relatives often receive less information and support from professional sources than do patients, although their anxiety may be almost as great.

EVALUATION

Assessment needs to be continuous and evaluations made after each interaction so that a picture of the patient's problems and support needs is gradually built up. Having explored how the patient is feeling, the next question is 'How is the patient coping?' What support is needed to enable her to cope better? Evaluation of patients' and relatives' needs for information and support during advanced illness requires great professional sensitivity and skill. There is an obvious need to address more than just the medical problems although physical distress must be treated promptly. Patients may present with physical distress and it is only when this has been brought under control that psychosocial and spiritual issues come to the surface (G R Nimmo, unpublished work, 1982). Many patients cannot separate their physical problems from other aspects of their lives and seek support for their total situation. Often, people fear dying rather than death, imagining they will have pain and other distressing symptoms, and fear a loss of dignity. They need us both to help them to realistically appraise these threats to their identities and to listen and understand as they express their emotions. Knowledge of patients' coping styles is important and requires careful reflection and evaluation by nurses. For example, Anna coped by putting her illness to the back of her mind, sometimes more successfully than others.

> *How long can you go on with not knowing – mind you part of me doesn't want to know – what's happening. When you think you've got over one bit, something else crops up. For a long time I worried. Then it sort of dawned on me that I was still here. It wasn't so serious. You could put it in the background. Then that stupid doctor made me feel that it was going to be my last Christmas. I wouldn't even see January. From then on it was difficult.*

She feared the prospect of dying. Contrary to her wishes, A GP insisted on discussing her prognosis.

> *She spoke to me as if I had minutes to go. She said, 'We'll have to rule out something much more serious.' She said, 'You do realise what's wrong with you?' She started telling me what was wrong. I said, 'I know as much as I want to know.' Things have progressed but I don't want to know any more. She insisted on telling me. I think if you don't want to know, it shouldn't be forced on you. I'm not ready to know any more because I'll go right over the edge. I don't see how her telling me was any help because it frightened the daylights out of me.*

Nurses may find the needs of some patients difficult to evaluate, for a variety of reasons. Stockwell (1984) found that nurses spent less time communicating with 'unpopular' patients because they were unrewarding, being unappreciative of what was done for them. Sometimes, in advanced illness, patients and relatives may become very withdrawn and uncommunicative and this may deter staff from spending time with them. At other times, patients and relatives are reserved about approaching staff and speaking to them, especially when they are perceived to be busy, and again may not receive the support they need.

PLANNING

In Chapter 1 of this book, Johnston describes the importance of valuing patients, entering their experiences, empowering them and helping them to find meaning in their situations. To create such therapeutic relationships between nurses and patients, I think it is important that a key worker is appointed so that there is continuity of dialogue and support for patients. Planning should be carried out with the multidisciplinary team and with the co-operation of patients, whenever their condition permits. Acting as a key worker can be emotionally demanding for the professional concerned. Sometimes, the key worker comes to be regarded more like a friend than a professional helper. This was Carol's perception of her relationship with her health visitor (Lugton 1994).

> Sheila doesn't feel like a health visitor. These people can make you feel so intimidated – officialdom! She doesn't make you feel like that at all. You can have a rare blether and a good moan if you like. She's not there waiting to pick holes in you. She's not waiting to report back, that sort of thing. She's really nice. It's like she's always been there. I've heard about her family as well. They don't feel like strangers. It's a nice feeling, a comfortable feeling.

As health care professionals, we are usually only temporary members of our patients' social networks. However, our support, especially in serious illness, can play a vital part in maintaining their identities and those of their relatives and friends. For example, many women with breast cancer found the support of health visitors very important to their coping (Lugton 1994).

Timing of interventions

Timing of support is important. People with advanced illness are likely to have passed through a series of crisis points during which they receive bad news, for example, at diagnosis, at recurrence or relapse and at cessation of curative treatment. At these times they need both professional and informal support to avoid negative thought and to encourage positive thinking. Professional support is important at times of transition. When people pass from one status to another, for example at diagnosis or on discharge from hospital, their identities are redefined by others and by themselves. It is at these times that they need both professional and lay support to avoid negative and to encourage positive self-concepts. In an earlier research study of the support of relatives of terminally ill patients (Lugton 1987), I found that the presumed finality of admission to a hospice was a major concern to both patients and relatives, being perceived as a 'rite of passage', which conferred, on those admitted, the status of 'the dying' in a unique way. Professional support was very necessary at this time. At the time of their admission, few patients saw themselves going home again from the hospice. One relative described her own and her mother's feelings.

> I thought once you were here that was it. My mother had that attitude too. Sheila (home care nurse) pointed out that some patients go home but my mother had that attitude that you walked in and you got sort of carried out, you know.

Many patients later expressed contentment with the hospice to their relatives; they gave 'individual attention' and 'personal care' as well as 'feeling safe and relaxed' in the hospice as the main reasons for their satisfaction.

Support is not effective if given after a crisis has passed. When patients have worked through their anxieties they do not want to discuss them again. How quickly should you proceed? Having assessed the patients feelings it is important to go at the patient's pace. Carol's health visitor had noticed the importance of going at Carol's pace to avoid her feeling frightened of the future.

With having advanced disease, Carol admits to being terrified. There have been all sorts of social, financial and practical type things which have been necessary but she's not always willing to accept them, being so independent. I've noticed if I've left it for a while she'll come back and ask.

Helping patients to appraise their situations

Nurses can play a vital role in helping people to assess their situations, what support is available to them and the adequacy of their coping resources. When breaking bad news it is important to find ways of giving hope and not promoting despair. A defined threat is usually less frightening because knowledge makes coping easier. Diagnosis of a terminal illness is stressful but usually less so than coping with uncertainty. When presented positively, information about the disease and its treatment and can help make these appear less threatening.

Coping support

Nurses can help to restore patients' ability to cope by helping them to clarify problems and deal with negative emotions. They can also provide practical help. People with advanced disease have to cope with continued uncertainty about the future and deteriorating health. Sometimes they are uncertain whether they want to know more, in case they cannot cope. Margaret had lived with her recurrent breast cancer for 18 years but seemed to be on a downward path.

I find the time between remissions seems to be shorter and shorter. I think that makes you very frightened. I found the last time I came to clinic I didn't take it in. Normally I would ask questions and ask for something to be explained to me and then I've got it. But I didn't. I was in a daze. I couldn't even remember what the doctor said to me.

Nurses can provide psychotherapeutic support, encouraging patients to explore and express their feelings, clarify problems, make plans and develop coping strategies. They can also assess whether patients are in an anxiety state or clinically depressed.

Learning new skills develops a positive self-image. Patients may have to cope with, for example, a new body image, wearing a prosthesis or stoma bag. Those receiving chemotherapy have to cope temporarily with caring for a wig. They need support from nurses to acquire these skills. Support needs to be balanced against the individual's needs to perceive themselves as coping. Sometimes, patients' family and friends can be overprotective towards them. This can affect their self-esteem and identity as independent people, capable of giving, as well as receiving, support. In a study of adjustment of individuals to heart attack, Johnson (1991) noted that:

If the informants believed they were incapable of reciprocating support, either now or in the future, they felt devalued as human beings. As the informants began to improve and gain strength in the immediate weeks following their discharge, their need for support diminished. If their family members were not cognisant of their improvements and continued to provide support in the same ways, without modification, the informants felt overprotected.

THE NURSES' ROLE IN MAINTAINING PATIENTS' IDENTITIES

To cope with serious illness, people usually need to both maintain and make changes to aspects of their identities. Most patients' main anxiety will be uncertainty about the future. Nurses can help patients cope with these anxieties, not with false reassurance, but by encouraging them to talk about their fears and by providing appropriate medical information. It is important that in the earlier stages of advanced disease, patients are able to put their illness into perspective, so that they can participate in other aspects of life. Nurses can help patients to think positively about the things they are still able to do. For example, many people with advanced disease struggle to remain involved with family and community life. Some will want to continue working for as long as possible. Joan wanted to remain active but had curtailed some activities.

> I've always been a very energetic person, doing three or four things a day. Now I curtail them. I really feel that one of the main things is to keep going and have as much interest as you can in things and not give in. I've been pretty involved in the church. I am an elder and I do my district and I really enjoy it. I go to the flower arrangement and I enjoy that.

Work is another way of leading a normal life, despite having advanced disease. In a study of women with breast cancer (Lugton 1994), nine of 14 women with advanced breast cancer were employed. Six managed to continue work, despite their illness.

The illness and treatment undermines patients' sense of their autonomy. As decision-making is an important aspect of autonomy, patients should be encouraged to be involved in decisions about their treatment and care.

Nurses should support patients' relationships and thus indirectly support the patients. We should spend time speaking to relatives and friends for whom this is a stressful time.

Knowing when to withhold unwanted information is also supportive. In contrast to nurses' support, which can be tailored to individual needs, media articles and programmes about various diseases are often unhelpful to patients, increasing their fears as they apply the scenarios to their own situation. Elizabeth was not helped by reading a book about cancer.

> Somebody gave me a book and I just opened it up and it said something like, 'Cancer spreads very quickly round the body'. I thought, 'That's the last thing. No, I'm not going to read anything.'

Patients often have anxieties about their treatments. The need for professional support at this stage has been researched. Anderson (1986) found that few of her respondents with breast cancer received explicit information about what to expect, emotionally or physically. Treatment can help people with advanced illness to feel in control of their lives. Joan was grateful to have a reasonable quality of life.

It was diagnosed here in the tummy [secondary cancer]. I had these pills for a while. I had these jags for about 18 months. It seems to have kept it at bay, which is great. I'm grateful to be here all these years.

Margaret needed to feel that some form of treatment would always be available.

Well I think it was about Easter this year I had the chemotherapy and then I started having problems about August. You think, 'I'm sure they should have started the treatment ages ago.' I don't think I could actually cope with not having any treatment for it.

Clare was also afraid that the doctors would run out of treatment options.

I'm kind of frightened in case they say, 'Don't take any more Tamoxifen.'
I'm getting to rely on it. It's worked for me.

During their treatment, people feel dependent on professional expertise, as effective treatments affect prognosis. Medical information is important in enabling people to make treatment decisions and for their coping during treatment. However, patients' vulnerable positions, as sick people with limited medical knowledge, may restrict the extent to which they feel able to be involved in decisions about treatment, especially if they think such decisions will affect their prognosis. It is therefore important to assess the extent of patients' desire to be involved in decision-making and to tailor medical information and responsibilities in decision-making to individual requirements. For example, some women with breast cancer wanted much more information about their illness and treatment than others (Lugton 1994). Angela, a finance consultant, wanted as much information about her treatment as possible, regardless of how the information might make her feel.

Dr A was always condemning me because I was asking her for statistics.
She says it's not something they volunteer because most people can't cope with that. I said, 'I would rather know.' There's no point in kidding yourself.

On the other hand, Jane and her family felt that it was unfair to ask patients to make decisions about whether to participate in clinical trials offering different medical treatments or whether to accept the current conventional treatment.

My husband didn't think it was very fair putting that onus on anyone. I said to Dr D, 'What do I know about radium?' I said, 'Nothing.' I know nothing about cancer. I said, 'I'm believing every word you're telling me about what you've done for me, but I don't know anything about cancer or radium.'

Time should be spent on explaining treatments and listening to patients' anxieties about treatments. Many treatments are conducted on an out-patient basis, so community nurses' role in enabling patients to cope with these is appreciated. Patients often need information and advice about medical problems, or treatment side-effects, and support to assess the significance of these problems. Informal support is important throughout treatment. Family and friends can play a role in discussing treatment options with the patient.

Preserving and promoting informal support

It is increasingly being realised that focusing care upon patients without considering their relatives and friends is an inadequate nursing approach. The behaviour of one family member affects the behaviour of another but not necessarily in a predictable or simple pattern. Sometimes, nurses need to give direct support to patients' relatives and friends to enable them to cope better with the patient's illness. In other cases nurses should provide support to patients by acting as their confidants when the patient feels unable to share anxieties about themselves or their network members with the latter. Patients sometimes need help in removing communication barriers between themselves and their relatives and friends.

Some patients may be reluctant to express their concerns about their illness to those closest to them, wanting to protect loved ones from anxiety. They need encouragement to talk to relatives about their feelings or opportunities and to express their fears about their illness to nurses who are not emotionally involved. Even in apparently good relationships, barriers exist. Patients' relatives can also create barriers, preventing them from supporting patients effectively. When possible, nurses should help relatives to discuss their feelings about the illness and how this may be inhibiting their support of the patients. The patient's partner sometimes wants information from nurses to enable them to understand more clearly what the patient is experiencing. In the community, relatives may want to be present during the community nurse's visit to enable them to hear their partner's worries at first hand and to express their own concerns.

Informal support should be encouraged because it is vital in helping people to cope with negative feelings about their illness. Professional and informal sources differ in their methods of providing support. Whereas a sick person's family, friends and neighbours rely on their personal knowledge of and relationships with her to provide help, professional health care workers use their medical expertise and experience with other patients.

An aspect of informal support, often mentioned in the literature, is its variety. In my research among patients with breast cancer I found that such variety was very important because many different types of informal support were needed (Lugton 1994).

Instead of encouraging patients with advanced disease to rely too much on professional support, nurses should aim to help them maintain and, if necessary, create, their own informal support during illness. This can include:

- Emotional support (concern and love)
- Companionship
- Practical help
- Opportunities for confiding
- Experiential support (sharing experiences with others in the same boat)
- Sexual identity support (usually from partners)
- Advocacy (accompanying the sick person to clinic appointments, etc.)

Spiritual support

A terminal illness can be perceived as being fulfilment of the journey through life or as an annihilation. Spiritual support encourages the development of hope, despite the difficulties of the circumstances. Staff should not feel hesitant about trying to give spiritual help and sharing their own beliefs if they feel that the patient is asking and that such a sharing would be appropriate.

■ REFLECTIVE PRACTICE 4.4   Types of support

Take a few moments to draw a diagram with yourself at the centre. Put three concentric circles, each larger than the last, around yourself as the central point in the diagram. Write the names of the people closest to you in the smallest circle so that they are placed nearest to you. Then write the names of the other people in your social network in the other two circles. What forms of support do you/have you received from these people:

• In crisis?
• In your everyday life?

Support in the community

Hospital discharge can be both stressful and pleasurable for patients. They no longer have the cushioning hospital environment, supported by staff and fellow patients. It can be difficult for those with advanced disease to acknowledge that they can now only receive palliative care, especially when they are attending a unit where other patients are receiving curative treatment. Professional support in the community is very important for them. However, they may now have less contact with hospital medical and nursing staff, except when attending clinics. GPs are usually busy people and the amount and quality of support they can give varies. If patients are not requiring practical help from district nurses, they may have little professional support between visits to the hospital consultant. Fortunately, cancer helplines and support agencies are increasingly considering the needs of people with advanced disease.

Community nurses with preparation and education in palliative care are in a unique position to provide effective support to these patients in the community. Such support, involving medical, psychological and social skills, cannot easily be provided by informal carers who, in any case, may need support themselves. It cannot always be given by other professionals, such as GPs, who usually lack the time for much home visiting. The availability of community nurses can be important in allaying patients' anxieties. For example, women with breast cancer mentioned the benefits of expressing their deeper worries to health visitors who were perceived as being 'outside' their normal social relationships and therefore detached from the patterns of obligations and expectations inherent within these relationships (Lugton 1994). Relatives themselves need support from professional staff.

Social support and nursing education

Nurses who want to develop skills in social support should focus initially on increasing their awareness of threats to identity, which can arise in advanced disease. In major illness, a patient goes through critical phases in redefining her identity and therefore needs a key worker whose relationship with her is sufficiently empathetic and continuous to provide appropriate support. Nurses should be aware that both professional and informal support are needed to enable patients to pass through these critical phases and reach self-acceptance, as these types of support work in different, but complementary, ways. As having a variety of support types and sources is beneficial, nurses should seek to keep patients' social networks as wide and effective as possible. Hospital and community nurses are also involved with care of the bereaved, who need help to develop a new sense of identity.

In devising a quality of life index for patients with cancer, Calman (1987) maintained that to improve their quality of life, the aim should be to try to help people reach the goals they have set for themselves. This means adopting a patient-centred approach to care. Calman's definition of quality of life has four implications:

1 It can only be described by the individual
2 It must take into account many aspects of life
3 It must be related to individual aims and goals
4 Improvement is related to the ability to identify and achieve these goals

Assessment of which aspects of patients' identities they are struggling to maintain against the threats posed by disease and disability, and which changes in self-concept they are trying to develop, would add an important fifth dimension to efforts to improve quality of life.

SUMMARY

As nurses, we should examine our own motives for feeling less attracted to supporting people with some conditions and in some situations than others. It may be that these conditions and situations threaten aspects of our personal or professional identities. For example, contact with patients with breast cancer may increase some nurses' perceived vulnerability to developing the disease. Being asked to care for such patients without education about or preparation for the role is likely to threaten their identities as competent professionals.

Support for patients with terminal illness can be emotionally draining and nurses need support from colleagues and managers. They need to develop teamwork and to learn to receive as well as to give support. They need to have some insight into their feelings and to be able to acknowledge when they are upset. They need to be aware of distancing strategies they can use in communication to protect themselves from pain. Personal experiences can influence our attitudes to work with dying people. Self-awareness is one of the qualities Egan (1990) considered necessary in effective counselling. Other qualities were empathy, genuineness and unconditional acceptance of others. A climate of trust is created, not only by what is said, but by the understanding shown in facial expression, tone of voice and gestures. Recognition and support come not only from colleagues but, perhaps surprisingly, also from dying people and their relatives.

By developing their understanding of the role of support in enabling terminally ill people and their relatives to pass through critical phases of their illness and bereavement to self-acceptance, nurses have a major role to play, both in providing sensitive, professional support and in promoting patients' and relatives' informal support networks.

REFERENCES

Anderson M J 1986 The nursing contribution to the aftercare of the mastectomy patient. Report prepared for the Scottish Home and Health Department, University of Edinburgh, Nursing Research Unit

Anderson M J 1988 Coming to terms with mastectomy. Nursing Times 84: 41–44

Bard M, Sutherland A M 1955 Psychological impact of cancer and its treatment. 4. Adaption to radical mastectomy. Cancer 8: 656–672

Benjamin A 1981 The helping interview, 3rd edn. Houghton Miffin, Boston

Bowlby J 1975 Attachment and loss, Vol. 2. Separation (anxiety and anger). Pelican Books, Middlesex

Calman K C 1987 Definitions and dimensions of quality of life. In: Aaronson N K, Beckmann J (eds) The quality of life in cancer patients. Raven Press, New York, pp 1–9

Combs A W, Snygg D 1959 Individual behaviour: a perceptual approach to behaviour, revised edition. Harper Row, New York

Dixon R, Lee-Jones C, Humphris G 1996 Psychological reactions to cancer recurrence. International Journal of Palliative Nursing 2: 19–21

Dunkel-Schetter C 1984 Social support and cancer: findings based on patient interviews and their implications. Journal of Social Issues 40: 77–98

Egan G 1990 The skilled helper: a systematic approach to effective helping. Brooks/Cole Publishing, California

Erikson E H 1965 Childhood and society. Penguin Books, Harmondsworth

Glaser B G, Strauss A L 1965 Awareness of dying. Aldine Publishing, Chicago

Henley N 1973 Power, sex and non-verbal communication. Newbury House, Rowely, Massachusetts

Hirsh B J 1981 Social networks and the coping process. In: Gottleib B H (ed) Social networks and social support. Sage, Beverly Hills, pp 149–171

Johns C 1996 Developing reflective models of nursing. Lothian College of Health Studies, 1st Biennial Nursing and Midwifery Conference, Edinburgh Conference Centre, Heriot-Watt University, Edinburgh

Johnson J L 1991 Learning to live again; the process of adjustment following a heart attack. In: Morse J M, Johnson J L The illness experience. Sage, London

Kelly M P 1991 Coping with an ileostomy. Social Science and Medicine 33: 115–125

Kelly M P 1992 Self, identity and radical surgery. Sociology of health and illness 14: 390–415

Lichtman R R, Taylor S E, Wood J V, Bluming A Z, Dosik G M, Leibowitz R L 1985 Relations with children after breast cancer; the mother–daughter relationship at risk. Psychological Oncology 2: 1–19

Lugton J 1987 Communicating with dying people and their relatives. Mosby, an imprint of Times Mirror International Publishers, London

Lugton J 1994 The meaning of social support; a descriptive study of informal networks and of health visitors' formal role in supporting the identity of women with breast cancer. PhD Thesis, Nursing Studies Department, University of Edinburgh, Edinburgh

Lynam M J 1990 Examining support in context; a redefinition from the cancer patient's perspective. Sociology of Health and Illness 12: 169–194

Maier S, Seligman M E P 1976 Learned helplessness; theory and evidence. Journal of Experimental Psychology 105: 13–46

Mead G 1934 Mind, self and society. University of Chicago Press, Chicago

Morse J M, Bottorff J, Anderson G, O'Brien B, Solberg S 1992 Beyond empathy: expanding expressions of caring. Journal of Advanced Nursing 17: 809–821

Northouse L L, Swain M A 1987 Adjustment of patients and husbands to the initial impact of breast cancer. Nursing Research 36: 221–225

Nouwen H J M 1979 The wounded healer. Image Books, Doubleday, New York

Nyhlin K T 1990 Patients' experiences in the self-management of diabetes mellitus. Umea University Medical Dissertations, New Series No. 288 ISSN 346–6612, Department of Internal Medicine, University of Umea, Sweden

Oakley A 1974 The sociology of housework. Martin Robertson, London

Perry B 1996 Influence of nurse gender on the use of silence, touch and humour. International Journal of Palliative Nursing 2: 7–14

Proctor S 1996 Fuzzy boundaries; multi-professional working and visibility in nursing practice. Paper for The Royal College of Nursing of the United Kingdom Research Society, Annual Nursing Research Conference, Newcastle upon Tyne

Sherif M 1953 Reference groups in human relations. In: Coser L A, Rosenberg B (eds) 1969 Sociological theory: a book of readings. Macmillan, New York

Stockwell F 1984 The unpopular patient. Croom Helm, London

Tait A 1988 Whole or partial breast loss: the threat to womanhood. In: Salter M (ed) Altered body image: the nurse's role. John Wiley and Sons, Chichester and New York, pp 167–177

FURTHER READING

Callaghan P, Morrissey J 1993 Social support and health: a review. Journal of Advanced Nursing 18: 203–210

Cohen S, Syme S L 1985 Social support and health. Academic Press, New York

Kelly M P 1992 Self, identity and radical surgery. Sociology of Health and Illness 14: 390–415

Morse J M, Johnson J L 1991 The illness experience. Sage, London

Norbeck J S, Tilden V P 1988 International nursing research in social support: theoretical and methodological issues. Journal of Advanced Nursing 13: 173–178

Wilkinson S 1991 Factors which influence how nurses communicate with cancer patients. Journal of Advanced Nursing 16: 677–688

Spiritual issues

Margaret Elisabeth Smith

5

SPIRITUALITY: 'DEALING WITH THE WHYS'

After years of lip service, spirituality is receiving increased attention. It is a buzz word in nursing circles. Published material in journals and books has increased, particularly UK writings. Varying degrees of attention are now allocated within educational curricula, but nurses struggle to understand spirituality and demonstrate difficulty in conceptualising it (Taylor et al 1994).

Spirituality has many meanings and different interpretations. This chapter provides an opportunity for readers to develop their own concepts and applications for practice. It will help nurses to identify how spirituality has developed (or not) within nursing and how it can be delivered by exploring different:

• Definitions and interpretations of spirituality
• Contexts for applying spirituality
• Phrases and terminology associated with spirituality

LEARNING OUTCOMES

The chapter addresses PREP categories of care enhancement, patient, family client and colleague support, and education development. At the end of this chapter, the reader will:

• Identify relevant definitions of spirituality
• Identify terms associated with spirituality

- Recognise and assess spiritual distress, pain, and isolation in clients
- Plan relevant care, nursing interventions and provide support in a spiritual context for clients
- Be aware of a range of resources to assist further development of knowledge and teaching spiritual needs in palliative care

WHAT IS SPIRITUALITY?

Spirituality is part of a person's life philosophy. Dependent on who uses the term, spirituality has many different definitions. These can be expressed in terms of religiousness or faith but each is indelibly linked to the nature and very being of man. Neuberger (1987) referred to the 'labelling' of people by their particular religion. This is not always straightforward and, to some extent, is anthropological. The same applies to the complexity of spirituality.

Definitions take on subtle inferences when applied in the context of nursing, especially palliative care. In this chapter, definitions for spirituality are examined within religious, secular, nursing and palliative care contexts.

THE RELIGIOUS DEFINITION OF SPIRITUALITY

The Concise Oxford English Dictionary (1982, p. 1023) states that spirituality is concerned with the spirit rather than 'matter'. It is 'of, or proceeding from God, holy, divine, inspired and concerned with sacred or religious things'.

Leech (1986) described Christian spirituality as a process where the individual is formed 'by' and 'in' Christ. He emphasised that spiritual formation was a process of 'Christ-ening', through confrontation, exploration and struggle. The goal is maturity in Christ and living a 'good' life within the guidelines and frameworks laid down by God and the Bible. This applies to any religion where there are holy being(s), the equivalent of a Bible (e.g. the Koran) and the goal for a 'good' life.

The 'good' life is not just one of 'actions' but one of 'feelings' – one of 'being', as guided by the religion's rules and beliefs. Reed (1986) identified the benefits of leading this 'good life' as the feeling of 'well-being', which can be interpreted in terms of a person's harmony and fulfilment of their spiritual life. McGilloway (1985a) records a common thread in recognised world religions being the goal of followers to pursue the living standards as set by a Supreme Being. Believers are expected to act in accordance with these standards and see this Supreme Being (or God), as the creator of their universe. There are defined rules for how followers should act towards their God. The ultimate outcome of any religion is for the individual to feel spiritually fulfilled, i.e. at peace and in harmony with nature and life.

The spiritual dimension of religion involves a believer following specific rites and practices. Neuberger (1987) explored different religions that are common in the UK today. She demonstrated that each religion has specific observances relating to how people carry out their:

- Daily lives – lifestyle, customs, prayer
- Dying rituals – mourning, etc.

If these are not recognised and observed, individuals can feel troubled, 'out of sorts' or 'at odds' with their usual pattern and standard of living. This creates fear and anxiety of a spiritual nature, which may cause spiritual problems or dilemmas resulting in distress.

Religion and spirituality

Religion is not all-encompassing of spirituality. It does not imply a specific, or one-track, view of life and therefore of spirituality. Burnard (1993) explored the possibility of separating 'God' from 'religion' as the two terms are not synonymous. He emphasised that people can oscillate between 'belief' and 'disbelief' in a God and in a religion. He believes that it is misguided and restrictive to see spirituality purely in terms of religion. Even when there is that specific link, it is not always straightforward or clear-cut. Furthermore, religiousness and religion through beliefs and practices will always differ between individuals, within and between different faiths. For example, although some claim to belong to certain religions, e.g. Catholic, Jewish or Muslim, they may not, in fact, be active followers or observers of that religion. Neuberger (1987) calls our attention to the fact that within a particular religion believers can disagree with certain of the practices.

The Concise Oxford English Dictionary (1982) defines faith as a reliance or trust founded in authority. This can involve a promise or engagement besides the usual accepted religious connotations. Faith is therefore not necessarily the attribute of a religion. Atheism and agnosticism are, in themselves, forms of faith. Atheists do not believe in a God. This does not mean that they do not have faith. Agnostics, on the other hand, believe that the reality of God can be proved neither true or nor false. This does not suggest a total abstinence from some religious practices or observances.

The spirituality of a person generally implies adherence to a specific ideology. This provides meaning in daily living and is expressed either as an established religion or as a personally constructed interpretation of a religion (Harrison 1993). The religious believer with spiritual problems can face situations whereby the very things, beliefs and observances that they have relied on, are challenged or threatened. They may then question their faith and what it has or has not done for them (Harrison 1993). 'Who' and 'what' they thought they were, can become jeopardised by illness, potential death or general life events. They may lose their way with the particular religion or with a specific aspect of that faith. Their framework for living, the principles that they have adhered to, can vanish, leaving them floundering or isolated from the familiar, and uncertain of what to do and believe in. In contrast is the need to change their religion. This means finding a new appropriate faith, causing a possible revolution in their lifestyle.

For the religious believer, spiritual problems can arise from the fact that suddenly his faith becomes more important and real than ever before. The person then calls into account the past actions he performed in defiance of, or in spite of, his faith. This causes stress, fear of retribution and the need to seek forgiveness and reacceptance. Lapsed believers sometimes quite suddenly return to their faith and this may be difficult or traumatic. Others can feel the need to find a faith – a 'God' – for the first time.

■ CASE HISTORY 5.1   Mrs Jack

Mrs Jack was terminally ill. She began having panic attacks and gradually isolated herself from people, in particular her relatives. Initially she refused talk but finally owned up to her worries. Thirty years earlier she had had affairs with two friends' husbands.

She was Catholic and believed that she would have to enter purgatory after death. Although a lapsed Catholic, and in many ways scathing of Catholic dogma, the fear of retribution became very real. She felt unable to discuss her fears with a priest. Eventually, nurses helped her talk though the issues and supported her in finding a priest who was empathetic towards her. Her fears became manageable and the panic attacks ceased.

■ REFLECTIVE PRACTICE 5.1   Spiritual distress

Mrs Jack's spiritual distress arose when she 'owned up' to past behaviour that was in conflict with the fundamental beliefs she had grown up with. Despite having had a good relationship with staff, she withdrew and found it difficult to speak to anyone about what troubled her, especially a priest.

• In your experience have you ever observed patients becoming withdrawn when previously there had been a good rapport with staff? Can you think of examples where the patient concerned was dealing with a spiritual problem?

• Have you known patients who claim to have a particular religious affiliation yet do not wish to speak with their religious leader? How often do you presume that a religious leader is required?

• From what you have read so far in this chapter what factors will you now consider when dealing with a physical symptom, which is either not resolving or does not have an obvious physiological cause?

Harrison (1993) used the phrase 'spiritual distress' as something emanating from spiritual problems. Some spiritual problems, for example, arise when one person questions the religion and others find this hard to accept. Burnard (1987) defined spiritual distress as an inability to invest life with meaning. This may manifest in one or more symptoms, such as pain or feelings of anxiety, guilt, anger, uncertainty, fear, loss, despair, isolation or alienation.

Religion itself may be a cause, or an ultimate solution to a spiritual problem or dilemma. Reed (1986), for example, found limited literature about the value of religion in assisting people to die an 'appropriate death'. Some see religion as a help or a significant resource in giving meaning, guidance and structure to life. She went on to research religion in terminal illness and found that the 'perceptions about the distance of self from death' (i.e. how near death was), was linked to how patients viewed themselves and religion. It was then either an aid or a hindrance to their comfort.

Often people presume that a nurse with a known religious affiliation is better at delivering spiritual care. Although this has been inadequately researched, several studies have demonstrated the opposite (Carson 1989, Taylor et al 1994). It is important for nurses never to presume what a person believes in. Such presumptions can cause confusion and engender a lack of trust in the nurse.

THE SECULAR DEFINITION FOR SPIRITUALITY

The idea that spirituality is wholly a religious concept needs to be challenged. Whoever people are, whether they believe in a specific God or faith, or not, they still have a need for spiritual well-being through living a 'good' life. The Concise Oxford English Dictionary (1982) provides a secular definition. Spirituality is concerned with: 'the higher qualities of the mind; or based on the spirit' (p. 1023). Stoter (1995) interprets this as being the spirit of man, the vital principle of man and the breath that gives life to the physical organism.

In some ways the non-religious definitions treat spirituality in its most simple sense. Spirituality means making sense of the questions: 'who am I?' and 'what am I?'. Secular spirituality centres around a unifying force that integrates and transcends the physical, emotional and social dimensions and searches for meaning in life. McGilloway (1985b) suggests that this search provides a common bond between individuals and is an essential element for human relationships. In this, spirituality represents the very nature of man and his relationships with others. The secular approach to spirituality is about treating and being treated by others as someone of worth and with feelings. Doing so, acknowledges, implicitly or indirectly, a person's spirituality.

Culture and spirituality

Having established that everyone has a spiritual dimension, irrespective of their beliefs, it would seem appropriate to now examine the influence of culture on spirituality. It has been stressed that spirituality incorporates the whole of a person's life's experiences: positive, negative, actual and observed. Culture is essential in people's unique make up, whether or not they are conscious of it. Sampson (1982) pointed out that tradition, folklore, history, national, local and regional customs, and education all make up a person's background. He urges us to explore these within any assessment of spiritual needs.

Cultures exist within cultures and this contributes to who an individual is and how he sees himself. In the present day pattern of changing populations and mixing of neighbourhoods, there is now a melting pot of traditions from which the potential for new customs and cultures are already emerging. Sampson (1982) sees this as a new challenge with a knock-on effect for how people develop and express spiritual meanings in their life.

Religious and secular perspectives compared

The secular aspect of spirituality brings out subtle differences from the religious contexts when identifying spiritual problems. There remains the challenge in what a person experiences through life-threatening illness, anticipation of death and the life events shared with or in isolation from significant others. The two perspectives contrast in terms of a person seeing himself as an independent worldly person, or in terms of a religion or God. This will be reflected in the language a person uses when expressing feelings, fears and concerns.

Facing a limited lifespan is a difficult human experience for the one dying and for those sharing the experience. Death and dying is an unfamiliar experience for many people today and for some this, in itself, may cause spiritual problems. For others, problems arise from the difficult process of making sense of, or the inability to rationalise what is or what is not happening to them and their threatened identity (Harrison 1993). Spiritual alienation occurs when someone feels isolated or cut-off from what has always been familiar and second nature.

■ CASE HISTORY 5.2   Mr and Mrs Young

Mr and Mrs Young had a 10-year-old son, Peter, who was dying. They were both atheists and were faced with supporting Peter through the dying process. Neither parent had previously been exposed to death and had always believed in the finality of death. They were, however, unable to tell this to Peter. This caused great distress. To add to this, all the materials available on the children's unit focused on the belief in some form of life after death.

Mr and Mrs Young, despite nurses' misgivings, decided to work from their own philosophy when talking to Peter. Although it brought some peace of mind in the short term, later they had misgivings. The difficulty appeared to be the parents' own lack of knowledge and conviction in what they told Peter. The nurses felt powerless but could only take the parents' lead and support the family.

■ REFLECTIVE PRACTICE 5.2   Belief system

A person needs to feel confident when their belief system or philosophy of life is tested. Sometimes people's beliefs and philosophy is based on 'living for today' without any real focus on death. When confronted with death these belief systems are put to the test.

Many adults find talking to children difficult because of a child's lack of experience or presumed inability to conceptualise. But given time, support, preparation and education, adults can usually vocalise and discuss ideas with children. It is usually the adults rather than the children's fears that intervene.

• How would you prepare parents/grandparents to help children prepare for their own death or that of a close relative? What do you think would be your initial feelings about this?

• What resources (human and other) can you access to help you with this. If you cannot list any, perhaps this is an activity that you could include in your professional portfolio.

In summary, the secular definition of spirituality speaks of finding meaning in life, in consolidating an identity, and making sense out of what happens to people as and when they face life crises.

Spiritual distress arises whenever the individual is unable to answer the questions: 'who am I?', 'why is this happening?', 'what have I done to deserve this?'. Situations that leave the individual unable to adequately answer these questions result in the manifestations of spiritual distress described as pain, fear, isolation and alienation.

SPIRITUALITY IN A NURSING CONTEXT

Nurses interact with patients and families in a variety of situations. The people they care for have a whole range of life experiences. These are influenced by the uniqueness of that individual and, hence, the uniqueness of his spirituality (Stoter 1995). Interpretations are made by nurses about patients and others based on the individual's:

- Need for care
- Source of the need
- Response – how and why that person is responding or not to what is happening

Harrison (1993) highlights the importance of spirituality for nurses by referring to the UKCC code of practice for nurses in which nurses are required to recognise and respect the uniqueness and individuality of each client. With regard to spirituality, this means ensuring that spiritual well-being is established in nurses' agenda for care. Nurses have access to personal details and private information about patients. This affords them a special opportunity to be with people and to establish a distinctive intimacy with patients. This can lead to a spiritual relationship, or can be seen as a spiritual relationship in itself. Such relationships usually happen rather than being fostered or planned.

Sampson (1982) recognised that nurses do not deliberately neglect patients' customs and spiritual beliefs. More often this happens because of ignorance. Different cultures, backgrounds, and hence spirituality, influence nursing interactions, whether or not this is consciously recognised. Misunderstanding 'who' and 'what' the patient 'really is' may cause nurses to unwittingly cause spiritual problems for some patients.

The importance of understanding different terms that relate to the concept of spirituality has already been identified. This is especially important for nurses who are involved in identifying spiritual needs and planning care within a multidisciplinary health care arena. Stoter (1995) refers to Maslow's hierarchy of personal needs and acknowledges that many of these are met in everyday life circumstances. Activities of living, such as breathing and eating, are part of an individual's natural make up and unconscious existence. These, like the aspect of being a spiritual person, can sometimes be taken for granted. It is an established fact that patients who require nursing interventions (for whatever cause), do not always require direct help or intervention with every need. This is often true of breathing and eating. Similarly, patients do not automatically need help with spiritual matters. This may be one area of need that they can manage more than adequately by themselves.

An important aspect in nursing is to recognise why needs arise and how they can be dealt with. Patients can often manage to deal with their own needs, provided the environment is right and guidance is given. For example, a person with breathing problems can cope well if assured of support, supplied with enough pillows and taught how to use an oxygen mask: patients with arthritis can manage to feed themselves if provided with the right equipment. The same applies to spiritual needs, i.e. providing access to relevant religious leaders if that is the requirement. A fundamental requirement in the provision of spiritual care is effective communication and the recognition of each patient as a unique individual with:

- The right of choice in his life
- A range of experiences that has got them where they are today

People develop their own perceptions throughout their lives. These may or may not be of a spiritual nature but, because of them, individuals form ideas about themselves within their immediate context, situation and lifestyle. Becoming ill does not necessarily alter these perceptions, although for some it may affect their spiritual development, either positively or negatively. Nurses must take this into account. In addition, nurses should recognise the potential influence that they may assert when a patient is questioning the meaning and value of his own life.

Spirituality is intangible – something that an individual might well be unaware of. This can make identifying spiritual problems difficult for nurses. Two important aspects of the nurse–patient relationship that can help in this context are:

- Acceptance of who the individual is, when and wherever he is
- Accurate recognition of problems

Nurses cannot solely rely on the patient to exhibit distress or voice spiritual concerns. They need to recognise different types of spiritual problems and whether these have a religious or secular focus. It then becomes simpler to decide who is best suited to help with the spiritual problems. Highfield (1992) reported that many nurses and families rated a family friend as the one most able to help when there was an actual problem. Within a nursing context, the responsibility is to help patients and their carers maintain their health status, to help them identify actual or potential problems and to plan appropriate intervention. A nurse can be the facilitator and many actions involved in resolving spiritual concerns and problems may be performed with or without intent.

■ CASE HISTORY 5.3   Julie Smith

Julie was 19 years of age and had decided to stop her chemotherapy. Her heart was set on attending the summer ball that the nurses were planning.

Julie's mother was worried about the outcome of such a decision but wanted to respect her daughter's decision, which might help her realise her last unfulfilled ambition. Julie became quite depressed. Both mother and daughter were afraid of how the staff would view Julie's decision and were reluctant to discuss the situation. Sister Jones knew them both well and she sensed a tenseness between the two. She took the initiative to approach Julie and her mother together.

With a straightforward honesty, built on the basis of knowing the two, together with her professional knowledge, Sister Jones was able to provide them with the confidence to pursue their decision. Julie attended the ball after which she announced that she was now ready to die, having achieved all her ambitions and goals.

Spiritual problems in nursing

Sampson (1982) and Burnard (1987) both refer to ways that spiritual problems arise in a nursing context. First, these can be mistaken for physical problems. A common example is when dealing with pain. Sadly, non-physical problems continue to be overlooked in the presence of unresolved symptoms. Second, spiritual problems may be ignored deliberately. This is because nurses may lack confidence, knowledge, skill or expertise in how to deal with them. Third, problems receive a low priority because of ignorance or limited resources to deal with them. Finally, nurses may fail to act on a spiritual issue because of the belief or the assumption that someone else will deal with it.

SPIRITUALITY IN THE PALLIATIVE CARE CONTEXT

Palliative care becomes appropriate when it is known that a patient's illness will culminate in death. Spirituality has been defined as a meaning of life and how people accordingly respond to different situations. Death is a central consideration in a person's spirituality. Spiritual problems can develop at any time in a person's life, but these are probably more sharply focused when certain death is confirmed. In palliative care, nurses meet death 'face on'. They therefore need to consider being prepared for it themselves and to understand and assist patients in the ways they deal with dying.

Undeniably, death is a major life event. It is, however, the least experienced but most feared. This inexperience and fear can generate spiritual problems. Kitson (1985) identified that people suffering from chronic and life-threatening illnesses must overcome a huge hurdle in coming to terms with the fact that a cure is unlikely. These individuals need to be viewed not only from a perspective of their functional ability (physical, mental and social) but also from the viewpoint of the illness' effect on their life philosophy as death comes nearer. Illness and the threat of death have the potential to encourage introspection and a person may consequently dwell overmuch on what his life means or has meant. Thinking about what has or has not been achieved in life can cause stress and fear, resulting in spiritual pain. Some patients need to be drawn out of their spiritual isolation and affirmed as living and living with worth.

Patients and families experiencing death want and need meaning, possibly more than at any other time. McGilloway (1985b) identified uncertainty, powerlessness and inadequacy as feelings that can emerge when people come face to face with situations in which medical and technical science fail. Spiritual care is essential to help people face and persevere through the crisis. Although death is the final outcome in palliative care, the patients being cared for are very much alive. Time is limited and therefore precious. The nurse should accordingly aim to use this time to the best advantage for a patient. This demands that fundamental issues are identified and prioritised.

There is always a danger in over-professionalising spiritual care in palliative care. It may be that a patient needs help to identify the problems or dilemmas facing him. The task is then to help that person come to terms with death, the associated fears, and his lack of experience and exposure, in a way that is positive for him. Kitson (1985) stresses that this requires absolute honesty, with self and others, in effective communication. It may be that a patient has spiritual problems, which he neither wants recognised nor interfered with. In such cases, acceptance and a sense of being valued is the most pressing need.

■ CASE HISTORY 5.4   Mr George Patterson

Mr George Patterson was a 70-year-old bachelor who had lived alone in a hermit lifestyle. He had little contact with his only brother. His living conditions were filthy. George was fiercely independent and very unkempt when admitted to the hospice. His one wish was to return home and be alone. The nurse's assessment of George presented him as intensely out of place in the hospice, lonely, in spiritual pain and 'messy': George did not seem troubled with his clothes being badly stained. He hated washing. He spoke only under tolerance or duress. When the nurses attempted to change his clothes by cajoling him he was distressed. He preferred to be left alone in his shabby state.

One day, he appeared to be particularly isolated, having been told that he would not be able to return home. He had been sleeping badly. Nurse Andrews felt he needed or wanted something so she asked George if he would mind her sitting with him. His look was strange, both wanting and rejecting the offer. He asked, 'Why?'. Nurse replied 'Sometimes patients like someone just to sit with them.' He gave nothing away. Nurse Andrews pulled up a chair and lightly put her hand on his shoulder. He neither tensed nor commented, but in his face there was acknowledgement. Gradually he began to relax. After 30 minutes in silence he fell deeply asleep.

■ REFLECTIVE PRACTICE 5.3   Spiritual problems and interventions

Often, spiritual problems and interventions are not verbalised by staff or patients. These may be dealt with in the course of 'normal care'. Some people, like George Patterson, appear to have spiritual problems. Their source may never be identified nor their resolution achieved. One can speculate that becoming a recluse had solved his difficulties, up to a point.

Prejudice creates a barrier, as does being rejected by a patient. There is sometimes the presumption that once rejected–always rejected and to approach such a patient is to test the reality of this. In this case a need was met, although what and how could forever be deliberated upon.

• Have you been involved in a situation similar to the one described – what did you do or not do?
• Looking back now, would you or could you have done anything differently?

In palliative care, spirituality is often a discreet entity. The true issues that worry the individual need to be precisely identified. There may be a need for death education – for example, what exactly happens when someone dies? How do people feel and react? Once individuals are informed, any real spiritual considerations that exist can be examined. There needs to be a balance in addressing death-related issues: those that are physical or knowledge-based and those that are spiritual by nature.

WHY DO NURSES AVOID THE SPIRITUAL DIMENSION OF CARE?

In their avoidance of death situations, nurses lose contact with the person and risk diminishing or negating what that person is experiencing spiritually. This is a neglect of who and what that person is. It is an evasion of spirituality as a concept and as a nursing responsibility.

Nursing was, and still is to many, heavily imbued with the attitude 'thou shalt not become involved with patients!' Implicit in this attitude is the belief that one should not touch on personal subjects that are likely to upset people. This particular attitude could well be the reason why, until recently, nurses have not felt or recognised the need for spiritual care. Although this attitude is one that is discouraged in nursing today, sadly, it still exists, despite the research that negates any of its supposed benefits (Burnard 1987, 1993, Carson 1989). In situations where people die, nurses will become 'involved', despite thinking that they will not and trying not to. Kiger (1994) noted that this conflict makes caring harder and less effective.

Nurses sometimes avoid active participation in spiritual care because of the genuine belief that chaplains and formal religious advisors are better suited to the task. This originates from linking spirituality purely with religion. Nurses can sometimes feel that they are the least appropriate people to intervene or advise on spiritual problems. In this chapter an attempt has been made to demonstrate that this is misguided. Spiritual care does not always require special or complicated interventions. Frequently, intervention is about listening to the person, being with him and accepting him as he is. The person providing the help requires the abilities to provide time, be willing to be with and to share in emotion.

Sometimes, nurses can be caught between patients and their relatives. Harrison (1993) reminds nurses to be aware of their own spiritual needs and problems. These are often overlooked and can develop from the nurse's feelings of her own inadequacy and isolation. Equally they can stem from a crisis of faith or from challenges to the purpose and point of being a nurse. Carson (1989) and Stoter (1995) reiterate that spiritual carers have to 'self-care'.

■ **CASE HISTORY 5.5   Nurse Brown**

Nurse Brown worked on a busy acute care of the elderly ward. She complained of frustration at not being able to do anything about what she perceived as spiritual pain of the elderly patients who were dying. They wanted the nurses to be with them but she was too busy to stay and chat. She knew within herself that this did not feel right. Having reflected on this for some time she came to the realisation that spiritual fear of dying alone was an acute problem for the patients and this needed to be a priority for intervention. She began to detail this in care plans, adjusting work priorities to manage time and care. Later she reported back that 'it feels better, patients are more settled – other staff are now doing it'.

■ **REFLECTIVE PRACTICE 5.4   Counselling patients – 'making time'**

One of the difficulties that nurses face on 'busy' wards is the fear or discomfort in talking about spiritual issues. It is easy to feel self-conscious when writing in care plans that this patient is worried about meeting God, or that patient wants you to help pray with him. Similarly, it is almost inbred in nurses that they must be seen to be constantly active; therefore 'just' sitting with a patient can be interpreted as 'slacking'.

- Is 'slacking' an accurate interpretation or an excuse?
- Can you think of situations when you have been the 'accused' and the 'accuser'. This may not have been actually verbalised, so in the first situation how did you come to the conclusion that you were being accused and, in the second, what made you want to accuse your colleague of 'slacking'?
- Looking back, would you think or behave differently given the opportunities to fully explore the situation from the patient's point of view?

Burnard (1987) believes the counselling of patients in spiritual distress to be a process of personal growth and development. Carers, however, can be profoundly affected. They may subsequently question their own beliefs. Such questions may not be satisfactorily answered. The stress involved in demanding spiritual problems, with the in-depth interventions required by nurses, can accumulate, causing them to withdraw from patients' spiritual problems. This raises the important issue of clinical supervision for nurses.

Some nurses become overwhelmed when dealing with death and dying. The greatest percentage of people in Britain die in hospitals. Palliative care units are designed for patients who have difficult and complex needs. Consequently, much palliative care is delivered in non-specialist units by staff who may not be able to prioritise the needs of patients who are dying but whose death is not imminent. The problem may be about expertise and competence in dealing with spiritual issues in palliative care. It is just as likely to be about scarce resources, making it difficult to prioritise time for the spiritual nature of problems that arise in this group of patients.

■ **CASE HISTORY 5.6   Mr and Mrs Clark**

Mr Clark was admitted in 'crisis' to the hospice. He had been diagnosed as being terminally ill. His symptoms were controlled and he could have led a reasonably active life. His wife, however, had latched on to the idea he would imminently die and consequently treated him as though he was helpless. Mr Clark led a 'double life'. During his wife's visits he was a passive gentleman. At other times he was alert, relatively active and a 'chatty' gentleman. This frustrated the nurses and they were unable to communicate the 'real' situation to Mrs Clark. Mr Clark accepted the circumstances as it seemed to help his wife and he also wanted it 'this way'.

Mrs Clark had never lived alone. She thought of herself as a practical woman. She was preparing herself for her husband's death by clearing his wardrobe and booking his funeral. This created a dilemma for the nurses but they settled for what the couple wanted rather than pursue a spiritual dimension to their care.

There is a mystique built up around spirituality in nursing. It is seen as something important yet an intangible dimension of care that must be provided. Nurses are sometimes unaware or uncertain as to what they should actually be doing. It is an aspect of care that no-one claims responsibility for.

Spirituality deals with the very 'core' of human beings. Bradshaw (1994) tells us that it demands that nurses have 'intimate and lengthy discussions' or, at the very least, explore pertinent and sensitive topics with patients. The increased recognition of necessary 'communication skills' and 'relationship building' in nursing has probably been one motivating factor in fuelling the demand for greater spiritual knowledge.

THE INTEGRATION OF SPIRITUALITY INTO NURSING PRACTICE

Spirituality formally appeared in the nursing domain with the introduction and application of nursing theories that underpin nursing models. Spirituality is a core element of nursing, as are physical, social and emotional dimensions of care.

Carson (1989, p. 6) characterised spirituality as:

... [it is] my being; my inner person. It is who I am – unique and alive. It is me expressed through my body, my thinking, my feelings, my judgements and my creativity. My spirituality motivates me to choose meaningful relationships and pursuits. Through my spirituality I give and receive love; I respond to and appreciate God, other people, a sunset, a symphony, and spring ... Spirituality allows me to reflect on myself. I am a person because of my spirituality – motivated and enabled to value, to worship and to communicate with the holy, with the transcendent.

Carson's (1989) definition provides a balance of all the aspects of 'spirit' – air, life force, psyche, soul, attitude, disposition, essence, outlook, courage, energy and mettle. Harrison (1993) suggests that people have within them a unique capacity to transcend themselves and reflect this with three basic needs – the need for:

* Self acceptance
* Relationships with others
* Hope in a positive future, however long that might be

When basic needs are not met, irrespective of the definitions used to interpret them, spiritual problems will ensue, resulting in spiritual distress.

According to Carson (1989) a human spirit cannot exist in a vacuum. It is housed in a human and physical body. She argues that throughout the history of nursing, nurses have believed in the need to care for patients in a way that ministered to all their needs. This ministration combines scientific knowledge and skill with the art of personal gifts and talents to share fully in patients' experiences. Taylor et al (1994) argues that spirituality is an essential dimension of 'person' and an important focus for nursing care. This is in line with the development of spirituality into the nursing theory of holism. The individual is described as: body, mind and spirit, dynamically interwoven.

Despite nursing being embodied in theories and models of care, application of knowledge to practice is diverse. The spiritual dimension in nursing, according to Highfield (1992) and Bradshaw (1994) has been the least understood and explored. Several reasons are offered. Spirituality is a very personal construct and it has religious connotations. Subsequent to the increase in research since the late 1980s, nurses have scrutinised their care and paid more attention to spiritual problems and more appropriate interventions with patients. Despite this, there is a presumption that spirituality is not adequately delivered in the majority of clinical nursing areas. Today, nurses face situations where there is the need for reinforcement of the theories of 'communication skills' and 'relationship building' (Burnard 1993). Spiritual care is an integrated part of everyday nursing care. Subsequently, there is a need for education about what is spirituality and what exactly particular spiritual care interventions are (Bradshaw 1994).

PROVISION OF SPIRITUAL CARE

There are several ways of examining how nurses can provide spiritual care. Campbell (1985) advocates that an important element in spiritual care is a willingness to find truth in a matter and not how the truth is reached. There must be an enthusiasm to help people and a willingness to share their spiritual pain. There is, however, no single or specific strategy for nurses to use.

Providing spiritual care means building on and adapting general care approaches and theories. It requires a framework of care planning wherein there is a focus on resources needed for providing spiritual care.

Spiritual care must be centred on the patient. Stoter (1995) described care as a shared journey for both the patient and the nurse and whoever else the patient deems appropriate. Whilst the nurse may feel frustration, it is the patient's dreams, hopes, goals, ambitions, and feelings and interpretations that are important.

Remember Mr Clark (case history 5.6)? The nurses were frustrated and restricted in their care. They were impelled to accept Mr Clark's circumstances and followed his lead. In the end they had helped him. The same was true in the example of Mr Patterson in case history 5.4.

Campbell (1985, p. 1) used the term pastoral care in a Christian context, writing that, 'Pastoral care is, in essence, surprisingly simple. It has one fundamental aim: to help people to know love, both as something to be received and as something to give'. This definition applies to the spiritual nursing care of everyone. Implicit in this is the belief that we are all worthy and with a valuable role in life and death. It reinforces the points made throughout this chapter about respecting the individual and helping him to make sense out of who he is, wherever he is, doing whatever he is doing. Any approach to spiritual care begins with the premise that an individual is someone with a spiritual dimension and spiritual needs within a holistic framework (Kitson 1985). By producing an environment and atmosphere of love and care, nurses will provide spiritual care. We saw this with Mr Patterson in case history 5.4. He was ultimately accepted as someone worthy and in need of constant attention.

Burnard (1987) and Taylor et al (1994) contend that that effective spiritual care happens when nurses are confident and at ease when talking about death, dying and spirituality. In tandem with this, an effective spiritual carer makes patients feel confident about themselves. Kitson (1985) examined nurses' exploration of spirituality and identified three important elements in nurses' communication skills. These were:

- Time spent with patients
- Level of interpersonal contact
- Ability to identify spiritual problems

These skills have been illustrated in the case histories described in this chapter. Sister Jones' knowledge of Julie and her mother prompted recognition of a problem (case history 5.3), Mr Patterson (case history 5.4) responded to the appropriate use of touch and Nurse Brown (case history 5.5) made a significant difference to the care of elderly patients in her care planning, by providing for spiritual support.

Dombeck's study (1991) of nurse–patient encounters examined what the nurse 'could be', 'mean to' and 'do for' the patient. The data from this study focused on communication skills. From this study a model emerged, incorporating:

- Communion
- Consideration
- Concern
- Comprehension

Care that is helping patients and significant others 'to cope', is central to nursing. Widerquist & Davidhizar (1994) refer to this caring and coping as the 'ministry of nursing'. Four nursing actions or interventions complied with the idea of responding to spiritual distress and ministering to patients. These were:

- Providing comfort and concern
- Finding meaning in suffering
- Providing hope
- Promoting expression of feelings

Widerquist & Davidhizar (1994) concluded that nursing, although described as a ministry, is not necessarily a religious one. Two of the above interventions are demonstrated in the case of Mr and Mrs Young (case history 5.2). Their lack of conviction in what they claimed to believe precipitated their distress. The nurses could not resolve the problem but helped the parents to cope. In taking the parents' lead they were able to care for the whole family.

Leineger (1984) states that 'Caring is nursing and nursing is caring,' and Roache's (1991) theory supports this idea: 'Each day when in contact and present with patients, nurses are *there.*' By being there, in the spiritual care context, nurses aim to empower, respect and treat patients as individuals. Caring, according to Leineger (1984), is the essence of humanity. It is a fundamental, yet most elusive, element of spiritual care in nursing. Caring encompasses all that a nurse does. It incorporates every aspect of the nurse's role, including: assessing, planning, delivering and evaluating care. It involves:

- Using initiative
- Being available and knowing when to refer to someone else
- Communicating with others
- Attending to patients' individual physical needs, such as nutrition, hygiene and elimination

Campbell (1985) subscribes to the belief that pastoral care is not the sole responsibility of a particular profession. As with any other aspect of care it is important to decide who within the team is best suited to help the patient identify and come to terms with his own particular spiritual concerns. If there is a particular religious dilemma, sometimes a neutral person may be more appropriate to help. This might be someone from a different religious persuasion, perhaps the nurse, hospital chaplain or another patient.

Alternatively, it may need a member of the same religion – whether a member of the clergy or laity – to help. Nurses have an important role in helping patients to make their own decisions and in facilitating access to relevant people. Their involvement might range from actually contacting, or having available, lists of appropriate personnel.

To deliver spiritual care, nurses must first have a clear, workable and practical framework to follow, incorporating:

- Specifically what must be identified
- Clear goals
- Which care interventions are appropriate
- What records must be kept
- A timeframe and monitoring system to evaluate what is being done

Assessment of spiritual needs

Neuberger (1987) advocates starting with assessment. Information should be brought together through:

- Observation
- Listening
- Talking
- Questioning, to include what individuals would like nurses to know and what nurses need to know

A checklist might be helpful. For example, when considering spiritual integrity, one would identify and assess spiritual pain, spiritual alienation, spiritual guilt/anger and spiritual loss/despair. Assessments should include practical details about a person's culture and religion; this should identify what the norms or standards are for that particular culture and religion. Information should also include what the person accepts or ignores about their culture and religion. It is important to know a person's views about the value and sanctity of life, her codes for living and expectations for the future (Neuberger 1987).

Boutell & Bozett's (1990) research showed that with spiritual needs, nurses most frequently assessed for fears, sources of strength and feelings of hope. Among the least assessed were: giving love to God, meaning in suffering and transcendence. Older nurses, with significant psychiatric nursing experience, were more competent in their assessment skills. A major criticism was that nurses rarely assess spiritual aspects by formal means. When assessments were made these were done instinctively or intuitively and were usually influenced by a nurse's personal experiences.

Highfield (1992) compared the assessments of spiritual health made by oncology nurses with those of the patients. There was a significant difference between the two. It needs to be recognised, however, that there is a difference between formal and informal assessment and identification of problems. It is possible for nurses to meet the spiritual needs of patients and avoid problems. This will be achieved through effective communication and by giving patients the assurance, from the first point of contact, that time, attention and respect will be provided. Boutell & Bozett's (1990) research concluded that availability of time and a sensitivity towards a patient's spiritual needs positively influenced assessment, planning, delivery and the overall effectiveness of care.

From the assessment data, nurses should be able to differentiate between problems that are actual or potential and those belonging to nurses, patients or significant others. An absence of problems should be clearly reflected in the initial assessment data and reassessments made to ensure that any new concerns or problems will receive attention. In contrast with other research, Highfield (1992) found, from the convenience sample studied, that there was a higher level of spiritual health rated by patients than is inferred in other studies. Her results indicated that nurses must remain open-minded about the absence and presence of spiritual needs. If there are problems then clear goals of care are needed.

Goals of care

A common primary goal of spiritual care is to help individuals achieve peace of mind (Kitson 1985). It must be clear, however, what the real problems are and who is best positioned to help. Depending on individual circumstances, the outcome of goals will focus on the problem itself or on the source, which might be revealed through deeper and lengthier exploration. Typical goals and appropriate intervention will aim to:

- Relieve distress
- Compensate for losses
- Reduce, prevent or stop pain, isolation and alienation

Intervention

Stoter (1995) described spiritual care as a journey and suggests that nurses must be prepared to accompany patients. Her analogy suggests a specified destination, well-packed baggage, luggage and sustenance. There will be visits en route, stopping and resting places, and companions. Once the journey starts there will be detours, accidents and/or obstacles to overcome. As the journey progresses there will be some sights that are unpleasant and some that are memorable. At the end, some of the companions will not have made it, others will have stopped, whilst others will have branched off in a different direction; the rest will be with you. This journey must then be evaluated, as all nursing care and interventions ought to be. Such interventions involve having the ability to recognise their own vulnerabilities and limitations. She provides the following directions for the journey:

- Helping people to come to terms with the fact that their life will end sooner, not later
- Knowing when to speak and when to remain silent
- Exploring with patients what they want and need
- Allowing patients 'to be'

Nurses require to have effective skills in assessment, ongoing exploration and implementation of appropriate interventions. This involves highly developed microcommunication skills, such as active listening, exploration, clarification, probing and confronting with the aim to encourage patients to speak and explore their feelings and to facilitate emotional expression. It has already been said many times in this chapter that effective communication is at the heart of effective care, be that care focused on the patient or their significant others and delivered by nurses, religious leaders or any other member of the team. One may be helping patients to access the knowledge or facts about beliefs, faiths or might be involved in helping individuals to pray or be prayed for. There is also scope to help patients identify their own coping mechanisms and direct care to support them.

Styles (1990) built a model of nurse–family relationships from her research findings. It can be adapted to provide spiritual care in palliative care. The five themes to consider whilst facilitating relevant cultural or religious practices are:

- Ways of being
- Ways of doing
- Ways of knowing
- Ways of receiving and giving
- Ways of welcoming a stranger

Another useful model to help nurses plan and record interventions in spiritual care is described by Highfield (1992). She summarised the spiritual dimension of persons as the unique human capacity to transcend self in the need for:

- Self-acceptance
- Relationships with others
- Hope in a positive future

Documentation

Care should be documented to show that it has been given and as a means of evaluating its effectiveness. Broten (unpublished work, 1991) explored the documentation records for the provision of spiritual care. Although some nurses and patients could verbally report some care, there was minimal formal recording of what was done, when, where and how. The few references made were restricted to religion and choice of clergy.

Evaluation of care

Nurses face difficulties when evaluating spiritual aspects amidst the enormity and diversity of care that has been given. It could be that spirituality is not something that is highlighted or easily extracted from the overall care delivered. How care is documented depends very much on the model used, if any, and the appropriateness and flexibility of the design of records. The onus for providing evaluation of care very much falls upon the individual nurse. This is a responsibility that must be reinforced through education, continuing practice and standards for practice. Regarding this, spirituality is no different from any other aspect of care. The onus, however, is with nurses to overcome self-consciousness when using the language of spirituality. This can sometimes appear long winded, effusive or clumsy. In the final analysis – something written is better than nothing at all.

EDUCATION

For many nurses, spirituality is synonymous with palliative and terminal care; hence with death and dying. Expertise in this area of care cannot be learned solely in academia. Several research studies have tried to identify what death education is offered to nurses (Cobb 1994, Field & Kitson 1986). Most agree that death education affects how nurses cope with death, but to what extent is unclear. Bradshaw's (1994) research concluded that spirituality needed more attention within educational curricula in both pre- and postregistration programmes. Whilst education curricula recognise the different component parts of caring for someone who is dying, the emphasis varies. In a subject-led curriculum, spiritual care is often at the end of a list dominated by the physical aspect of care or general communication issues and listed as a subtopic. Alternatively, spirituality may be a theme running through the whole curriculum and, as such, ought to be included in all relevant topics, for example, sociology, nursing studies and adult nursing. Those teaching palliative care must insist on opportunities to teach spiritual issues in a time-limited curriculum.

Cobb (1994) stresses that palliative care is a sensitive topic. It is one that brings home many personal issues and should be taught as such. When taught in didactic mode to large groups it is not possible to facilitate exposure to the emotional and spiritual aspects which bring about meaningful learning. Education is important to build the foundations for spiritual care. An important aim in education about spirituality is to make it challenging but not divisive. Through education, nurses need to be challenged about themselves and about spirituality. This does not imply that nurses have to know or learn all the answers. They do, however, require to be supported as they develop confidence in being challenged and as they develop their understanding of spirituality and what/who they are. A realistic educational outcome would be for the nurse to respond effectively to difficult and complex spiritual circumstances presented by patients.

Language is important when speaking about spiritual matters. There is a need to use or develop clear unambiguous terms when exploring spiritual well-being, disharmony and so on. Taylor et al (1994) stressed that all too often nurses linked spirituality with vague concepts and transmitted unease to patients. Unfortunately, nursing aimed at the spiritual needs of patients can appear vague or superfluous to other carers. Nonetheless, it is integral to patients' well-being and can overtly or discreetly be the difference between acceptable care and excellent care. To be effective in this area of care, nurses require to be alert to their own attitudes and approaches to spiritual well-being and the impact that these might have on a patient's spiritual well-being. Education and dissemination of good practices have a vital role in this.

Resources for learning about spirituality

There is a variety of material available to support learning about spiritual issues. The quality, quantity, accessibility and applicability, however, varies. Most literature makes many valid points, which substantiate each other, but there is a strong repetitive element between and within particular writings. This is partially unavoidable because of the complexity of spirituality. The number of textbooks has increased over recent years. Much of the research data seems to indicate that the level of knowledge and expertise in spiritual care has altered little over time. It also implies that there has been little transfer of knowledge to clinical practice. Some books, such as 'Nursing and spiritual care' by McGilloway & Myco (1985) are written at an introductory level but are quite vast and diverse. In contrast, 'Lighting the lamp' by Bradshaw (1994) is more theoretical. Common to many books is the exploration of spirituality in different contexts. These invite readers to expand their viewpoints, but can also be very complicated. The complex nature of spirituality often leads to concepts being explored in religious, anthropological, health care and in layman's terminology. Spirituality introduced as a chapter within a general book, or as a subheading within a chapter, can have the potential to mislead or undermine the importance of spiritual care.

Other good sources of literature about spirituality include books of poetry, which facilitate the expression of spiritual distress and comfort. Novels, biographies and autobiographies provide specific examples of people experiencing spiritual trauma, spiritual care and spiritual healing. These can help to give concrete meaning and concrete expressions to nurses, and sometimes to patients and their carers, who are searching for understanding.

Journal writings are probably the most prolific resource for reading about spirituality. Many of them are complex and most cover a wide range of facts within a finite word limit. They can be categorised into two general groupings. Those which:

- Regard spirituality purely as a religious phenomena
- Are based on extensive literature reviews

Journals that include substantial articles on spirituality have mainly a research, oncology-related or educational focus. The majority of research articles are either concerned with nurses' and patients' perceptions of spiritual care, or attempt to identify means of assessing spiritual needs. Relatively few examine specific care interventions. The education journals tend to provide reports that highlight educational requirements and critically identify the shortfalls or limited nature of existing programmes. This pattern has not altered since the articles first appeared with frequency during the early 1980s. Articles are predominantly American. Although these have a great deal to offer UK nurses, they must be read and appraised bearing in mind differences in both American culture as a whole and the nursing culture that facilitates care.

Major research works, e.g. theses, are again predominantly American, and a significant number are not easily available. Several of these remain unpublished and in the professional literature domain. Reasons for this vary. It is an enormous task to reduce complex material into a short article or it may be that the motivation for the research has been purely personal. One could, however, argue that academics have a responsibility to publish their findings in professional journals, especially when the data emerging has the potential to change clinical practice.

Readers wishing to explore spirituality further will find the following texts useful.

• 'Spiritual aspects of health' by Stoter (1995) examines spirituality from a multidisciplinary perspective.

• 'Spiritual dimensions of nursing practice' by Carson (1989) and 'Nursing and spiritual care' by McGilloway & Myco (1985) focus primarily on spirituality through nursing history, theories and care planning.

• 'Lighting the lamp' by Bradshaw (1994) is useful for in-depth exploration of spiritual theories and research.

Nurses intending to write literature reviews are strongly advised to use CD-ROM facilities, such as CINHAL. This provides a rich source of materials ranging from theoretical perspectives to care planning and interventions. Writers referenced in this chapter would be a good starting point. When reading and reviewing material, especially research data, it is crucial to give yourself sufficient time to read, understand, assimilate and interpret the rationale behind the research, the methodology employed, the data generated and the application which the author makes.

Teaching spirituality

A range of activities can be used within the teaching or learning setting. The best are those that encourage participation. Simple exercises that are relatively non-threatening involve examination of:

• Pieces of prose
• Excerpts from biographies
• Poetry

Such activities encourage nurses to explore what the authors could have meant. This can lead to reflecting, as far as they feel able, to identify with the situations described. Suggested material include:

• Lewis (1961) 'A grief observed'
• Elliott (1994) 'The longest journey'. An anthology of poetry and prose for the sick and terminally ill
• Whittaker (1994) 'All in the end is harvest'. An anthology for those who grieve

Another technique is to discuss a book and then watch a film or video excerpt based on the same book. An example would be Lewis's 'A grief observed' (1961) followed by the film 'Shadowlands', which was based on it. Films such as 'Philadelphia' and 'Whose life is it anyway?' generate many spiritual and ethical themes for consideration. 'Philadelphia', for example, has scenes that show how two partners may have different goals and interpretations of care. It highlights the imagery of how people can express emotions. It shows concisely how moments for talking and sharing can be lost. One particular scene shows how we can forget the person and family behind the illness. Television soaps are yet another media for illustrating spiritual pain, distress, isolation and alienation relating to individuals, family, neighbours and the community as a whole.

Many nurses are frightened by experiential exercises and to enforce these would negate the potential for learning. When engaged in experiential activities it is always important to set ground rules and to obtain full agreement and co-operation from the group about the activity and regarding confidentiality of information. The difference between discussing process and content of information must be clearly understood. Such activities may have to be postponed until group members come to know and trust each other. The emphasis of exercises in palliative care is focused on the meanings of death and the spiritual feelings it engenders. This can then be dissected for feelings of spiritual loss, spiritual comfort and pain relief. Facilitators must be prepared, as with all experiential exercises, for strong and emotional expressions to surface within and between each group member. It is wise to keep groups small and, whenever possible, to have a co-facilitator in the group. This ensures that the process and the content of the group work can be effectively dealt with.

A standard exercise is a questionnaire, which group members complete about personal and professional death experiences (age when first exposed to death in personal and professional contexts, then how/when/where would you like to die). Even simpler is the lost item; each member of the group, sitting in a circle, selects a belonging that has some particular meaning for them. They are asked to examine it and then hide it under their chair, or it can be collected in a box and the box taken out of the room. Individually, they are asked to describe the item, how they are feeling and what the loss means to them.

A similar exercise is picture cards. A series of pictures with different images are placed on a surface. The pictures can depict varied nature scenes, people, 'disturbing' images, whatever. Each group member is asked to pick a picture that they identify with. In turn they each describe what they actually see in the picture, then what it means to them and why.

The facilitator taking part in exercises should try always to come fresh into them, selecting different personal items or pictures each time. How in-depth, far-ranging or simple the information and feelings uncovered, will depend on the skills of the facilitator and his relationship with the group. Afterwards it is important to reorientate and debrief the group to the present situation and time but to allow further discussion on a group or individual level, whatever they need or feel to be appropriate.

The vital element of these, and any exercises in exploring spirituality, is the need to talk and exchange ideas between nurses. Personal thinking time is important but the verbalisation of ideas and understandings are essential for effective learning and translation into real practice.

SUMMARY

In this chapter, spirituality has been presented as a concept and an aspect of nursing care that cannot be undervalued. Both nurses and patients feel self-conscious about discussing spiritual matters. Sometimes, more attention than necessary is paid to issues that patients may not want to explore. Nurses must make a definitive effort to ensure that they formally document spiritual care in having a more co-ordinated approach to its assessment, planning and evaluation. Spirituality is an aspect of care that must be given its own individual merit and attention within educational programmes at both preregistration and postregistration levels. Clear, if only broad, general guidelines must be established as to what spirituality is and what spirituality can comprise. These definitions and interpretations must not be exclusive or restrictive.

REFERENCES

Boutell K A, Bozett F W 1990 Nurse assessment of patient's spirituality: continuing education implications. Journal of Continuing Education in Nursing 21: 172–176

Bradshaw A 1994 Lighting the lamp. Scutari Press, RCN, London

Burnard P 1987 Spiritual distress and the nursing response: theoretical considerations and counselling skills. Journal of Advanced Nursing 12: 377–382

Burnard P 1993 Giving spiritual care. Journal of Community Nursing January 6: 16–18

Campbell A V 1985 Paid to care? SPCK, London

Carson V 1989 Spiritual dimensions of nursing practice. W B Saunders, Philadelphia

Concise Oxford English Dictionary 1982 Guild Publishing, London

Copp G 1994 Palliative care nursing education: a review of research findings. Journal of Advanced Nursing 19: 552–557

Dombeck M T 1991 The contexts of caring, conscience and consciousness. In: Gaut D A, Leineger M M (eds) Caring, the compassionate healer. National League for Nursing Press, New York, pp 19–36

Elliott 1994 The longest journey: an anthology of poetry and prose for the sick and terminally ill. Dovecote Press, Devon

Field D, Kitson A 1986 Formal teaching about death and dying in the UK nursing schools. Nurse Education Today 6: 270–276

Harrison J 1993 Spirituality and nursing practice. Journal of Advanced Nursing 2: 211–217

Highfield M F 1992 Spiritual health of oncology patients; nurse and patient perspectives. Cancer Nursing 15: 1–8

Kiger A M 1994 Student nurses' involvement with death: the image and the experience. Journal of Advanced Nursing 20: 679–686

Kitson A 1985 Spiritual care in chronic illness. In: McGilloway O, Myco F (eds) Nursing and spiritual care. Harper & Row, London, pp 143–157

Leech K 1986 Spirituality and pastoral care. Sheldon Press, London

Leineger M M 1984 Care, the essence of nursing and health. Wayne State University Press, Detroit

Lewis C 1961 A grief observed. Faber & Faber, London

McGilloway O, Myco F (eds) 1985 Nursing and spiritual care. Harper & Row, London

McGilloway O 1985a Religious beliefs, practices and philosophies. In: McGilloway O, Myco F (eds) Nursing and spiritual care. Harper & Row, London, pp 23–36

McGilloway O 1985b Spiritual care: the potential for healing. In McGilloway O, Myco F (eds) Nursing and spiritual care. Harper & Row, London, pp 74–87

Neuberger J 1987 Caring for dying people of different faiths. Lisa Sainsbury Foundation, London

Reed R G 1986 Religiousness among terminally ill and healthy adults. Research in Nursing and Health 9: 35–41

Roach M S 1991 The call to consciousness: compassion in today's health world. In: Gaut D A, Leineger M M (eds) Caring: the compassionate healer. National League for Nursing Press, New York, pp 7–17

Sampson C 1982 The neglected ethic. McGraw-Hill, London

Stoter D 1995 Spiritual aspects of health. Mosby, New York

Styles M K 1990 The shining stranger: the nurse–family spiritual relationship. Cancer Nursing 13: 235–245

Taylor E J, Highfield M, Amenta M 1994 Attitudes and beliefs regarding spiritual care: a survey of cancer nurses. Cancer Nursing 17: 479–487

Whittaker A (ed) 1991 All in the end is harvest: an anthology for those who grieve. Darton, Longman and Todd, London

Widerquist J, Davidhizar R 1994 The ministry of nursing. Journal of Advanced Nursing 19: 647–652

Body image and sexuality: implications for palliative care

6

Norrie Sutherland   Richard Gamlin

Those people denied physical intimacy and tenderness, due to mutilating surgery and chronic or life-threatening disease, are extremely vulnerable to depression. Likewise the partner of the patient might need support and help to explore new ways of expressing love and gaining sexual satisfaction.
[Fallowfield 1990]

INTRODUCTION

In this so-called permissive society it might seem strange that a chapter like this needs to be written at all. There is an assumption that people learn about their gender and their sexuality at an early age, and that they grow up with a healthy acceptance of who they are and what their bodies do.

In spite of all the early education there still seems to be a problem surrounding sexuality, which continues into the professional life of health care professionals. In a recent, unpublished survey, 53 nurses were asked how confident they were in dealing with a patient's sexuality needs. Only four responded that they felt comfortable in dealing with the topic and had sufficient knowledge to give support and advice to patients and their relatives (N Sutherland, unpublished work, 1995). Other responses include statements like 'It's none of our business' (n = 14), 'I would be too embarrassed' (n = 32) and others stated that they had insufficient knowledge about expressing sexuality as an activity of daily living. This is really interesting when one considers that all those surveyed use the Roper et al (1980) model of nursing, which has, as one of its activities, 'Expressing sexuality'.

This chapter is an attempt to assist those less confident nurses to gain some insight, information and, through the use of the exercises, some practice in dealing with these sensitive, personal issues, as they relate to the field of palliative care. Yes, dying patients and their partners have needs too! The authors will address sensitive issues by talking about sex and sexuality rather than simply opting for the safety of 'body image'.

LEARNING OUTCOMES

This chapter meets the aims of PREP by discussing care enhancement, patient and family support, practice development and education development. It will assist those nurses who are less confident to:

- Extend their knowledge about the broad range of issues associated with body image
- Gain some insight into their clinical practice through the use of the exercises in techniques of communication and assessment of client needs
- Empower their clients to raise sensitive personal issues of sexuality as they relate to the field of palliative care

LEARNING ABOUT SELF

Children learn about themselves from a very early age. The process of learning includes sucking, touching and smell. Mothers sometimes mistake a baby's attempts to gnaw her fists as a sign that the infant is hungry, when in reality she is making a discovery about herself. Shape, texture, wet and dry can be discovered orally and provide immense satisfaction for the infant. In the same way, she uses her fingers to explore the things around herself, including her own body. Genital play is quite normal but parents may become anxious about this if they do not understand its purpose. This, in turn, may lead to smacking the child for being naughty, which, besides upsetting the child, also informs her that she should not touch her genitals and this is not the way to gain approval. She learns that there are some areas of the body which are more acceptable than others.

If disapproval in relation to sexuality is repressive and restrictive throughout her growing years, the child may develop a negative view of herself together with poor self-esteem. On the other hand, if she is given approbation and allowed to continue healthy discovery of herself, she is more likely to grow up with a more positive picture of her 'self' and with good self-esteem. There is a very strong argument for censorship to protect and nurture our young people from pornographic materials, but if children and adolescents are 'protected from' materials that have a sexual content because of parents' inability to face these issues, they receive powerful messages about sex and sexuality. Clearly, parents must always try to act in their children's best interests while providing them with a sound education.

Our difficulty in facing things sexual persists into the education of health care professionals. One of the authors (RG), was sent to the library while his fellow female students attended a lecture on the anatomy of the female reproductive system. This implied that he did not need to know this information to be a nurse and that the female reproductive system was somehow embarrassing. We are delighted to report that the theory/practice gap has been bridged and he is the proud father of two daughters. He hopes to complete the theoretical component when health care education is ready for this. Many readers are no doubt thinking that this was a long time ago, and indeed it is. In 1996 the same author was asked to present a sexuality workshop for a group of male palliative care volunteers. The female volunteers had already completed their workshop without their male counterparts.

ADULTS AND ILLNESS

Regardless of how self-confident people are, serious illness may affect and distort this positive self-image. A look in the mirror reveals someone with a different shape, bald, with skin and colour changes, clothes that are too big and whose looks are generally unappealing. The effects of illness, its treatment and medication take their toll on the patient. Linked to other stressful factors, such as loss of earnings, strained relationships and a diagnosis of an incurable illness, she may become depressed, lethargic and socially isolated.

EXPRESSING SEXUALITY IN SERIOUS ILLNESS

Good communication skills are essential for the support of patients throughout the period of illness. Areas of her life that have not been problematic until now may become a source of concern, anxiety, fear and distress. Expressing sexuality may be one of these concerns. If not addressed by professional carers, the patient and her partner may assume that this is an aspect of their life together that is now at an end. This assumes that professional carers know what the potential problems may be, and that they have the prerequisite knowledge to discuss these confidently with the patients! It may be useful to look at where the difficulties lie for nurses. If it is a belief that it is 'none of our business ...' who else will provide the patient with the relevant information? There appears to be an assumption that the patient will know intrinsically how to resolve these issues and that nurses should not interfere. However, the patient may also assume that because no-one has discussed sensitive issues with her, it is because this is an area of her life that is now at an end. She, too, is likely to be embarrassed and may not provide the relevant cues or ask questions about her situation.

If carers do not discuss issues owing to embarrassment, this may say more about how they perceive these areas and may reflect their upbringing and socialisation processes. Nurses carry out some extremely intimate tasks for patients, in spite of their embarrassment, because these tasks are not sexual in intent. However, there does seem to be a lack of knowledge amongst female carers around the issues of male arousal. Contrary to popular thinking, male patients do not deliberately have an erection while having an intimate task carried out. This occurs as a result of normal physiological processes that are beyond the control of the person involved. To then be castigated or ridiculed for an event that was not premeditated is unhelpful and may prevent the patient from asking questions relating to intimacy.

Although the practice of men nursing women is becoming more acceptable, many male nursing staff find themselves prevented from nursing women. They are told that this is for their own good because a female patient might accuse the male nurse of rape or some other sexual misdemeanour. Of course this is possible but important issues arise from this. First, female nurses are not discouraged from nursing male patients. This is largely for practical reasons as men only account for 8% of the UK nursing workforce. It is assumed that female patients do not like being cared for by male nurses because they will be embarrassed. It is also assumed that male patients will not be embarrassed but actually enjoy having intimate, invasive and uncomfortable procedures performed by female nurses. Again, practicalities must be considered but it is time this cyclical and ridiculous argument was laid to rest. Patients – male and female – will meet nurses – male and female. While preserving patient choice, it is time that we stopped restricting certain nursing tasks to male or female nurses. Nurses should be prepared for the challenges of caring for patients, complete with their worries, fears and sexual hang-ups.

Ignorance on the part of the professional carers is easier to address if they are otherwise willing to discuss intimate issues with patients. An understanding of male and female sexual responses, and the effects of illness on these, will assist the nurse to provide care and support in this area. It is also necessary to understand the effects of medication on libido as this can influence the advice that is given.

MALE AND FEMALE SEXUAL RESPONSES

It is not the intention of this chapter to deal with male and female sexual responses in great depth but rather to select areas that will assist understanding at a very basic level. For more detailed information see 'Suggested reading' at the end of this chapter.

EFFECTS OF ILLNESS AND TREATMENT ON LIBIDO

Depleted energy reserves

Patients who are seriously ill have depleted energy reserves. The normal tasks of breathing, eating, grooming and excreting become onerous and difficult. Physical and mental fatigue may in themselves prevent any sexual activity, particularly penetrative intercourse, from taking place. However, research has shown that patients do enjoy being hugged and cuddled, even when seriously ill and dying (Leiber et al 1976).

Explanations may need to be given to partners who may themselves be feeling miserable and rejected. It is often assumed by professional carers that patients in an older age group do not require this advice as they are no longer sexually active. There are studies to show that many couples continue to have satisfying sexual relationships well into old age (Kaiser 1992).

There may be several reasons for reduced levels of energy in seriously ill patients. Excessive weight loss, as in cancer cachexia, causes extreme fatigue. Infection, especially when accompanied by an increase in body temperature, reduces the notion for physical intimacy and sexual contact. Even the common cold can prove to be a hindrance to the most ardent of lovers! Patients and their partners may be fearful and anxious about the outcome of their illness, or about whether they can tolerate the treatments for the illness, and these fears and anxieties may also reduce libido. If the couple stop communicating with each other as a result, then their ability to show affection may be reduced.

Effects of treatment

This extract from 'Cancer ward' by Solzhenitsyn (1968), gives a graphic and moving account of the reactions of a young lady who discovers that she has breast cancer and must have a mastectomy.

■ BOX 6.1

Effects of treatment for illness

Asya and Dyoma had been friends through school. Dyoma was in hospital while his leg was operated on and Asya because of a breast lump.

'What is it, come on tell me?' asked Dyoma. 'They are going to cut it off,' she cried. Dyma tried to comfort Asya saying, 'Maybe they won't have to.' 'They will on Friday,' replied Asya ... 'What have I got to live for?' she sobbed ... 'Who in the world will want me now!' Dyoma tried to console her. 'People get married for each other's character,' he said. 'What sort of fool loves a girl for her character?' she replied angrily. 'Who wants a girl with one breast?'

Dyoma mumbled, 'Of course, you know, if no one will marry you ... well of course, I will always be happy to marry you.'

'Listen to me Dyoma,' said Asya, looking straight at him with wide eyes. 'Listen to me – you will be the last one! You are the last one that can see it and kiss it. Dyoma, you at least must kiss it, if nobody else!'

Asya pulled her dressing gown apart and Dyoma kissed her doomed right breast. Nothing more beautiful than this gentle curve could ever be painted or sculpted. Its beauty flooded him. 'You'll remember? ... You'll remember won't you? You'll remember what it was like?' Asya's tears kept falling on Dyoma's close-cropped hair. When she did not take it away, he returned to its rosy glow, softly kissing the breast. He did what her future child would never do.

Today it was a marvel. Tomorrow it would be in the bin. [Solzhenitsyn 1968, pp. 422–425]

After surgery, particularly quite mutilative surgery, the apparent change in body image may result in the person not wishing to be seen by their partner and not wishing to participate in sexual activity. Sometimes women are encouraged, soon after mastectomy, to let their partners see the scar. There is an assumption that the partner actually saw her breast, which may be quite wrong. There are many couples, young and not so young, who undress in the bathroom or in the dark, and who make love in the dark and who have never seen each other naked. Any insistence, however gentle, that the partner be shown the scar, may have the effect of preventing other questions being voiced, which would assist in promoting positive self-esteem and the coming to terms with altered body image.

Men who have had surgical treatment for bladder cancer or who are ostomates have had the nerve pathways disrupted, leading to an inability to have an erection. It may be possible for a prosthesis to be used, although at present in the UK there does not appear to be a wide acceptance of prostheses. However, there are many ways of giving and receiving sexual gratification if penetrative intercourse is neither possible nor desirable. There are booklets and books available from Relate (partner counselling) that can provide clear, factual information if there are no staff available or able to give such advice. The simplest advice of all is that if it feels OK to both partners, do it. Touching and discovering areas of each others' bodies that are responsive and which is enjoyed by both may seem relatively easy to do, but sometimes 'official' permission is required for this to happen, particularly if doing something different is thought of as rather naughty. One of the authors of this chapter (NS) was involved with a lady who had particular problems with sexuality. She was a deeply religious lady with strongly held beliefs and needed to be reassured that what was being suggested would not require her to have to make a confession. She was pointed in the direction of the Song of Solomon in the Old Testament and was greatly surprised to find that the Bible was so explicit.

Deep X-ray therapy and chemotherapy also have effects on libido, feelings of well-being and changed body image. Some chemotherapeutic agents cause total hair loss and hair loss is also associated with radiotherapy to the scalp areas. After chemotherapy the hair generally grows back in but, with radiotherapy, patchy hair loss may remain. These situations cause distress to men and women and, coupled with other effects of illness and treatment, may reduce the patient's desire or ability to be involved with her partner. Radical pelvic radiotherapy may lead to permanent vaginal fibrosis if no instruction is given on how to keep the vagina patent. If a vaginal dilator is given, it is often wrapped in a disposal bag. The message being given here is that the use of such a piece of equipment is 'dirty'. Instructions on how to use it may be unclear and it could lead to painful injury if the patient is not entirely sure which orifice is her vagina. It is the authors' contention that such an item should be gift-wrapped with simple, clear instructions for use and provided with a diagram that cannot be misunderstood.

■ **CASE HISTORY 6.1   Irene**

A true story although names have been changed

Irene is a 42-year-old district nurse. She had a routine smear test and was shocked to discover that she had extensive cancer of the cervix and uterus.

She had been having heavy, irregular bleeding but had put it down to the menopause, as her mother and sister had both experienced an early menopause. She was greatly supported by nursing and medical staff throughout her treatment and felt that they had always been open and honest with her. She had had surgery, chemotherapy and radical pelvic radiotherapy, and her partner had been a great help during the emotionally turbulent times. Jeff was 56 years old and they had been together for 4 years. There were no children. On discharge from the hospital Irene was given a vaginal dilator with the instruction 'use it regularly'. Irene had never worked in a gynaecology unit and she was not sure what to do with it. She kept it in the medicine cupboard in the bathroom. She and Jeff had been given no advice about resuming intercourse and decided to wait until Irene had a check-up at the hospital 6 weeks later. No pelvic examination was carried out at this time although Irene was asked if everything was all right. There was still no advice about resuming intercourse so she and Jeff continued to abstain. She had to cancel her next appointment as she had a wedding to attend and it wasn't until several months after her treatment that she was seen again. By this time she had developed pain and discomfort in her vaginal area. On examination there was extensive fibrosis.

■ REFLECTIVE PRACTICE 6.1 Irene

How would you, as Irene's nurse, have provided her with the information that would have prevented further problems from developing?

Simple instructions for using a dilator are as follows:

- Choose a time when there are unlikely to be interruptions
- Using Astroglide or KY-Jelly, lubricate the dilator and place into the vagina while lying down in a comfortable position – this should be done very gently, but the dilator should be inserted as far as possible
- Leave the dilator in place for about 10 to 15 minutes, after which it should be removed and carefully cleaned and washed with unperfumed soap and water
- Do this daily until advised to discontinue

It should be said that if the couple both wish it, and if great gentleness is used, the partner's gloved fingers can be used, instead of the dilator, to assist the process. We suggest gloved fingers to prevent damage (and possible infection) to the very sensitive vaginal mucosa. The other possibility is that if fingers or dilators can be inserted into the vagina, then so can the penis. Again, great gentleness should be used and some couples may find it more comfortable to lie on their sides, just quietly, together. The use of appropriate lubricants can be discussed, which would avoid the really sticky creams and ointments being inserted into the vagina. Saliva, Astroglide and KY-Jelly are all appropriate, although saliva tends to dry up more quickly. Vaseline, baby creams and oils and vaginal sprays should be avoided. Vaseline was never intended to be used for internal lubrication and other creams, oils and sprays can set up irritation in the vagina, causing pain, itching and distress.

■ REFLECTIVE PRACTICE 6.2   Use of a dilator

- Is there an age 'cut-off' point for this kind of information?
- What if the lady is single and elderly?
- What if the lady is married and elderly?

Medication

Some medications have an effect on the nervous system, which is responsible for heightening sexual arousal, leading to a loss of libido. The potion affects the notion! Explanations can be given to both partners, so that there is understanding on both sides. The man's inability to have an erection may be directly associated with the drugs he is taking, rather than with the illness itself.

Sexuality represents a complex interaction between genetic, physical, psychological, social, cultural, spiritual and racial components. Although the literature contains many definitions, defining such a complex issue is difficult and perhaps restrictive. The terms 'body image' and 'sexuality' are frequently used interchangeably although they are not the same. Body image is used instead of sexuality because of our difficulty and uneasiness with matters sexual.

According to Lion (1982), nurses who are comfortable with their own sexuality and the sexuality of others, who have a sexual health knowledge base and who cultivate sensitive and perceptive communication skills, can effectively integrate sex into the nursing process.

IS SEXUALITY A COMPONENT OF PATIENT CARE?

It is easy to assume that a patient with an advanced or advancing illness may have far more important things than sexuality to concern herself with, but it is possible to be wrong about this. The patient may have a number of concerns about sex/sexuality. For example she may worry about her appearance and whether her relationships with others will be affected by her illness.

■ CASE HISTORY 6.2   Robert

Robert was 26 years old and had worked on a building site as a joiner's assistant. He played football, went swimming and at weekends spent his evenings in the pub with his friends. He had a steady girlfriend with whom he had a sexual relationship. Apart from childhood illnesses, Robert had no experience of serious illness. Both parents were alive and kept well. Robert began to feel lethargic and weary and was too tired to take an active part in sport. Eventually his mother persuaded him to see the doctor, thinking he might have anaemia. Robert had been too embarrassed to tell either of his parents that his testicles were swollen and sore. His GP suspected testicular cancer, which was confirmed by tests. Treatment, including orchidectomy, was undertaken but Robert's illness was quite far advanced, prior to diagnosis, with metastatic spread to lungs and liver. Robert and his parents and girlfriend had been advised of his prognosis and knew he was dying. Robert was very preoccupied and staff assumed he was trying to come to terms with having a life-threatening illness. He had been told that he could go home at the weekend. Robert was reluctant to go and asked if he could stay longer. Katy, his girlfriend, was really disappointed and asked the nurse to speak to him. The nurse chose a time when the ward was reasonably quiet and asked Robert if he had any unanswered questions about his illness. He became very embarrassed and said he knew all he needed to know about his disease but, after some hesitation, he said, 'It's Katy – she might want sex and I don't know if I can! And she might not want me near her at all and I couldn't bear that!' This particular nurse was not very comfortable discussing sexual matters but was able to suggest that she would talk to Katy if Robert wished. She also offered the services of the stoma nurse who was 'more into that sort of thing!' The outcome was that Robert went home to his parents' house and Katy went too.

It is possible to become so taken up with the diagnosis that, as professionals, we relate everything else about the patient to her disease.

Questions and thoughts that may go through the mind of the patient may include:

- I look so awful
- She will not want to see me like this
- I used to look so good in these clothes
- Am I still attractive?
- I just want to be held – I don't want sex
- If we have sex I might pass it on
- My past sexual behaviour may have caused this
- I just can't face making love, it reminds me that we soon won't be able to do it any more
- I cannot bear the thought of her starting a new relationship when I die
- Am I allowed to have sex?
- Should I feel like this?
- Where can we go?

Questions and thoughts that may go through the mind of the partner may include:

- Will I hurt her?
- I don't find her as attractive as I used to
- I was going to leave her but it will look awful if I leave now
- If we have sex I might catch something
- My past sexual behaviour may have caused this

- I could never start another relationship when she dies
- I need sex and she is just using this illness as an excuse
- I have needs as well
- How can I convince her that I still love her?

Many jokes are based on sex and sexuality and most health care staff are reasonably comfortable listening to or making jokes about sex. Sometimes, patients attempt to discuss their sexual concerns with staff. This may be done in a direct way, or may be presented in the form of cues, which staff are supposed to be able to pick up. The following are examples of the latter.

■ BOX 6.2

Patients' attempts to discuss sexual concerns

- Ian, a 40-year-old gentleman with advanced cancer was sitting talking to his doctor who asked him how he was feeling. Ian replied, 'Well I now find that I bend in the middle, doctor. What are you going to do about that?'

- John was a patient in an orthopaedic ward following a road traffic accident. He was making a good recovery and expected to remain in hospital for another 3 weeks. One night while speaking to Julie, his primary nurse, he told her he felt sexually frustrated. Julie felt a little embarrassed but she did not take this as a sexual advance. She related John's comments to Chris, the senior house officer, who marched into the ward and said in a loud voice, 'Which horny git wants the bromide then?'

- Brian was 46 years old and suffered from cancer of the penis. While in the bath one day he said to Sam, his nurse, 'I've been made redundant you know, Sam.'

- Sally, a 68-year-old lady with lung cancer looks in the mirror and says, 'There's definitely something wrong with this mirror. It gets worse every time I look in it.'

- Bill, a 28-year-old man with multiple sclerosis who is about to go home on weekend leave says, 'Well, we'll see if everything is working OK tonight.'

In reality it seems that patients' worries are rarely discussed in a meaningful way in wards, departments or the community, despite the fact that a patient's sexuality is likely to be affected by advancing illness. Nursing models usually address sexuality in some way and the 'Activities of living model' (Roper et al 1996) is perhaps still the best known to nurses in the UK. The following comments were made by a student nurse in 1987.

We use Roper's model. We go through all of them in class and in theory it's all very good. One of these of course is expressing sexuality and that's important. But when it comes to doing it in class, what do you talk about? Helping women to look better after they've had a hysterectomy so their husbands will want to have sex with them? You spend ages on breathing then you get down to the end of the list, dying and expressing sexuality, and how we should talk to patients and get them to discuss their feelings, and that's it! No-one ever does it! We write in our care plans, 'Encourage patients to express their feelings and anxieties' but it's never really approached. [Savage 1987]

Although this quotation appeared in a 1987 publication it is reasonably safe to assume that things have not changed very much. It is interesting to note that some NHS Trusts that adopted the 'Activities of living model' have completely removed the section on 'Expressing sexuality' or have sanitised it by renaming it something less explicit (and less threatening?), such as 'Bodily appearance'. An examination of a range of nursing care plans reveals entries such as, 'Mary likes to dress according to her sexual orientation' or 'Likes to wear own clothes and aftershave after his shower'. Then again, there is the ubiquitous 'No problems expressed'. Such entries suggest that these nurses have little awareness of the meaning of the concept and perhaps felt compelled to make an entry in the nursing assessment for the sake of completeness.

The following entries suggest some understanding, but the reader is left wondering what and how the patient was told, and what the patient's understanding was following such comments:

- 'Worried about stenosis following radiotherapy. Told to get a vibrator!!' [The exclamation points are the authors']
- 'Counselled re sperm banking'
- 'Told about complications of treatment, including possible impotence'
- 'Given "Safe Sex" leaflet!'

It appears acceptable to some health care professionals to talk to or give information to selected groups of patients. It seems acceptable and advisable to talk to patients postmyocardial infarction, before the return home where they may resume sexual activity. Anxiety may be unnecessarily high in both patients and partners who fear reinfarction or death as a result of sexual intercourse. Thompson (1990) cites Ueno (1963) who claims that coitus accounts for fewer than 0.6% of cases of sudden death, most occurring in extramarital relationships. Overcoming the methodological challenges in such a study is difficult, but anecdotal evidence would suggest that the risk is low. It is worth reflecting on how many patients you have come across with postintercourse emergencies.

Men and women who have had cancer treatment, which will affect their primary or secondary sexual organs, may receive information. Ladies who have had a mastectomy or hysterectomy and men with testicular, prostatic or penile cancer may receive information, and possibly support, but it appears that although cancer and cancer treatment can profoundly affect sexuality, support is not often offered. Fallowfield (1990) goes further to suggest that:

… ignoring such issues as sex in studies of patients who have undergone gynaecological or genitourinary or bowel surgery might result in a very incomplete assessment of the impact of treatment.

The authors agree with Fallowfield and suggest that ignoring issues of sexuality in patients who have undergone any form of treatment for cancer might result in a very incomplete assessment of the impact of treatment.

When visiting a colleague in hospital, who had undergone surgery for a hysterectomy a few days previously (she did not have cancer), I jokingly asked her if she had been given the 'predischarge chat'. She then proceeded to show me the leaflets and booklets she had received, and I asked what advice she had been given about resuming sexual activity. She told me that she had been advised not to have sex for at least 4 weeks and that, during that period, she should not become aroused. I (RG) suggested that it was time for me to leave in case my presence aroused her, as neither of us knew what would happen if we broke that hospital rule!

What prevents nurses from initiating discussions – and whose responsibility is it? Initiating a discussion about sex or sexuality is difficult to do for many reasons. Bor & Watts (1993) suggest that embarrassment, lack of training and a belief that sexuality is not relevant to a particular disorder, prevent staff from approaching the subject with patients. In addition, Waterhouse & Metcalf (1991), citing Gross Fisher (1985), suggest that anxiety and conservative attitudes are significant factors. Not much has changed in the last 10 years according to Sutherland's unpublished survey (1995). There is clearly an important role for education if things are to improve. Perhaps the most important issue in this debate is that nurses and other health care professionals expect the patients to initiate any discussion of this nature, while the patients expect that the staff will do the initiating. This is supported by Baggs & Karch (1987), Jenkins (1988), Krueger et al (1979) and Waterhouse & Metcalf (1991). The debate is also clarified by these authors who clearly conclude that there are patients who do want staff to talk about sexual matters and who do want staff to initiate discussions.

Another useful opt-out for the nurse is that the patient is too old or too ill but, as Lieber et al (1976) point out, there are some patients who have neither the ability nor the urge for sexual intercourse, yet intimacy and close human contact are desired. Their study concluded that patients with advanced cancer experienced, simultaneously with their spouses, an increased desire for physical closeness and a decreased desire for sexual intercourse. In a study concerning sexuality and the older cancer patient, Kaiser (1992) found that 63% of patients wanted more information on the impact of cancer on sexuality and that 54% wanted to discuss the issue with their physician. Patients rarely found that this need was met despite the fact that loss of libido, impotence, decreased arousability and orgasmic difficulties may occur in patients with cancer.

It cannot be assumed that all patients share these feelings but the literature is both helpful and challenging. It is helpful in that it shows that we should consider initiating discussions and challenging in that it does not tell us how to do it. Approaching a patient with a prearranged script is unlikely to be particularly helpful, but considering how a discussion could be initiated might reduce anxiety for the nurse and increase the benefits for the patients. This means that nurses should at least have some solutions for some of the problems that can arise.

PROBLEM-SOLVING APPROACH

Below are problems about which most nurses could give very simple information, which would assist in ameliorating them if they themselves were aware of some solutions. It is not possible to make the bad things that have happened in patients' lives, because of the illness, become 'good' but information and advice may help with the process of adaptation and help to minimise some of their current distress. In providing information to health care professionals the authors are not implying that all couples should be sexually active in the middle of crises that illness thrusts on them. However, we do think that it is reasonable that if both partners wish it they should be given clear, appropriate, information that is not confused with myths and old-wives' tales.

Ways of helping

The patient with the large abdominal wound could be advised to adapt the preferred position for intercourse so that there is neither weight nor pressure on the wound. If this is not possible, then a total change of position may be required if the couple wish to have intercourse. Advice about stroking and caressing other areas of the body should be included.

There are many myths about radiotherapy and the partner becoming radio-active is just one of them. It may come as a disappointment to her that she will not glow in the dark! To prevent this kind of situation becoming a problem, when the patient is informed that she will be having radiotherapy she should be told at the same time that this will not affect her partner in any way.

In lovemaking, legs are used for balance and for erotic stimulation. As well as the assault on body image and self-esteem, the loss of one or both legs can profoundly affect the physical relationship. To achieve and improve balance, cushions and pillows may be used. Pretty covers and soft textures may enhance the experience, and caressing other areas of the body can greatly increase erotic stimulation, provided that it is what both partners enjoy.

Again, there are many myths surrounding hysterectomy, especially the one that says a woman can no longer have intercourse after hysterectomy. For some women, this may be seen as a blessed release. If they have never really enjoyed sex with their partner, they may be quite glad that this is an aspect of their lives which has 'legitimately' ended. The nurse who tells the husband that 'Of course it's OK to have sex with your wife' will not be popular! In the first instance, discussion should take place with the wife, on her own, at the time surgery is planned and her decision respected. However, it is the experience of this author (NS) that women can be helped to enjoy sex if they and their partners have more information on aspects of foreplay and fun. If the illness is not immediately life-threatening, this is the kind of situation that could be referred to a marriage counsellor or therapist, provided it is what the patient wishes.

Pain is a powerful deterrent to physical intimacy. If it is constant, it should be reassessed to discover the cause and to find if there are ways of reducing it. The use of cushions and pillows to provide support for aching joints and limbs may help, and, while it may rob the act of lovemaking of some of its spontaneity, it may be possible to 'plan' for it. This would allow for analgesia to be effective and to reduce the experience of pain afterwards. If the act of sex is associated with pain, it will rarely be anticipated with pleasure. Do encourage couples to tell each other what they like and what they don't like. This applies to all the situations discussed. Partners are not all intuitive and may need direction from their spouse, especially in changing circumstances.

The gentleman who is unable to have an erection may well prefer to discuss this with a woman rather than a man [verbatim discussion with two psychologists]. This is a result of the fact that there is less of a threat to his manhood than there might be in discussing his situation with a man. This is not a law, it is an approach to consider. Adapting to this problem takes some time, particularly if the possibility of impotence was not discussed in advance. It may be that his main concern is in not being able to sexually satisfy his partner, rather than the permanent droop. This is a situation requiring a very sensitive approach and is not one that I would recommend for using to try out the skill of discussing sex for the first time. A wide knowledge of other ways of giving and receiving sexual gratification is needed, otherwise, if only one suggestion is made and the patient or his partner do not care to try it out, they may be left thinking that there is nothing else for them. If, however, there are health care professionals reading this who are sufficiently confident to further develop their skills, they might wish to discuss issues around mutual masturbation and caressing and fondling. There are couples who have found that since there is now no pressure to 'perform' they can take their time and both can have an extremely enjoyable time doing so.

■ REFLECTIVE PRACTICE 6.3   Helping patients with sexual problems

Take some time to be as creative as possible in finding some ways in which the patient and her partner could be helped in the following scenarios.

- The patient has a large abdominal wound
- A husband fears that he may become radioactive if he has intercourse with his wife who has just completed a course of radiotherapy
- A patient has an above-the-knee amputation
- A lady who has had a hysterectomy believes she can no longer have sexual intercourse
- The patient has pain
- A gentleman who has been treated for prostatic cancer is unable to have an erection. He did not appreciate that this would happen as a result of his treatment

Discuss these situations with a colleague and consider what advice could fairly easily be given and which situations are more difficult to deal with. What is it that makes a difficult situation 'difficult'? Would you consider referring any of the above to a specialist? If so, why and to which specialist?

Prostheses and implants may have a place for some patients, while others may find that glyceryl trinitrate patches sited at the penile–scrotal junction gives enough of an erection for vaginal penetration to take place. Papaverine or alprostadil injected into the corpus cavernosum may also be appropriate for some patients. Specialist advice will be required for some of these.

However, the important thing in all these situations is the relationships involved. Assisting couples to talk to each other may be far more effective than advice on the nitty-gritty of sex. Keeping a sense of humour and using humour appropriately while giving advice can reduce the embarrassment to both patients and staff. Avoiding the trap of being coarse and crude, and remaining professional, can make the situation quite acceptable to couples.

■ **REFLECTIVE PRACTICE 6.4** **Learning exercise**

Think of a patient you have known and cared for over a period of time. You are in a quiet, private environment where you will not be disturbed. The patient has made good progress in hospital and is to be discharged tomorrow. You have discussed all the usual matters like diet, exercise, out-patient appointments and resuming work, and you know that it would be in the patient's best interests if you gave her an opportunity to discuss any concerns about sex/sexuality.

What will you say to your patient to initiate the discussion? You might say something like:

- 'Is there anything else worrying you?' This is very general indeed
- 'How are things between you and your partner?' This is a bit more specific
- 'Are you having problems of a sexual nature?' This may be too direct for many patients
- 'Some patients with a condition like yours have some questions/worries/ concerns about sex/sexuality. I was wondering if you had any questions that you might like to discuss with me or someone else?' This question is gently direct and might be met with 'Mind your own business, you smutty offensive person …' or 'Well … there is something but it is a little embarrassing… !'

It is very important that you do not attempt to memorise these approaches as if they were scripts, but instead you should consider how you would approach sexuality. After all, if you do not pick up the patient's cues or broach the subject yourself, there may be no opportunity to consider this aspect of life.

SEXUALITY AND CONFIDENTIALITY

All health care staff are taught the importance of confidentiality throughout their work and are told that it is a fundamental human right. Although rights are never absolute, the issue of confidentiality and sexuality merit special consideration. It is usual for a nurse to share most information, which she receives from a patient, with her colleagues. This practice is considered to be valuable in that it helps all staff to be aware of their patient's problems and needs. While caring for a patient a nurse may learn about that patient's worries, concerns, anxieties and fears about sexuality. Before sharing such information with her colleagues, it is essential that the nurse considers these two questions:

- Do I need to write this down?
- Do I need to tell my colleagues this information?

The 'knee-jerk' response to both these questions may be, '… Yes … I must record all information and I must tell my colleagues so that they can provide holistic care for the patient.' After careful consideration, it may be decided that the patient told the nurse of her feelings and that there is nothing to be gained from telling the rest of the ward team. Such answers are rarely straightforward and the following scenarios could be used as a team-based learning exercise.

■ REFLECTIVE PRACTICE 6.5   Scenarios for a team-based learning exercise

Jim is a 48-year-old sales executive who has been admitted to your ward with chest pain and hypertension. While talking to him in private one day, he tells you, his primary nurse, that he is worried he will not be able to satisy his wife anymore. During a long discussion with him, you explain that his chest pain is not a heart attack and that with a change in lifestyle he should soon start to feel much better.

- Should the nurse write this down in the patient's notes?
- Should the nurse discuss this with her colleagues?

Mary is a 64-year-old lady who had a mastectomy for breast cancer 6 years ago. She remained very well until about 6 months ago when she developed multiple bony secondaries. While caring for her at home one Friday, she tells you how desperate she feels because her husband does not want to make love to her anymore. You acknowledge her concerns and because of a very heavy schedule you apologise and tell her that you do not have the time to stay and discuss this with her now. You promise to return on Monday morning.

- Should the nurse write this down in the patient's notes?
- Should the nurse discuss this with her colleagues?

Feedback

Patients can expect that, in general, confidences will be kept, but confidentiality as an absolute right is debatable. What is important in the above examples is that the nurse receiving such personal and sensitive information must consider the consequences of keeping or of not keeping such confidences. As a patient, one might expect that information about sexual matters should not be discussed openly unless it will be of benefit to that patient to do so. If the nurse feels the need to discuss such issues with another member of the care team, there must be justification in doing so. In short, it may not be necessary to record or share information about sexual matters or concerns. If it is thought to be necessary, it should be done in the interest of the patient.

After the ice has been broken

As previously acknowledged, initiating a conversation about sex and sexuality is likely to be difficult and embarrassing. Once the discussion has begun it is likely that the patient will want to express feelings and will perhaps want to ask for some information and advice. Responding to the first need requires good listening skills, which are discussed elsewhere in this book. It is very likely that you will be able to respond to the patient's informational needs without further assistance.

THE PLISSIT MODEL: A CONCEPTUAL SCHEME FOR THE BEHAVIOURAL TREATMENT OF SEXUAL PROBLEMS

The PLISSIT model (Annon 1976) can be helpful when caring for a patient who requires information about sexual matters, although it was originally developed for patients following myocardial infarction. This model has four aspects.

• Permission. This involves the nurse giving permission to the patient to talk about sexual matters, either by raising the subject or by being available and accessible. It is very important not to assume that a patient will want a partner to be present, and it is vital that the patient's permission is gained before other persons are involved. Two contrasting examples illustrate how a nurse may give permission.

Andy is a 43-year-old man with AIDS who is receiving palliative care. Jim is Andy's primary nurse. On a quiet evening after visiting time, Andy says to Jim, 'Carrying on a relationship when you've got this isn't easy, you know.' Jim says, 'I'll have a word with the doctor and perhaps we can get the social work appointment brought forward.'

On a similar duty, Kathy is in charge:

Kathy invites Andy to a quiet area of the ward and asks him if there is anything on his mind. 'Well things have been getting me down recently, you know, but it's a bit personal,' Andy replies, rather tentatively. 'It's a bit difficult for you to talk about some of your concerns but if there is anything at all that's worrying you, I would like to see if I could help,' replies Kathy.

Jim, for whatever reason, did not give Andy permission to voice his concerns. In contrast, Kathy indicated that it was permissible for Andy to tell her anything he chose. Clearly, if Andy were to respond, his relationship with his carer must be based on complete trust.

• Limited information. Factual, general information about the patient's treatment and condition and how this may affect sexuality, should only be offered after permission has been granted. This should include information being given in a positive rather than in a negative way. For example, 'It is perfectly safe for you to sleep in the same bed …' 'There is no problem in having family and friends nearby …' 'You will not harm your partner by kissing and cuddling, and it may help you to adjust to the shock you have both recently suffered …'

General information about lubricants should be included. KY-Jelly may be part of the professional's vocabulary and of senior house officer-leaving party armoury, but it is not part of everyone's vocabulary!

• Specific suggestions. This will depend on the questions and concerns voiced by patients and their partners and on the particular illness. These responses are best if not prepared. You may need a knowledge of relevant anatomy, physiology, pathology and psychosocial responses to help with specific suggestions. There is no problem if you do not have every answer at your fingertips, so long as you find out quickly.

• Intensive therapy. Occasionally, because of complex or pre-existing problems, a patient may require specialist help. A patient may have suffered from a delayed sexual response or impotence before the illness was diagnosed and may benefit from the help of a sex counsellor or sex therapist. A clinical psychologist may be the best person to offer advice, while it is important to impress upon the specialist that the patient's prognosis is limited. However, it is important to be aware that long-standing sexual problems may not be resolved rapidly.

HOMOSEXUALITY

The aim of this chapter is not to discuss the morality of homosexuality or any other sexual practices, but to acknowledge that homosexuality exists. If asked how many homosexual patients you have cared for, you would probably answer, 'Not many' or 'I have no idea' or 'Why do you ask me such a question?' The number of homosexual patients you have encountered is unimportant. Rather, the question has been posed so that the reader may begin to think about how a homosexual relationship may affect the care of a dying patient and her loved ones.

The health care system with its architecture, rules, boundaries, hang-ups and schedules is not generally welcoming to any couple who wish to demonstrate their affection or their love for each other. It may be valuable to consider how much more difficult it is likely to be for a couple in a homosexual relationship. Although it is the 1990s, gay men and women risk criticism and contempt from their fellow patients, other visitors and from staff members, because of loving behaviour that remains unacceptable and distasteful to many.

HIV and AIDS

Over the years, more and more people are dying from acquired immune deficiency syndrome (AIDS). This population and their partners, their families and their friends represent a part of the community who require some consideration because of the problems they face during their illness and into bereavement.

Many lay people and health care professionals automatically assume that the patient with AIDS is gay. Clearly, this is by no means the case, but the person with AIDS is powerless to remove this label, which has been firmly attached by society and which has been attached where the patient is unlikely to see it. If they escape the 'gay' label they are just as likely to pick up the 'promiscuous' label, when in fact neither may be true.

Our society recognises and values the concept of kinship and its apparent hierarchical relationship to the intensity of grief. The member of staff who has been bereaved is likely to be awarded compassionate leave according to their relationship to the deceased, even though the personnel policy states that such leave is at the discretion of the manager. No account is taken of the actual relationship, therefore survivors from non-traditional (heterosexual) relationships can have great difficulty in finding understanding and support from their friends, their families and from professionals. Thus, they are at risk of developing a complicated or unresolved grief reaction. When a gay person dies, the survivor may be excluded from the funeral and from inheriting from the deceased's estate.

Buckman (1988) offered these helpful words intended for lay people who are helping a dying friend. They are equally helpful to those professionals who feel challenged when caring for a patient who has a different sexual orientation from their own.

> It should be your objective ... to help your friend to let go of life in his own way. It may not be your way and it may not be the way you read about it in a book but it is his way and is consistent with the way he lived his life. You can and should help your friend achieve that. [Buckman 1988]

■ REFLECTIVE PRACTICE 6.6   Let's look at attitudes

It is widely acknowledged that education must consider skills, knowledge and attitudes, and that attitudinal change can be extremely difficult. A prerequisite of attitudinal change is awareness and exploration. Before embarking on this exercise it is important to be aware that challenging attitudes can expose lack of knowledge and deep-rooted prejudice. It therefore requires considerate facilitation and respect for others. This exercise may be used in wards, departments, and community settings. It does not assume or require any particular knowledge. It can be used in a unidisciplinary setting but has greater impact if a variety of disciplines can be encouraged to join in.

The exercise

It is best to begin by setting your own ground rules around issues such as confidentiality, use of strong language and respect for others. It is important that the group is not interrupted during the exercise.

Each group member is given some (three to five) 3" × 5" index cards and asked to write a few words that sum up any thought, feeling or attitude to sexuality, which are present in society, in the home or in the work environment. Anonymity can be enhanced if everyone uses a pencil and prints their statements. There are no constraints about what may be written on the card, except that 'vulgar' language may only be used for a clear purpose. Some participants will appear puzzled, so you may wish to give some examples such as:

- Where I work, sexuality ...
- The thought of two men ...
- Sex is a private affair and should be left well alone ...
- If they want our help they will ask ...
- People should be allowed to ...

The individual does not have to believe or 'own' the statements, nor should the cards be signed. All the cards are then collected and shuffled thoroughly. Group members are invited, in turn, to select and read one card from the pile. They are invited to respond to the statements on the cards as they wish. If they would prefer not to respond to particular statements, regardless of the reason, they may return these cards to the bottom of the pile, without any explanation or justification, and select another one instead. When one person has responded, the remaining group members are invited to respond to the statement on that card as they wish. Supportive challenging is to be encouraged if the ground rules permit. As the exercise progresses, many attitudes will be discussed. Some group members may be surprised at their own and the others' reactions to the statements. The exercise should be brought to a close by generating an action plan which emerges from the preceding discussion. Each group member is given a 'Post-it' note and asked to write one action for the group to pursue. Again, a few examples may help:

- Invite the health care adviser from the genitourinary medicine clinic to speak to staff about the latest AIDS statistics
- Collect up-to-date literature
- Attend a study day
- Contact health education department for current information on ...
- Redesign our care plan
- Talk to one patient about sexuality

If the action plan is ever to become a reality it is important to include a time frame and to agree on responsibilities.

Example
Invite the health care adviser from the genitourinary medicine clinic to speak to staff about the latest AIDS statistics.

Action:

Peter James	*Contact health care adviser. Suggested date: week commencing 4/10/99*
Sarah Winter	*Organise duty rota and book seminar room*

This may seem blindingly obvious, but remember, goals left to chance have no chance!

When you have finished the exercise you can collect the cards and use them with subsequent groups. You may like to invite the next group of medical students, complete with consultant and entourage, to participate in this exercise over their post ward round coffee and biscuits. It could well be worth it, even if you have to buy the coffee and biscuits!

SUMMARY

Health care in the UK has a long way to go before double beds become the norm in health care institutions and where sexual matters are openly discussed. Most of a couple's sexual relationship is, and will remain, deeply private. Health care professionals must be prepared to create opportunities for patients and their partners to express their concerns and to deal with them with skill, sensitivity, tact and diplomacy. We owe it to the dying to enable them to make the best of the life that is left and, to the partners who will soon be bereaved, we owe the opportunity for cherished memories.

REFERENCES

Annon J 1976 The PLISSIT model: a proposed conceptual scheme for the behavioural treatment of sexual problems. Journal of Sex Education Therapists 2: 1–15

Bor R, Watts M 1993 Talking to patients about sexual matters. British Journal of Nursing 2: 657–661

Baggs J G, Karch A M 1987 Sexual counselling of women with coronary heart disease. Heart and Lung 16: 154–159

Buckman R 1988 I don't know what to say – how to help and support someone who is dying. Macmillan, London

Fallowfield L 1990 The quality of life: the missing measurement in health care. Souvenir Press, London

Gross Fisher S 1985 The sexual knowledge and attitudes of oncology nurses: implications for nursing education. Seminars in Oncology Nursing 1: 63–68

Jenkins B J 1988 Patients' reports of sexual changes after treatment for gynaecological cancer. Oncology Nursing Forum 15: 349–354

Kaiser F E 1992 Sexual function and the older cancer patient. Oncology 6(suppl.): 112–118

Krueger J C, Hassell J, Goggins D B, Ishimatsu T, Pablico M R, Tuttle E J 1979 Relationship between counselling and sexual readjustment after hysterectomy. Nursing Research 28: 145–150

Leiber L et al 1976 The communication of affection between cancer patients and their spouses. Psychosomatic Medicine 38: 378–389

Lion E M 1982 Human sexuality and nursing. John Wiley and Sons, Chichester

Roper N, Logan W W, Tierney A 1980 The elements of nursing. Churchill Livingstone, Edinburgh

Roper N, Logan W W, Tierney A 1996 Learning to use the process of nursing, 4th edn. Churchill Livingstone, Edinburgh

Savage J 1987 Nurses gender and sexuality. Heinemann, London

Solzhenitsyn A 1968 Cancer ward. Penguin Books, London

Thompson D 1990 Intercourse after myocardial infarction. Nursing Standard 4: 32–33

Waterhouse J, Metcalf M 1991 Attitudes towards nurses discussing sexual concerns with patients. Journal of Advanced Nursing 16: 1048–1054

Ueno M 1963 The so-called coition death. Japanese Journal of Legal Medicine 127: 333–340

FURTHER READING

Andrew C, Andrew H 1991 Sexuality and the dying patient. Journal of District Nursing November

Comfort A 1989 The joy of sex. Quartet Books

Gamel C, Davis B D, Hengeveld M 1993 Nurses' provision of teaching and counselling on sexuality: a review of the literature. Journal of Advanced Nursing 18: 1218–1227

Gillan P 1987 Sex therapy manual. Blackwell Scientific Publications, Oxford

Greengross S 1992 You're never too old. Journal of District Nursing May

Greengross W (undated) Lifestyle and your ostomy – love and sex. Abbott Laboratories

Kolodny R C, Masters W H, Johnson V E 1979 Human sexuality. Little, Brown, Boston

Salter M 1988 Altered body image. Wiley

Savage J 1990 Sexuality, privacy and nursing care. Nursing Standard June: 37–39

Stanway A 1995 Sexuality and cancer. Bacup

Wennerdahl C 1981 Counselling those with sexual problems. The Christian Counsellor's Journal 3: 18–23

Also various leaflets from: The Association for the Sexual and Personal Relationships of the Disabled, 25 Mortimer St., London W1N 8AB, UK.

Complementary therapies

7

Brenda Bottrill   Ishbel Kirkwood

INTRODUCTION

In recent years there have been wonderful technological and pharmacological advances, which have gradually given nurses a more clinical approach to their patients. Therapies such as homeopathy, reflexology, massage therapy, acupuncture and aromatherapy have captured the interest of some nurses as a way of re-establishing a hands-on, caring approach. The choice of term 'alternative' to describe these therapies was unfortunate as it created a division between the orthodox and holistic approaches. Currently, we employ the term 'complementary therapy' showing that we work as a team for the benefit of the patient.

To palliate is to make the patient's condition seem less harsh by easing the symptoms without curing. The therapies included in this chapter adhere to that. They include relaxation, massage, aromatherapy and reflexology as these are the therapies best known to the authors. We will, however, mention other therapies and topics, allowing a wider appreciation of the possibilities for patient care.

LEARNING OUTCOMES

- The creation of a peaceful, relaxing environment in which to perform complementary therapy
- Recognition and treatment of stress
- Understanding of relaxation for use with patients and for self-care
- Ability to convey simple, relaxing techniques to patients for self-care at home
- An understanding of the most commonly used therapies: relaxation, massage, aromatherapy, reflexology
- Immediate comforting ideas with a few touch techniques
- A basic understanding of psychoneuroimmunology
- Guidelines for nurses wishing to train in a complementary therapy

The basic principles and aims of complementary therapies are shown in Box 7.1.

■ **BOX 7.1**

Basic principles and aims of complementary therapies
- Relieve tension, pain and other symptoms
- Relax, revitalise and nurture
- Improve circulation and balance energy flow
- Support psychoneuroimmunological responses
- Release negativity and affirm the positive

CREATING AN ENVIRONMENT IN WHICH TO WORK

It is helpful to create a peaceful environment when conducting complementary therapy, taking account of all the senses. The ideal is a quiet room, decorated in light colours, with comfortable, supportive chairs and foot rests so that patients can sit or lie back with their feet raised. It can be enhanced by books, a music centre and an outlook onto a garden, so that plants, trees and birdsong can be appreciated. If patients are confined to bed, make them as comfortable as possible, well supported and warm. Relaxing music can be used if the patient wishes. If the window looks onto a garden or trees, a little fresh air accompanied by nature sounds is helpful in achieving relaxation. The patient's choice is paramount. These are only suggestions.

The senses can be stimulated or calmed by the environment:

- Sight. All colours have an effect on how we feel and have helpful attributes and vibrations. Some of these effects are listed in Table 7.1.

Sunlight through the window is welcoming, flowers are always available and are uplifting, a tank with fish has a calming effect.

Table 7.1 Attributes of colours

Colour	Attributes
Brown	Grounding and nurturing
Red	Physical energy, blood stimulant
Orange	Courage
Gold	Uplifting as in sunlight
Pink	Love
Green	New life
Blue	General healer
Turquoise	Protective
Indigo	Mental clarity
Yellow	Emotional balance/wisdom
White	Purity
Purple	Meditation

• Smell. Aromas can evoke memories and feelings and are therefore very personal. Aromas of food, toiletries or cleaning fluids can affect a patient's emotions as everyone perceives smells differently. This subject is discussed in more detail below.

• Hearing. Music can be helpful in creating any mood, e.g. quiet and peaceful, uplifting and bright, sombre and deep. There are various relaxing musical tapes available; also the therapist's own relaxation tapes, which I have found useful for group members to use on their own. The familiar voice of the therapist helps when it is more difficult to relax without the support of the group. Some patients prefer nature sounds, e.g. water falling, waves rushing inshore, whale sounds, bird calls, wind rustling leaves. Songs can sometimes be too emotionally evocative to create a quiet mind. Generally there is a vast choice of easy listening and light music from which to choose. Peace and quiet is sometimes preferred.

• Touch. Touch to the patient is discussed in more detail below. Touch by the patient is very important and is demonstrated by the number of soft toys and favourite items that patients have beside them. The soft touch of an animal's coat has a relaxing effect and some patients gain comfort from stones, crystals and talismen.

• Taste. In creating a particular space for peace, taste is perhaps not a relevant point but it is very much part of the hospital stay. Nutrition plays a key role in palliative care and appetite is so often poor when patients feel low. It is important to stimulate taste buds with small portions of enticing and nutritious food. Smell and colour play their role in this also.

STRESS

In palliative care, nurses often help patients to cope with a slow deterioration, probably interspersed with acute episodes and hospital admission. This ongoing situation brings with it extra problems and stress relating to family, home, employment, finance and mobility. Symptoms of stress are shown in Table 7.2.

Table 7.2 Symptoms of stress

Physical	Mental	Emotional
Nausea/diarrhoea	Panic attacks/loss of control	Fear: of the unknown, of death
Tachycardia, hypertension	Racing thoughts	Shock
Eating disorders	Anxiety/depression	Exhaustion
Hot or cold sweats	Loss of concentration	Emotional withdrawal
Headaches	Paranoia	Anger
Muscular pain and tension	Memory loss	Loss of self-esteem/ confidence
Tachypnoea/dyspnoea	Disorientation	
Dry mouth and throat, loss of voice, grinding of teeth, insomnia	Poor coping strategies	Guilt, grief

Stress may be intermittent or persistent. It can be described as anything that makes abnormal demands on the human body. It is not inherently bad and a certain amount may enable us to reach goals, develop abilities and discover our strengths (Selye 1974). The problems occur when stress and tension become 'distress' and, under this now destructive force, breakdown occurs.

In the past the energy triggered by adrenalin secretion was used to fuel the 'fight or flight' response, thus allowing the body to quickly return to normal resting function, i.e. sympathetic–parasympathetic balance. The stresses mentioned above still trigger the production of adrenalin but this 'fight or flight' response is inappropriate and the energy has no physical outlet, leaving feelings of frustration with all the attendant symptoms (Table 7.3).

It is in this state that patients can benefit from practising relaxation techniques or receiving relaxing therapies, giving the body a chance to recover.

Table 7.3 Patients' experiences of stress release

Physical	Mental	Emotional
Increased energy	Able to cope with illness/ treatment/domestic affairs	Feeling renewed
Relief from nausea/relief from muscular tension	Relief from anxiety and racing thoughts	Feeling soothed, calmed & reassured
Pain relief	General well-being	Pampered feeling
Improved breathing technique	Relief from panic attacks	Self-confidence restored
Improved sleep pattern	Pleasant dreamlike thoughts	Happier brighter
Improved circulation and warmth	Relaxed/refreshed	Hopeful

RELAXATION

Relaxation techniques go back to ancient times. In recent medical history the work goes back to Edmund Jacobsen in the 1920s and 1930s.

He connected increased emotional stress to muscular contractions and tension. His work concluded that conscious relaxation of muscles would quieten the emotions. This is also a principle of yoga. Jacobsen started the technique called 'Progressive muscle relaxation' of consciously tensing and releasing muscle groups in a sequence through the body (Jacobsen 1938). Other studies have been carried out, but Benson and Klipper are best known for continuing this work. In 1976 they published 'The relaxation response', basing their method on yoga and inducing a state similar to that achieved in meditation. Figure 7.1 illustrates the general direction of relaxation.

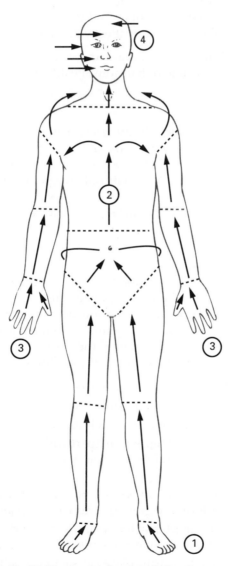

Fig. 7.1 The general direction of relaxation.

Relaxation activities

Try the relaxation activities described below.

Thought patterns

Experiment with the power of thought over the physical and emotional body sensations.

- Recall an event or a personal encounter that was difficult for you
- Remember your feelings at that time and observe your bodily reactions
- Don't dwell on those thoughts for too long. Let them go and recall another situation where you were really happy. It may have been in a place you enjoy and/or with friends
- Again, observe the bodily reactions and the change in feelings. Be aware of how your thought patterns can affect your bodily functions and feelings

In practices of relaxation, meditation and visualisation, we are using this knowledge to achieve a state of harmony, health and well-being.

Using the breath

- While sitting in your chair, take an easy breath in and sigh your breath out. Feel the letting go as your body sinks and relaxes into the chair
- Go on breathing normally. Your body has spontaneously relaxed and the following inhalation will be naturally deeper because of the deep exhalation
- Try not to slump too much because good posture for breathing creates space for each breath

Energy block release

Benson and Klipper's (1976) method of progressive muscle relaxation is popular in medical circles. I prefer to practise the short sequence known as 'energy block release' prior to relaxation because it not only begins to unlock tight muscles and joints by gentle movement and stretch, but also allows energy (life force) to flow within the body.

The sequence of energy block release is as follows:

1 Take shoes off and let your feet feel free. Stand up.

2 Flex and extend ankles and do slow rotations.

3 Alternate rising on to the ball of each foot (as if treading grapes).

4 With parallel feet, stand hip-width apart with knees bent as far as comfortable. Place hands on thighs. Circle knees slowly clockwise, then anticlockwise.

5 With parallel feet, again hip-width apart, bend knees alternately as if walking but keep heels on the ground. This eases hip joints.

6 Legs slightly wider apart than hip width, feet turned out ten to two. Knee bends alternately from side to side eases ankles, calves, knees and thighs.

7 Rub hands till really warm, place on sacroiliac joints then do pelvic circles one way then the other with feet hip-width apart.

8 With arms hanging loosely, feet hip-width apart, rotate spine keeping head and neck in line.

9 Keeping feet hip-width apart, bend sideways using the out-breath to bend, letting go into the stretch. Inhale to come up, repeat on the other side.

10 Breathe in, shrugging shoulders to ears, then sigh out and drop shoulders to release.

11 Dropping the head so that the chin rests towards the chest, very easily roll the head round to listen to the right shoulder then return through the centre point to listen to the left shoulder, then return to centre. Breathe in and lift the head back into a comfortable upright position.

12 Gently shake arms and hands.

13 Think of the trunk of the body as the trunk of a tree with the feet as roots and the branches as the nervous and circulatory systems flowing out to the fingertips. Cross your hands at your wrists and gently raise your arms as if taking off a sweater and, as they comfortably stretch above your head, feel the height of your trunk and spine and visualise the flow of sap within the tree as if flowing within your spinal column and see yourself as a newly sprouting and flowering spring tree. Use your sigh out to let your arms float down again a little in front of you, being careful not to stress the shoulders. Stand and breathe gently, observing how you feel; observe any changes in yourself. Repeat once or twice, resting, breathing, observing in between each stretch, then sit down comfortably.

Notice that the sequence has deepened and expanded your diaphragmatic breathing naturally. People also express that they notice warmth in their hands and faces, a feeling of silence and calmness with a glow, and worrying thoughts beginning to leave them. These exercises usually bring spontaneous laughter from patients, helping the relaxation process, and can be varied with patients according to their medical condition, mobility and comfort.

Visualisation

Visualisation is used by therapists to help patients form clear pictures within their minds when in a relaxed state. Gentle music can be helpful in evoking the images. Although guided visualisation has a place, we find that patients' own spontaneous visions are so varied and personal that they are more powerful in achieving the end result of relaxation, aiding their coping abilities.

Examples of images that people have found helpful are mostly taken from nature, e.g. water, sea, sand, trees, birds and mountains. Some experience free movements, such as dancing, swimming and flying. Happy childhood memories are also recalled. Images of health have been used as an aid to recovery. In cases of tumours some people find it helpful to use a focused image, such as lymphocytes attacking and defeating the tumour, others do not. Alternatively, one can imagine a light switching on, dispelling the darkness, using positive thought and giving no energy or space to negativity. This feeling of well-being after relaxation is produced by the release of endorphins in response to positive thought and pleasant images. For those who find visualisation difficult, self-suggestion by words (affirmation) is an alternative, e.g. 'I am lying in a silk cocoon and nothing will disturb me.'

Affirmation can help and support patients in gradual steps towards their goals. These must be attainable in reality or disappointment and negative feelings arise.

Deep relaxation

Nurses should try this technique for themselves before helping patients to achieve this deeper level of relaxation. It can be carried out sitting in a chair or lying on the floor or in bed. Make sure you are warm and comfortable and your body is supported. A pillow under your head is helpful to bring the neck in line with the body and a pillow under the knees helps release both the hips and lumbar spine when supine. Allow a few moments to breathe gently and naturally.

1 Take the hands to the solar plexus and diaphragm area and focus on that area for a few moments, enabling the upper abdomen and lower chest to rise and fall in diaphragmatic breathing.

2 When you have done this for a few moments take your hands back to any position that is comfortable and let your breathing be gentle and natural. Use this natural breathing as you move through the body, trying to make it feel more comfortable following the out-breath. Let go a little bit more as you go through each muscle group, starting at the feet and moving up to the head.

3 Take your awareness down to your toes, feet and ankles. Move them only as much as you need to make them comfortable and on the out-breath release tightness and experience softness and warmth as if the feet were melting into the floor or bed.

4 Repeat this sequence throughout the whole body, moving gradually upwards to the head and face. Experience the feeling of well-being as the face glows.

5 Enjoy this relaxed feeling for a few moments and then begin to reawaken the body. Starting with hands and feet (you may feel them very light or heavy), gently bring them back to life. Have a lovely soft stretch like a cat on a sunny windowsill. Stroke your eyes and face with your hands. If you are lying down bend your knees and curl up on your side before you sit up. If you are sitting have another stretch. Open your eyes and give your limbs a gentle rub, taking plenty of time to reawaken.

Coping with emotions during relaxation

During patient relaxation sessions there can be a resistance to relaxing because some people are afraid of letting go, thus releasing feelings and becoming tearful. This occasionally happens and the nurse or therapist must be prepared for and sensitive to the release of emotions, e.g. crying, hysterical laughing or nervous coughing. This can happen in a group or in a one-to-one situation. It is for this reason we prefer that group relaxation sessions should be led by two facilitators: one to lead and take care of the group and the other to meet individual needs and supply emotional support. Sometimes people can become uncomfortable or wake up suddenly and need to be reassured of their surroundings. We are often called to see patients following the delivery of bad news and our part is to provide a private and soothing environment while the patient comes to terms with the shocking reality of their diagnosis/prognosis. Relaxation is not appropriate when intense, volatile emotions need an outlet. However, such emotions need to be expressed, not repressed, and patients attending counselling alongside relaxation make good progress.

■ **CASE HISTORY 7.1   Wendy: a 54-year-old lady who was treated for carcinoma of the breast**

Wendy was referred by the nurse counsellor some time after discharge and attended the relaxation class. The following is her own description of relaxation.

After having been in hospital my biggest problem was insomnia, something I had never experienced before and something that began to take over my life. I dreaded going to bed at night and panicked because I wasn't sleeping. I wandered around doing household chores. There seemed to be nothing else for it other than the dreaded sleeping pills. However, this was a road I did not want to go down. Then there was a glimmer of hope. It was suggested that I go to a relaxation class. Sceptical at first, I attended my first class and the benefits were immediate. Here was something I could do for myself after all. I could never have believed that I could be so relaxed, I didn't even know where my hands were. Everyone in the group had different experiences, all positive. As the music played, afterwards I became very light and flew like a bird over the waves and soared on the air currents. I visited happy haunts and danced there. My sleeping pattern has improved tremendously, and I don't need pills anymore. I don't dread going to bed or panic if I'm awake. Part of my daily routine is to take my tape to a quiet corner and relax with it for half an hour. To be able to do this is a gift that I have been given which I'm sure will sustain me in all kinds of situations throughout my life. Every cloud has a silver lining.

■ **CASE HISTORY 7.2   Maureen: a 47-year-old lady with ovarian cancer**

Maureen was shocked by her diagnosis of ovarian cancer. She attended the relaxation class while receiving chemotherapy.

I was told I had ovarian cancer, and a course of chemotherapy would follow. After the initial feeling of devastation, I decided that I wanted to help myself and not leave it all to the medical profession. I joined the relaxation class 3 weeks after my operation. The relaxation was of great help, giving me a feeling of great happiness. At night sleep came more easily as the relaxation tape helped to switch off my anxieties. I also used it instead of painkillers, both for headaches and postoperative pain. I used the relaxation technique twice daily for the first 8 weeks. After that my great need for relaxation

> *appeared to diminish, i.e. pain had disappeared, sleep came more easily and I had started to live again. I still continue to set aside time to relax deeply at least twice a week, often using the tape. I believe a healing process takes place during this period of great peace.*

We recognise that from a medical point of view these cases follow a radical programme of treatment. From the complementary therapy angle we do not expect to effect a cure, therefore our input can also be termed palliative as we are helping to allay symptoms and aid the patient to control the ongoing stresses of life.

TOUCH

Few nurses consider what may be conveyed by touch. It can help alleviate tensions and anxieties associated with illness, either as a means of communication or relaxation. In the UK, touch is rarely used outside personal or familial relationships. In the past, nurses touched those in their care more than they do today. The increase in technology has meant that nurses are more in contact with equipment than with patients. The touching that does take place is often associated with a procedure or task rather than to show feeling or help comfort a patient. In palliative care, touch is particularly relevant as patients may have faced the ravages of modern-day treatment creating an altered body image. It is important, however, that nurses recognise individual differences in tactile communication and consider the patients' need for space and privacy if they so wish. Barnet (1972) identified groups of patients who benefit most from touch. These include people with altered body image and lowered self-esteem, those who are dependant, anxious or dying. Touch is in itself a form of communication, which enhances verbal communication, conveying empathy. Watson (1989) states:

> *It is an expression of the nurse's participation in the other's experience of suffering.*

In our experience, some patients with tumours have expressed feelings of being unclean. This highlights the importance of touch to support the undermined self-esteem. It is particularly so in clinically isolated patients who benefit from the reassurance of hands-on care. There are, however, those who have created barriers against the spontaneity of bedside touch. They may accept more easily the idea of premeditated touch, in a structured way, in the form of a massage. The action then is less likely to be misconstrued, ambiguity and anxiety are reduced and the touching is fully accepted.

MASSAGE

References to massage are numerous in Greek and Roman literature. It grew in popularity in the 19th century through the influence of Per Henrik Ling, whose system of Swedish massage has lasted right up to the present day. In 1894, the Society of Trained Masseurs was formed. They were the founder members of the Chartered Society of Physiotherapy (Hudson 1988). However, massage was used less by the physiotherapists with the advent of more fashionable electrical apparatus and modern drugs. Its use was thought to be pampering rather than therapeutic. Today the value of massage is gradually being recognised as a complement to conventional medical treatments. Massage, like touch, is a means of comforting someone who is ill, helping to relieve any unpleasant symptoms. Instinctively we 'rub better' an injured area of the body as a mother would do to her child who had fallen. The simple act of rubbing or massaging increases the blood flow, relaxes tense muscles and conveys to the person, non-verbally, that you care. Gentle massage strokes are soothing, help the patient to relax and improve the quality of rest and sleep. In a relaxed state the release of physical tensions can lead to the release of emotions that may relate to the illness or anxieties associated with it, which have been stored for a long time. In our experience, this letting go of the emotions occurs when the muscles that tighten to hold in the emotions are massaged; for example, the muscles in the shoulder girdle, lower back and face, when the 'stiff upper lip' relaxes. The whole body can be relaxed by massaging a small area; for example, the hands, face, head or feet. Nurses who have worked in haematology will appreciate that treatment, including bone marrow transplant, can last for several months with regular hospital admissions. It can be very hard on the patients who become neutropenic and are low in body and spirit. They must be nursed in near isolation for many weeks at a time. They need a great deal of encouragement to keep going and I am moved by their courage and determination. It is a distressing time for the relatives who try to keep cheerful for the patient's sake. My role as relaxation therapist is to help patients through this treatment regimen. Because they are neutropenic they cannot attend a group session so I work individually with them using primarily a gentle way of touching feet (following ward protocol). This technique has an extremely relaxing and calming effect on the whole body and can ease pain in the back, limbs and head. I always notice a change in their breathing pattern part way through the session, when a spontaneous sigh occurs and the deep, rhythmical, relaxing diaphragmatic breathing takes over. Sometimes they choose to have soothing music and sometimes peace and quiet. The patient's own moisturing lotion is used to massage the feet so that nothing foreign is introduced into the controlled environment. One drop of lavender essential oil is sometimes placed on tissue to give a subtle aroma. Its properties are antiseptic, relaxing and balancing. These patients are very vulnerable to infection and the chemotherapy leaves the skin, especially on the hands and feet, very dry.

Personally I have fallen asleep only once during massage. It was a hand massage. The hands, feet and face contain many acupressure points which, during massage, will receive a gentle stimulus.

As with all relaxation therapies, a quiet room is preferable but it is possible to create a pleasant environment at the bedside. Nurses with no massage qualifications can simply hold and stroke the forehead, hands or feet. Using oil or lotion, allow the hands to gently mould to the area being touched. A gentle circling motion, using the pads of the fingers, can be introduced using only light pressure. Relaxation can be assisted by ensuring that the patient is warm. A heated towel wrapped around the feet is beneficial. Encourage the patient to slow the breathing by placing a hand on the solar plexus.

Byass (1988) suggests that massage can have a positive effect on relationships between ill people and their relatives or friends. Communication barriers can develop for many reasons, ranging from a fear to a desire to protect each other from the truth of the situation. To teach a family and friends the basic massage strokes can promote rebonding and empathy between giver and receiver. Overeagerness to be able at last to do something could mean touching too deeply or firmly. Therefore, nurses or therapists should check their touch on themselves. When tight muscles are touched for the first time, the temptation to touch deep and hard should give way to a gentle hold, allowing the warmth from the hands to reach the muscles and help to relax them. If a patient is discharged with a carer or relative to give gentle massage, it is wise for them to keep in touch with the nurse or therapist trained in massage. Time spent teaching carers is time well spent. Passing on the skills of massage empowers them to enter the healing process, whether the healing is into life or death.

Contraindications for massage

Although massage is possible in the majority of consenting patients, there are some conditions where massage would be inappropriate. These include areas receiving or recently treated with radiotherapy or whole-body irradiation prior to bone marrow transplant, areas that have infectious skin conditions (because of the risk of spread), areas that have still to heal or have recent scar tissue, which is very fragile, and areas with diagnosed or suspected tumours. Patients who have deep venous thrombosis, petechiae or purpuric spots are also unsuitable for this treatment. Massage would be possible with medical guidance if the following conditions existed: jaundice, low blood count, thrombocytopaenia, skin rashes or cardiovascular conditions; for example, varicose veins.

Potential problems during massage

In ward situations, nurses should be aware of problems that may arise during massage so that these can be avoided.

• Intimate or private conversation should be avoided. Suggest a quiet period without conversation to facilitate the massage benefits. However, before some people can deeply relax it is a necessary part of the therapy that they have freedom to express their anxieties.

• Always state which items of clothing are to be removed.

• Try not to massage in an isolated or locked room; check that someone knows your whereabouts.

• Personality clashes can sometimes happen between nurse and patient, therefore such a combination would certainly not create a relaxed state.

• Although trained to deal with difficult situations, nurses are not counsellors, therefore seek help if you are unsure of how to deal with a patient's revelations during massage. However, a necessary attribute of the nurse or therapist is to be a good listener.

Although there are countless articles on the benefits of massage, nurses require good, sound, research-based studies on which to build their knowledge. The lack of co-ordination in nursing research has meant that opportunities for building on previous studies have been lost. However, as research projects are entering the lives of most nurses, it gives everyone with an interest in complementary therapy care an opportunity to prove its worth. Work based on single case histories is now accepted as valid evidence.

■ **CASE HISTORY 7.3   Helen is a 45-year-old lady, recently diagnosed with acute myeloid leukaemia. She writes:**

When I was admitted to hospital and diagnosed with acute myeloid leukaemia, the doctors and nurses I spoke to all emphasised how helpful a positive mental attitude would be in assisting my recovery. As I am generally quite optimistic, I was prepared to fight the illness and work on maintaining a positive attitude but it can be very hard work. There are times when inner resources become depleted. When I was offered the opportunity to have a relaxation foot massage on the ward, it seemed worth trying. As a regular, twice-a-week event, it became a very useful way of recharging my batteries and, especially on a bad day, brought a sense of perspective to all that was happening to me. It has also been pleasant to have someone non-medical, but still knowledgeable, to talk to. The use of aromatherapy oils (one drop) enhanced the massage process. The scent made the whole room a therapeutic place for some time after the massage session. I feel that relaxation has definitely helped me get through my treatment in a much better mental state.

Helen was admitted for two courses of harsh chemotherapy and continued to practice her own relaxation and health-promoting lifestyle to aid her recovery between visits. She is now in remission and hopeful.

■ **CASE HISTORY 7.4   Grace is a 37-year-old lady. She writes:**

When I was first given my diagnosis of breast cancer, I was an emotional wreck, having panic attacks, with very little self-confidence and experiencing a feeling of doom and devastation. In the ward, whilst recovering from my operation, I experienced having my feet gently massaged. It is like someone pulling the plug out and letting your worries disappear down the drain. I was left feeling so relaxed that I almost couldn't have cared less what was happening around me. My body felt heavy but light at the same time and I felt myself entering a peaceful space, tranquil and yet energising at the same time. Whatever thoughts had been spinning around my head had stopped, the butterflies in my stomach had disappeared and I felt an incredible inner strength. I changed over a very short time from a nervous wreck to a calm, relaxed, composed patient. Words do not do this amazing treatment justice. It has to be experienced to realise the full potential. (It has been noted that the difficulties experienced by the staff cannulating the veins of patients was made easier when patients received a relaxation foot massage.) I also attended the relaxation group and was helped by the techniques and the calming voice of the therapist. I have changed into the positive and self-assured person that I now am. Whilst in hospital I also practised Tai Chi, which strengthened my calmness and helped me to cope better.

Grace also described her fear of the 'dreaded chemotherapy' and needles, which she also had to undergo, and how using her relaxation tape she became so relaxed during this procedure as to appear asleep. Staff were amazed at the transformation. She also participated in a weekly support group, addressing issues of an emotional and psychological nature, during the course of her treatment. She still attends the weekly relaxation class for patients who have returned to work and, recently, very unluckily had to undergo a biopsy and received a second diagnosis of melanoma. She admitted that her ongoing relaxation practice and receiving the foot massage was helping her through this second trauma.

A year ago I could not have coped so well. I would have gone to pieces but I am managing to stay calm and positive.

As a complementary therapist I work under the instructions of medical and nursing staff and in concert with them. New knowledge on the safe and beneficial marrying of complementary therapies with conventional medical treatments is constantly coming to light.

AROMATHERAPY

Aromatherapy is a popular therapy for nurses to use. It is truly holistic, using essential oils from plants, in a controlled manner, as a form of treatment. We will give a general overview of this therapy before applying it to palliative care.

The essential oils are concentrated liquids extracted from the leaves, stems, flowers, fruit, bark and roots by several methods (Worwood 1992). The most common methods are distillation and simple pressure.

If an essential oil would be adversely affected by distillation, it is subjected to extraction by solvents or, more recently, condensed carbon dioxide, which produces a more true-to-nature fragrance. All essential oils are very volatile. They are, therefore, stored in little glass bottles with a dropper fixed in the neck. This facilitates measurement, acts as a safety device and helps to prevent evaporation.

Rene Gattefosse, a French chemist who coined the phrase 'Aromatherapie' in 1928, became fascinated by therapeutic properties of essential oils after discovering, by accident, that lavender essential oil was able to rapidly heal a severe burn on his hand. He also found that many of the essential oils were more effective in their totality than were their isolated active ingredients or their synthetic substitutes. This rings true in today's health care where the side-effects of modern drugs are an ever-increasing problem.

Marguerite Maury brought aromatherapy to the UK, applying the research of Dr Jean Valnet to her beauty treatments. She created an aromatic complex adapted to the client's temperament, health and lifestyle. This personal prescription is still used today, matching the therapeutic properties of the oils to the patient's condition. It is therefore important that the nurse therapist using aromatherapy should be familiar with the patient's past and present medical history.

Aromatherapy can be used in several ways:

- Vaporisation. This is an effective way of dispersing the aromatic molecules into the atmosphere. A small burner used in a room with the appropriate oils can create a relaxed or invigorating atmosphere or ease breathing in chest infections. I generally vaporise a blend of oils to create a relaxed atmosphere, which usually provokes an immediate response from the patient entering the room. As well as being enjoyable, it creates a talking point for the nervous or anxious person who may be unfamiliar with the therapy.

- Baths. This is one of the most pleasurable ways of using essential oils, adding between three and six drops of the oil of your choice when the bath is full. Again it can be relaxing or stimulating, depending on the oils used. Mixing the essential oil with a tablespoonful of milk before dropping in the water aids dispersal.

- Shower. Oils can be applied in the shower after the wash. Between one and three drops of oil dropped onto the wet flannel and rubbed on the skin are a substitute for those who don't have the luxury of a bath.

- Steam inhalations. These are used mainly for chest, sinus and throat infections. Two drops of essential oil are dropped into a bowl of almost boiling water. The head is bent over the bowl with a towel covering it to hold the steam in. This vapour is breathed for up to 5 minutes.

- Neat application. This is not usually recommended but there are a few exceptions. Lavender oil can be applied directly onto burns, insect bites and cuts. Tea Tree oil can be applied neat to spots, athlete's foot and verrucae. Lemon oil is effective in the treatment of warts.

- Internal use. Internal use of essential oils is not recommended in the UK at present. This means of application is, however, prescribed and used by medical aromatherapists in France.

- Massage. This is the method of application favoured by aromatherapists in the UK. Massage training is included in aromatherapy training. A blend of essential oils suited to the patient's condition is mixed with a base or carrier oil, preferably cold pressed to retain nutrients that are destroyed during the refining of some vegetable oils. In their raw, natural, unrefined state, oils such as olive, almond and sesame seed contain vitamins, minerals and essential fatty acids which in themselves nourish the skin.

Aromatherapists would use one to three drops of essential oil in 5 ml of base or carrier oil as a recommended concentration. In palliative care, one drop of essential oil in 5 ml of base oil is recommended. If the patient has sensitive skin, a little patch test of the blend can be carried out on the inside of the arm and observed for reddening or itching. If there is a reaction within 10–15 minutes, the patch test should be removed with plain vegetable oil. Massage with essential oils allows the skin to absorb the aromatic molecules, which are transported in the circulation to the system or organs for which the oils have an affinity.

Essential oils chemistry

Lawless (1992) noted that essential oils chemistry, in general, consist of chemical compounds that have oxygen, hydrogen and carbon as their building blocks. They are subdivided as follows:

- Hydrocarbons, which are almost exclusively made up of terpenes
- Oxygenated compounds, which are mainly esters, aldehydes, ketones, alcohols, phenols, oxides, acids, lactones, sulphurs and nitrogen compounds

The common terpene hydrocarbons include:

- Limonene, which is antiviral and found in 90% of citrus oils
- Pinene, which is antiseptic and found in pine and turpentine oils
- Chamazulene and farnesal, which have outstanding anti-inflammatory and bactericidal properties
- Esters, which are probably the most widespread group found in essential oils, with fungicidal and sedative qualities
- Aldehydes, which have a sedative effect with powerful antiseptic properties that are generally found in lemon-scented oils
- Ketones, which are some of the most toxic constituents of essential oils. They give the oils their potency and must therefore only be used by someone familiar with the chemistry. Ketones are often found in plants which are used for upper respiratory complaints to ease congestion
- Alcohols, which have good antiseptic and antiviral properties with an uplifting quality
- Phenols, which are generally bactericidal and strongly stimulating, but can be skin irritants
- Among the oxides, by far the most important is cineol, which stands in a class of its own with a powerful expectorant effect and is the principal constituent of eucalyptus oil

An understanding of essential oils chemistry is a necessary part of professional aromatherapy. Essential oils are the life force of the plants from which they come. The many therapeutic properties attributed to a single oil attracts scepticism but this diversity of properties and actions reflects the chemistry of the oil. When two or more oils are blended together, the synergy created is more than the 'sum of parts', i.e. the chemistry from each plant join, enhancing their effect and make the blend more active than when used singly.

Essential oils and chemotherapy

At present, the use of essential oils with patients having chemotherapy is not recommended. This contraindication has not been substantiated by any research but while no-one seems to know what chemical interaction takes place between essential oils and chemotherapy drugs, it is wise to err on the side of caution. McNamara (1994) suggests:

> It seems most unlikely that essential oils could override the impact of cytotoxic drugs, and therefore inhibit the body's response to chemotherapy.

As mentioned above, the current practice is to avoid massage on areas receiving radiotherapy. Two oils have been researched in French hospitals by Penoel & Franchomme (1990) with positive results. Niaouli and Tea Tree oils were applied as a thin film over the area to be irradiated; this helped to prevent burning and scarring. This is one of the areas where the application of essential oils without massage could be useful. Many patients enjoy the aroma and indeed their interest in the oil has led them to enquire about it and to purchase their own. The aroma from an oil burner or electric vaporiser may not be agreeable to other patients in a shared room. Therefore, a drop of oil suitable to the patient can be dropped on the nightclothes or pillow without invading the others' privacy. Because of their potent aromas, the essential oils can evoke memories already mentioned above, in 'senses'. These memories can be pleasant or otherwise and therefore their use on patients is a personal experience. Some orthodox treatments can disturb the olfactory system, and smells that have been enjoyed in normal circumstances can now be perceived differently. With over 150 oils to choose from, it shouldn't be difficult to select one that will give pleasure. Most patients welcome the pleasing aromas as a diversion to the everyday routine aromas experienced in hospital. Aroma alone can have a subtle but real effect on the mind and, via the mind, on the body. Inhaling the oils also has a direct effect on the body, as some part of the oil will be absorbed via the lungs and into the bloodstream. The oils in Table 7.4 are shown only for interest and not as guidelines for patient use.

Essential oils are now sold quite freely to the general public. There is no way of knowing the source of the oil, or its chemistry, and whether it has been adulterated to meet minimum standards. Cheap oils usually indicate poor quality. Therefore, it is wise to find a retailer where the oils come from

Table 7.4 Actions of essential oils

Regulators	Sedatives	Stimulants	Euphorics
Geranium	Roman camomile	Peppermint	Grapefruit
Bergamot	Lavender	Rosemary	Ylang Ylang
Frankincense	Sweet marjoram	Eucalyptus	Clary sage
Rosewood	Neroli	Juniper	Jasmine
Rose	Sandalwood	Tea Tree	Patchouli
	Vetiver		

a reputable supplier. Oils are like wine. There are good years with a healthy yield and bad years with a poorer yield. A reputable supplier will use his specialist knowledge to supply the best oils available.

■ CASE HISTORY 7.5 Christine a 57-year-old woman with breast cancer

Christine was a 57-year-old retired shop manageress. She was single but had a supportive manfriend whom she saw each week. Her sisters were very close and extremely supportive.

Christine had breast cancer. Initially a lump was removed; this was followed by a mastectomy. Two years later a lump was removed from the other breast and chemotherapy followed for 2 years with biopsies to check on condition. Her room in the hospital was easy to find by the aroma from her essential oils, which she loved. This love of the oils led her to me for therapy. The oncologist agreed to Christine's therapy and her treatment began in January, and continued almost every 2 weeks until her death in July.

Usually, I massaged where Christine felt her need was greatest, often on her upper back, arms, hands, face and feet. The massage was always carried out using a gentle technique with holding, stroking movements. The selection of oils I used were Bergamot for its uplifting qualities, Roman camomile for its antispasmodic and stress-reducing properties, Sandalwood for relaxation and tonic to urinary tract and Lavender as a general mood enhancer and to improve her sleep pattern. Neroli was always used on the face as she enjoyed the perfume and it has good rejuvenating qualities. The dilution was 1%, with one drop to each 5 ml of carrier oil. Christine enjoyed her visits and looked forward to them. She listed what she thought the benefits of her sessions were:

- It gives me a a definite sense of well-being
- It makes me feel more relaxed and less anxious about my own condition
- I felt I was doing something positive for myself and getting benefit from it
- It took about 4 weeks to really feel good but now I feel totally different
- It has helped to bring back my confidence
- The relaxed atmosphere while aromatherapy is being done is helpful

Christine always left with a feeling of well-being, which I shared also.

Research into the use of essential oils and massage

Research into massage, with or without aromatherapy was initiated by Dr Susie Wilkinson in Liverpool's Marie Curie Centre (Wilkinson 1995). The Rotterdam Scale Check List (RSCL) and State–Trait Anxiety Inventory were used. Post-test scores for all patients improved. These were statistically significant in the aromatherapy group on the RSCL physical symptom subscale, quality of life subscale and state anxiety scale. Responses indicated that patients consider the massage or aromatherapy to be beneficial in reducing anxiety, tension, pain and depression.

A quasi-experimental study compared the effects of massage, with or without the addition of a blend of essential oils, on patients undergoing cancer treatment (Corner et al 1995). This study's findings suggest that massage has a significant effect on anxiety and an even greater effect where essential oils were used. Massage was reported to be universally beneficial by patients in assisting their relaxation and reducing their physical and emotional symptoms.

A study by Stevenson (1994) showed that in a group of patients, foot massage using Neroli essential oil and vegetable oil lowered clients' blood pressure and their heart rates.

A study by McNamara (1984) examined the use of massage for people with cancer. They used 24 trained practitioners and results suggested that appropriate forms of massage were safe, soothing, relaxing and beneficial. Ferrel-Torry & Glick (1993) explored the use of massage as a nursing intervention to modify anxiety and patients' perceptions of cancer pain.

At present, insufficient research has been conducted to fully explain these results but in our experience there is usually a reduction of patients' distress and an increase in their well-being. Preliminary results of a recent randomised study investigating the benefits of the use of hand massage or a relaxation tape showed significant reduction in preoperative anxiety of women with breast cancer. Both therapies appeared to offer similar relaxation benefits but 97% of patients preferred the hands-on therapy/massage (Kirkwood et al, 1998).

REFLEXOLOGY

How beautiful upon the mountains and the feet of him that bringeth good tidings that publisheth peace. [Isaiah 3:7]

Few people pay much attention to their feet, which take a severe beating in their path through life. They are delicate structures a fraction of the body size, which support and transport the entire body weight. Little notice is given to self-inflicted foot problems, which can cause problems elsewhere in the body (Dougans & Ellis 1992).

Many reflexologists believe that reflexology originated in China some 5000 years ago, although concrete proof is evasive. Perhaps this knowledge was left aside in favour of acupuncture, which emerged as the stronger growth. This knowledge of foot reflex therapy may have been lost to antiquity had it not been for the enquiring medical minds of the late 19th century and early 20th century. The Europeans expanded on the research of their predecessors but credit must go to the Americans for putting modern reflexology on the map.

Dr William Fitzgerald, an American ear, nose and throat specialist, found, through knowledge that he gained in Europe and in his own research, that pressure he applied to the fingers created a local anaesthetic effect in the arm and shoulder right up to the face, ear and nose. This enabled him to perform minor surgical procedures using his pressure technique. He divided the body into 10 zones longitudinally (Fig. 7.2). A line is drawn down the centre of the body with fine corresponding zones on each side of this line. The zones are of equal width and extend through the body from front to back, his theory being that parts of the body within a zone will be linked with one another by the energy within that zone. Dr Fitzgerald gave lectures on his zone theory and gathered around him a circle of practitioners. Unwittingly, he gave American Indian Folk Medicine respectability. Diagrams of the zones of the feet appeared in the first edition of his book.

Eunace Ingham, an American masseuse, charted the zones in relation to the effects on the rest of the body, until a map of the body evolved on the

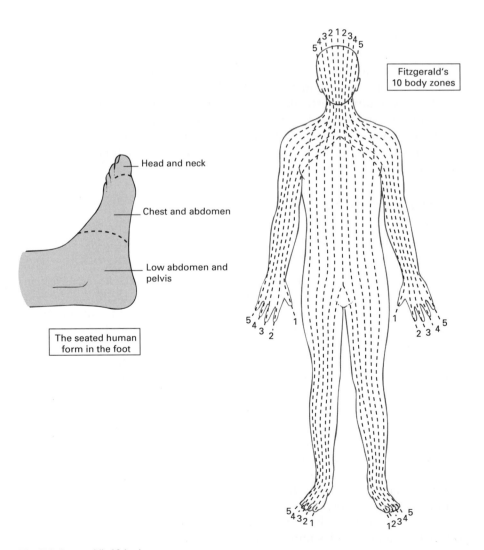

Fig. 7.2 Fitzgerald's 10 body zones.

feet. She developed a special subtle method of massage, which is now taught as the cornerstone of this work. To date, most reflexologists work on the theory of the zones described by Dr Fitzgerald but there exists a strong link between reflexology and acupuncture. As acupuncture and reflexology are concerned with balancing energy flow to stimulate the body's own healing potential, a greater number of therapists are now combining reflexology with meridian therapy to provide a more comprehensive and effective treatment.

Performing reflexology

Reflexology can be performed with the patient lying or sitting. Most therapists face the soles of the feet and prefer the head to be raised slightly so that facial expressions can be observed. The therapist should be aware of the patient's medical history, medications and general health state. The feet are observed for deformities, calluses, bunions and enlarged toe joints. As already mentioned above, the feet represent a microcosm of the body and every bump or crevice aids the therapist in building a health picture. The initial touch of the therapist's hand is important, it is reassuring to the patient. A gentle massage before treatment relaxes and warms the feet, allowing the patient to become accustomed to and feel comfortable with the feet being touched. Treatment consists of finger pressures traversing across the zones on the feet. The thumb is the finger mainly used but the index finger can also treat smaller areas. The treatment usually starts on the toes and works downwards on the foot until all the systems and organ-related zones have been worked on. Some discomfort may be felt in a zone; this can vary in intensity from a pinprick sensation to a deeper, intense pain. It is detected by the finger in various ways; for example, a change in tissue tone, a small pea under the skin, or granules like sugar. It is usual for the therapist to move away from a painful zone to allow the patient to relax but return later in the treatment to give that zone a gentle stimulus to help rebalance the organ or system that is out of tune. Some people are extremely sensitive to reflexology, experiencing light-headed sensations or discomfort in the organ or system being treated. The therapist is alert to these symptoms and holds the feet gently until the sensation passes.

Benefits of reflexology

Reflexology is ideally suited to patients who are shy, private people or whose lifestyle has no space for touching another individual. The feet being distal to the body makes treatment less invasive. I feel that I am secretly performing body maintenance.

Reflexology treatments can improve the quality of life of terminally ill patients. Alleviation of pain makes the patient feel more relaxed and comfortable. There is functional improvement of the organs of excretion, including the skin and lungs, and improvement of bowel and bladder sphincter control. It is a therapy that is acceptable to patients who have a poor body image through radical surgery, obesity or emaciation, or, who, for one reason or another, would prefer to keep their clothes on.

Reflexology rebalances and maintains body energy via the feet which, over the years, have lost out in the popularity stakes. However, with increasing interest in holistic healing practices comes the realisation that feet play a fundamental role. There are several, published, successful case histories of patients having reflexology, but no research studies to date. This current lack of validated research into the therapeutic values of reflexology and the mechanisms involved in its efficacy need to be addressed if its full potential is to be realised.

Limitations of reflexology

Reflexology does not discriminate. People of all ages can derive benefit from it. However, as with all therapies, it has its limits, beyond which its practice is ineffective. There are some conditions that contraindicate its use, for example, deep venous thrombosis, acute infectious diseases, conditions where surgery is indicated, gangrene or extensive mycotic infections of the feet and an unstable pregnancy. In insulin-dependent diabetes, blood glucose checks should be performed following reflexology as treatment can stimulate the pancreas, thus reducing the insulin requirement. Children are receptive to the therapeutic stimuli, as are elderly people, whose bodily functions are toned with treatment.

THE PRACTICE OF YOGA IN ANGINA PATIENTS

Yoga was introduced into palliative care as part of a lifestyle change and stress-management programme for patients suffering from angina. The facilitating team include a clinical psychologist, cardiologist, physiotherapist, nurse, dietitian and yoga/relaxation teacher.

The practice of yoga – postures, breathing control, relaxation, chanting, meditation and visualisation – all play their part in returning the body to health, happiness, wholeness, balance and well-being. Individuals can learn to practice yoga for themselves or be taught in groups as a therapeutic experience. The improvement in blood oxygen saturation is significant in angina patients who practice yoga.

Testimonies of angina patients attending weekly yoga classes

Below are some comments from three men on the benefits to their well-being of attending yoga classes.

A. Since taking yoga class I feel more able to relax on a bus or at a meeting or when walking – I now 'walk tall' with shoulders relaxed. Even more beneficial, I have changed [at the age of 70] my breathing pattern and through this I can counteract my 'stress' feelings more easily. I feel quite rejuvenated after the class and enjoy the company too.

B. As a regular in our group I reach total relaxation very quickly. On return [from complete relaxation practice] I have a deep feeling of warmth, peace and well-being with all previous stress and worry completely gone. It is difficult to believe that only 30 minutes have elapsed. The reaction is also evident in the others because there is a general sense of contentment and reluctance to get up and go home.

C. I have attended the weekly class for yoga, relaxation and meditation for the last 4 years. I can truthfully say that this class has done wonders for the angina from which I suffered and also for my general health. As a result I am a far more relaxed person and able to cope better with the stresses of everyday life. The feeling of well-being, experienced after a class, is quite remarkable and I am now able to do things that I thought were completely gone. For example, 4 years ago I could hardly lift a golf club and now I play regularly, two rounds per week, which is only an example of the benefits from the yoga, relaxation and meditation class.

The original angina management course that these patients attended for 10 weeks is a lifestyle change course of which yoga and relaxation is only a part. Aerobic exercise with a physiotherapist, and stress management and pacing strategy learnt with a psychologist, played a major part in the physical and mental tasks and recreations that patients are able to achieve. This course is based on work by Dr Dean Ornish (1990).

Clinical areas where complementary therapies could be beneficial are shown in Box 7.2.

■ **BOX 7.2**

Areas where complementary therapies could be used
- Stroke units
- Intensive therapy units
- Geriatric departments
- Pre- and postsurgery
- HIV units
- Antenatal care
- Respiratory units
- Rheumatology
- Oncology
- Hospice units
- Rehabilitation units
- Cardiovascular units

PSYCHONEUROIMMUNOLOGY

The autoimmune system is an area in which new knowledge is continually being developed. We are particularly interested in the recently named study of psychoimmunology. This is the effect of thought patterns on the immune system. Where these thoughts are stress related, complementary therapies are relevant on account of their relaxing and uplifting effect.

In his book, Dr Bernie Siegel (1986) states:

The immune system is controlled by the brain either indirectly through hormones in the bloodstream or directly through nerves and neurochemicals. Our state of mind has an immediate and direct effect on our state of body. We can change the body by dealing with how we feel.

He uses two major tools to change the body state, namely emotions and imagery. We would like to suggest that by working with the body using complementary therapies, yoga and relaxation, one can effect a change in negative patterns of emotion and thought.

Deep diaphragmatic breathing can also have an effect on the immune system by stimulating the flow of lymph. The cisterna chyli (deep receptacle for lymph from the lower body) is sited deep in the body at the diaphragm and can be touched by deep breathing, which stimulates the flow with an inner, massaging effect. Other ways of stimulating lymph flow are exercising the limbs, skin brushing, drinking plenty of water and special lymph drainage massage techniques; for example, the Vodder system of manual lymph drainage (Wittlinger & Wittlinger 1990). Using a selection of these tools, a feeling of well-being is achieved, which would scientifically be expressed as the natural release of endorphins, triggered by positive thought and action.

Dr Carl Simonton (1978) first used positive visualisation therapy with good effect on cancer patients. Louis Proto (1990) stated:

There is a connection between low energy states and disease.

This underpins the belief that stress depletes energy and therefore the body's normal ability to resist infection or breakdown. Dr Lawrence Le Shan (1989) discussed psychological changes necessary to mobilise the immune system. He moved from asking what was wrong with the patient to what was right with the patient. What was their most natural way of being, relating and creating? What kind of life and lifestyle would make them glad to get up in the morning and glad to go to bed at night? What would give them the maximum enthusiasm and zest for life? Some patients following this programme successfully increased their life expectancy. In a study that was carried out over 15 years, Greer et al. (1990) found strong evidence that women who responded to cancer with a 'fighting spirit or denial' were significantly more likely to be free of recurrence for a longer period than were women showing other responses.

We have moved from a consideration of how stress can depress the immune system to a discussion of mental, physical and emotional strategies that boost and mobilise the immune system. As we have seen, complementary therapies play their part in this. Both Le Shan (1989) and Gawler (1984) utilise and pursue the practice of meditation in healing. This brings us full circle back to our therapies of gentle yoga, relaxation, breathing and meditation.

SELF-HELP FOR THE NURSE

All carers need to care for themselves if they are to deliver a good standard of care to their patients. We each come to work with our life's experiences, ups and downs, and it is especially hard to be focused if our own life is disturbed. Experience has shown that those who tire easily do not take care of themselves. Be aware of the need for methods discussed above, always remembering to use the breath. Exercise also helps to dissipate the stresses encountered. It need not be strenuous. Walking briskly, taking in plenty of fresh air, swimming and badminton, are all pleasurable ways of exercising.

Perhaps you choose to relax in less active ways, such as reading, listening to music, going to the theatre, even taking a hot bath or receiving a relaxing massage. Some hospital trusts are now providing entrance to leisure complexes for employees. With target deadlines and high standards to be met, stresses can build up all too easily.

Therefore, employers should encourage their employees to make use of these facilities. Whichever you choose for yourself, taking care of your own needs helps to keep your life in perspective, ensuring that there is a balance between giving and receiving.

PATIENT SELF-HELP

In palliative care, patients feel at the mercy of medical intervention, whatever their disease. Empowering them in their own care helps to restore their self-esteem. Patients could be encouraged to do some gentle exercises, such as those described above, keeping within the boundaries of their capabilities.

Walking each day when the weather permits tones muscles, eases joints and improves the circulation. Relaxation can be undertaken either in a group setting, as some hospitals have, or at home, following the nurse's or therapist's guidelines. Again, some hospital units have complementary therapists available on a day care basis. If a patient wishes to have a particular therapy and the health care team agree that it is an appropriate adjunct to care, the patient will have an appointment on a regular basis and progress is monitored and reported. Information is given to patients about support agencies, all of whom employ caring staff who will respond to the level of need. Often, patients' appetites are impaired and sensible eating within their own limitations is advised. Social activities can again be picked up, as mingling with others whose company is enjoyed can both relax and stimulate. Laughter shared in company can reduce anxiety levels (Mallett 1995, Robinson 1977).

Dr Patch Adams promotes laughter as a therapy in the USA. He demonstrates this by taking a group of volunteers to less fortunate areas of the world dressed in comic suits; building bridges through laughter.

There are many other therapies available and those wishing to do so can refer to the the section on further reading at the end of this chapter.

GUIDELINES FOR NURSES IN USING COMPLEMENTARY THERAPIES

Any nurses interested in training for complementary therapy should enquire if the courses are recognised by the governing body of the particular therapies and if proof of completion is provided. The standardisation of training in aromatherapy, reflexology, hypnotherapy and homeopathy is currently under review, so it would be wise to gain the best qualifications possible. The RCN indemnity insurance lists activities for which a nurse is covered, provided satisfactory training has been undertaken. It includes aromatherapy, reflexology, massage, acupuncture and homeopathy.

The practice of a complementary therapy by any nurse should follow the UKCC guidelines set out in the UKCC (1992a, b) publications. There may also be local guidelines set down by whichever authority you work for.

As nurses are the professional carers most suited to providing complementary therapies, consideration must be given to the time-consuming aspect. Therefore, gaining the full support of peers, line managers and medical personnel is essential. It would be sensible to have agreed times with colleagues set aside for the therapy where the nurse can be fully attentive to the patient without anxiety about the ward workload. On the other hand, employing a professional therapist would free the nurses' time for other essential ward duties, which may benefit the patient. This might be better than trying to incorporate a complementary therapy into an already busy schedule. The authors represent both aspects of this care – one being a nurse and complementary therapist, the other a practising complementary and relaxation therapist. Last, but not least, consider whether the proposed therapy is in the patient's best interests and is an appropriate adjunct to care. If so, gain informed consent from the patient and relatives. In the present climate of litigation, nurses must be aware of the consequences of their actions. Therefore, research-based material to reinforce the therapy and provide evidence of its benefits would help nurses to justify their actions, should it be necessary. To date, the demand for therapists has overtaken the amount of research currently available that proves their validity. The small-scale pilot studies undertaken have failed to build on earlier work, leading to duplication in many cases. The way forward is for nurses to ensure that their therapy is research based, or to be involved in a research study using their own therapy. Proof of a therapy's efficacy will turn the trend towards its increased use.

The RCN have a Complementary Therapies Special Interest Group. It provides newsletters so that the committee can make contact with the membership, report on activities and share information. There are workshops and conferences nationwide, which are well attended by an ever-increasing membership. At the time of writing, membership is 8789. It has published guidelines for nurses who wish to train in a complementary therapy and a Statement of Beliefs for those practising.

This chapter is intended to stimulate interest in complementary therapies, giving an insight into their roots and into the potential for their use in palliative care. We hope to inspire nurses with a holistic awareness to bring touch and the associated therapies into nursing practice, hopefully helping patients to a better quality of life throughout their illness.

REFERENCES

Barnet K 1972 A theoretical construct of the concepts of touch as they relate to nursing. Nursing Research 21: 102–110
Benson H, Klipper M Z 1976 The relaxation response. Avon Books, New York
Byass R 1988 Soothing body and soul. Nursing Times 84: 39–41

Corner J, Cawley N, Hildebrand S 1995 An evaluation of the use of massage and essential oils on the wellbeing of cancer patients. International Journal of Palliative Nursing 1: 67

Dougans I, Ellis S 1992 The art of reflexology. Element Books, Dorset

Ferrell-Torry A T, Glick O J 1993 The use of therapeutic massage as a nursing intervention to modify anxiety and the perception of cancer pain. Cancer Nursing 16: 93–101

Fitzgerald W, Bowers E F, Zone Therapy, Health Research, California.

Gawler I 1984 You can conquer cancer. Hill and Coutent, Melbourne

Greer S, Morris T, Pettingale K W, Haybittle J L 1990 Psychological response to breast cancer and 15 year outcome. Lancet 335: 49–50

Hudson C M 1988 The complete book of massage. Dorling Kindersley, London

Jacobsen C 1938 Progressive relaxation, 2nd edn. Chicago University Press, Chicago

Kirkwood I et al 1998 Unpublished research carried out at Western General Hospital, Edinburgh

Lawless J 1992 Encyclopedia of essential oils. Element Books, Dorset

Le Shan L 1989 Cancer as a turning point. Gateway Books, Bath

Mallett J 1994 Humour and laughter therapy. Complementary Therapies in Nursing and Midwifery 1: 73–76

McNamara P 1984 Massage for people with cancer. The Cancer Support Centre, London

Ornish D 1990 Programme for reversing heart disease. Ballantine, New York

Penoel D, Franchomme P 1990 Aromatherapie exactement. Jallais, France

Proto L 1990 Self healing. Piatkus, London

Robinson V 1977 Humour in nursing, 2nd edn. In: Carlson C E, Blackwell B (eds) Behavioural concepts and nursing intervention. J P Lippincott, Philadelphia, pp 191–210

Selye H 1974 Stress without distress. Hodder & Stoughton, London

Siegel B 1986 Love, medicine and miracles. Arrow, London

Simonton C, Simonton S, Creighton J 1978 Getting well again. Tarcher, Los Angeles

Stevenson C 1994 The psychophysiological effects of aromatherapy following cardiac surgery. Complementary Therapies in Medicine 2: 27–35

UKCC 1992a Scope of professional practice. UKCC, London, paragraphs 1–7, pp 4–5

UKCC 1992b Standards of administration of medicines. UKCC, London, paragaphs 38–39

Vodder E 1990 Textbook of Dr Vodder's manual of lymph drainage, Vol. 1. Haug, Heidelberg

Watson J 1989 Human caring and suffering. A subjective model for the health sciences. Colorado Assoc. University Press, Colorado

Wilkinson S 1995 Aromatherapy and massage in palliative care. International Journal of Palliative Nursing 1: 21

Wittlinger H, Wittlinger G 1940 Textbook of Dr Vodder's manual lymph drainage, Vol. 1: Basic course. Haug K F, Heidelberg (translated, revised and edited by Harris R H 1990)

Worwood V 1992 The fragrant pharmacy. Bantam Books, London

FURTHER READING

Davis P 1988 Aromatherapy A–Z. C W Daniel, Saffron Walden, Essex

Gawler G 1995 Women of silence. Hill & Coutent, Melbourne

Hewitt J 1977 The complete yoga book. Rider, London

Keable D 1985 Relaxation training techniques: a review. Part 1, What is relaxation? Occupational Therapy April: 99–101

Keable D 1985 Relaxation training techniques: a review. Part 2, How effective is relaxation training? Occupational Therapy July: 201–204

Munro R, Nagarathna R, Nagendra H R 1990 Yoga for common ailments. GAIA, London

Price S 1991 Aromatherapy for common ailments. GAIA, London

Price S, Price L 1995 Aromatherapy for health care professionals. Churchill Livingstone, Edinburgh

Rankin-Box D 1995 The nurse's handbook of complementary therapies. Churchill Livingstone, Edinburgh

Siegel B 1990 Peace, love and healing. Rider, London

Wilson A, Bek L 1981 What colour are you? Aquarium Press, Wellingborough

Wright S G 1995 The competence to touch: helping and healing in nursing practice. Complementary Therapies in Medicine 3: 49–52

ADDRESSES

Association of Reflexologists
27 Old Gloucester Street
London WC1 3XX

British School of Reflex Zone Therapy
Marks Orchard
Whitbourne
Worcester WR6 5RB

Bristol Cancer Help Centre
Grove House
Cornwallis Grove
Clifton
Bristol BS8 4PG

Complementary Therapies Special Interest Group
Royal College of Nursing
20 Cavendish Square
London W1M 0AB

Maggie's Centre
The Stables
Western General Hospital
Crewe Road
Edinburgh EH4 2XU

International Society of Professional Aromatherapy
ISPA House
82, Ashby Road
Hinckley
Leicester LE10 1SN
Life Foundation School of Therapeutics

Body, Heart and Mind Technology
15 Holyhead Road
Upper Bangor
Dyfedd
North Wales

Royal Marsden Hospital
Fulham Road
London SW3 6JJ

Wordsworth Cancer Support Centre
P.O. Box 20–22
York Road
London SW11 3QE

Support for family and carers

8

Rosemary McIntyre

■ CONTENTS

The chapter that follows will draw on the author's recently completed doctoral study (McIntyre 1996). It is acknowledged at the outset that a chapter of this length will not permit more than an overview of the work. In light of these constraints a decision was taken to report the findings from a practical perspective. Accordingly, the emphasis is on sharing some insights gained into the relatives' and professional carers' experiences of advanced illness. A number of key themes and illustrative exemplars was selected from the analysis for discussion and for the insights they could offer.

LEARNING OUTCOMES

This chapter will address PREP requirements for care enhancement and practice and education development and will enable the reader to:

- Gain insight into relatives' and professional carers' experiences of advanced illness
- Enhance care for patients and relatives through a quality assurance framework
- Appreciate how action research can change practice
- Recognise the opportunities for reflective practice arising from team workshops

INTRODUCTION

When a patient's illness reaches the stage where curative efforts are no longer deemed to be appropriate, considerable demands are placed on the whole family. Whilst coping with their own profound emotions, those closest to the patient commonly report having had to provide support from the onset of symptoms through the stage of diagnosis and various treatments until, finally, a shift to a palliative mode of management had to be faced. Consequently, by the time the terminal stage of the illness is reached, the whole family may have travelled a long and difficult road and are likely to be vulnerable and in considerable need of support.

The author's own experience of providing care, in both hospital and community settings, has offered persuasive, albeit anecdotal, evidence that close relatives of dying patients often have unmet needs for support. Impressions gained in both care settings also suggest that within the complex structures of hospitals, where the number and range of patients and carers are greater, supporting the dying patient's family can present particular difficulties for staff.

Undoubtedly it can also be painful for health professionals to be regularly confronted with death and to be faced with the grief of others. Experience in nurse education highlighted issues that concern many nursing students as they approach the end of their pre-registration education. Whilst students commonly report a degree of diffuse anxiety about their future role as staff nurses, a specific and recurrent concern that students frequently voice relates to how they should deal with the patient's family around the time of death.

From all of this it seemed clear that staff who provide palliative care in hospitals need to know more about what it is that relatives of dying patients require from nurses. There also seemed to be a need to establish what factors make supporting the dying patient's family so difficult for nurses and what support they might need in order to care for the relatives with less distress to themselves.

STUDY OUTLINE

To address these key issues, a research study was conducted. It was based in eight wards in two major Scottish hospitals. The aims of the study were twofold. First, to explore and describe the needs of relatives of cancer patients who were dying in acute hospital wards and to identify the concerns of the nurses involved in providing their care. Second, to use the research data to design, implement and evaluate quality assurance standards for improved care and support of families of patients dying in hospital.

Brief overview of approach and methods

The study had two phases that were separated by an intervention. Samples taken from eight study wards comprised 16 staff nurses and 47 relatives of dying cancer patients. During the course of the study a total of 80 semi-structured, tape-recorded interviews were conducted. The interviews were transcribed and interpreted using interpretive textual analysis processes that generated themes, exemplars and paradigm cases.

During phase one of the study, interviews were conducted with the relatives and the staff nurses to elicit their views, needs and concerns. In the intervention period that followed, the staff nurses attended a 2-day workshop where the phase one findings were presented. The nurses then used the data to design quality assurance standards for improved care and support of dying patients' families in their wards. During the very active period that followed the workshop, the nurses worked closely with their ward teams to implement, monitor and audit changes in practice.

In phase two of the study, a second sample of relatives was recruited and interviewed and the nurses each had a second interview. Data from these phase two interviews were compared with the phase one findings to evaluate the impact that the intervention had had on ward practice.

■ REFLECTIVE PRACTICE 8.1   Ethical issues

- Explore the ethical issues that might arise when embarking on a study which includes dying patients or their relatives
- Suggest ways in which the rights of vulnerable research participants may be safeguarded

Readers are advised to consult one or more of the following:

Aranda S 1995 Conducting research with the dying: ethical considerations and experience. International Journal of Palliative Nursing 1: 41–47

Clarke J 1991 Moral dilemmas in nursing research. Nursing Practice 4: 22–25

Raudonis B 1992 Ethical considerations in qualitative research with hospice patients. Qualitative Health Research 2: 238–249

Thompson I E, Melia K M, Boyd K M 1993 Nursing ethics, chapters 1 & 2. Churchill Livingstone, Edinburgh

---

EPIDEMIOLOGY

Scotland holds the unenviable record of ranking top in the world for lung cancer deaths and of being second highest in overall female cancer mortality. Statistical data also confirm that in 1994 deaths from cancer represented around 25% of all deaths in Scotland (Registrar General for Scotland 1994).

Table 8.1 presents the 1994 Scottish cancer mortality figures. It includes data about the place of death, confirming that in Scotland, in 1994, the majority of cancer-related deaths occurred in hospitals.

Table 8.1 Number and place of cancer deaths in Scotland

All places	Home	NHS hospital	Non-NHS hospital hospice	Homes for the elderly and disabled	Other homes
15 488	4045	9774	1507	129	3
% Total	26.17	63.23	9.75	0.83	0.02

Source of information: Registrar General for Scotland (1994).

Changes in demographic and disease patterns over the past three decades and a shift from acute to chronic illness as a cause of death, have led to a steady growth in the demand for specialist palliative care services (Eve & Jackson 1994, Ford 1994, Higginson 1993, Seale 1993).

Palliative care represents the active total care of patients for whom curative treatment is no longer possible and for whom control of physical, psychological, social and spiritual problems are paramount. Effective palliative care should therefore provide a support system that will enable patients to live as actively as possible until death and should help the family cope during the patient's illness and with their bereavement (WHO 1990). Terminal care refers to the care given during the very late stages of the illness where there is a steady deterioration in the patient's condition and death is judged to be very close (Scottish Partnership Agency for Palliative and Cancer Care 1995).

DEVELOPMENTS IN CARE PROVISION

The development of specialist care in the UK can be traced to the 1960s when severe shortcomings were highlighted in institutional care for dying patients (Glaser & Strauss 1965, Sudnow 1967). In response to these reported deficiencies, Cicely Saunders developed an approach to care that emphasised symptom control, psychosocial support and a more open style of communication about death. This approach was to become the hallmark of future hospice care.

There is now a growing recognition of the need to extend the philosophy and principles of palliative care, laid down by Cicely Saunders, into community and hospital settings where the majority of patients still die (see Table 8.1). To this end, hospital and community staff are increasingly seeking access to advice and support from specialist symptom control teams and home care teams.

Nursing developments in palliative care were spearheaded by such organisations as Macmillan Cancer Relief and Marie Curie Cancer Care who provide support, counselling and home nursing services. More recently an increasing number of nurse specialists have been appointed in hospitals, hospices and regional cancer centres to provide specific nursing expertise and to enhance continuity of care between hospital, hospice and community settings.

Whilst it is confirmed in Table 8.1 that over 60% of patients in Scotland currently die in hospital, it should be recognised that most of these patients will have received care in other settings during the course of their illness. For example, 81% of the deceased patients studied by Cartwright (1991a) were found to have spent most of the last year of life in their own homes being cared for by close family members. Also, when compared with 1969 figures, Cartwright found that more dying people currently live alone or with only a spouse, and there are now even greater numbers of dying patients over 75 years of age (Cartwright 1991a, b). These figures have clear implications for service provision, both within the community setting and in hospital.

THE CANCER JOURNEY

A number of authors use the analogy of a journey to illustrate the stages which the family go through when a progressive illness strikes one of their members (Janes 1992, Kristjanson & Ashcroft 1994, McIntyre 1996).

It should be recognised that this journey can start long before the diagnosis is ever reached. This is particularly so when there has been a gradual onset of symptoms accompanied by a growing realisation, on the part of the patient and the family, that all is far from well. During this prediagnostic period, those closest to the patient can experience significant stress as their loved one undergoes a range of investigations and news of the diagnosis is anxiously awaited. Difficulties faced by the patient and family during this difficult time can be compounded when patients have been required to pass through the hands of a number of health care professionals, often in different settings and departments and sometimes even in different hospitals. In such situations continuity of care can be compromised, the quality of communication can suffer and the patient and family can be left feeling very badly in need of support.

An example of how the impact of the diagnosis, and the subsequent cancer journey, can be experienced is revealed in the following exemplar in which a husband describes the path that his 36-year-old wife's illness has taken since her ovarian cancer was diagnosed.

> *At first there were no symptoms at all of the cancer being there. Normally there is swelling of the stomach but there was nothing of that with Amy. She always had a good figure … she was always slim. She has had some gynaecological problems in the past so they thought maybe she had fibroids in her womb. When they brought her in initially what they expected to find was an ovarian cyst or fibroids in the womb. If it had been one or the other they were just going to remove the affected part. Unfortunately that wasn't the case. When they opened her up they discovered a massive tumour.*

> *Over that period … until after she finished her 6 months of chemotherapy the only side-effects she had were that she was sick after the first two doses. After she got a course of steroids, within a couple of days she got her appetite back and her quality of life came back. Everything was basically normal. Every 6 weeks she came in for her chemotherapy and steroids, with maybe one day of sickness – but milder than it had been. That was okay.*

> *They did an exploratory operation in October of that year and they discovered no trace of the tumour at all. The great news was that there was nothing there. Then for 2 years it was great. Two years ago at this time we were on holiday in Majorca but when we came back she wasn't feeling too great. She seemed to be going up and down. She went for a scan but nothing showed up. Then a month or 2 months later she came back for tests and there was a trace of … Obviously some rogue cells had been left and the tumour had continued to grow. It's just been a steady decline ever since. More so in the past year.*

In other situations where the seriousness of the diagnosis had perhaps not been anticipated, the bad news can be experienced rather 'like a thunder-bolt', leaving the family deeply shocked and vulnerable. The shocking impact that the diagnosis can have is illustrated in the following quote.

It was on Christmas Eve that the doctor told me that they had drained his lung and that they felt sure that he had cancer. I just said 'No … that's not true.' But on Boxing Day I had another word with the doctor and he told me then that Joe had only a few weeks to live. He said 'If you have any family abroad you should get in touch.'

Whilst the experiences of each family, and indeed of each individual family member, will be unique, a number of common factors have been found to influence family members' experiences of terminal illness. Such factors include the stage of the disease, the age of the patient, the ages of different family members and the roles and relationships that operate within the family. During a progressive illness, such as cancer, shifts and negotiations in family roles tend to occur and difficulties can be encountered by family members as they try to respond to fluctuating and often quite subtle changes in the ill person's physical and emotional condition. This fluidity and adaptation of family roles and relationships involves considerable hard work and negotiation, often resulting in significant stress within the family. Families best able to adapt to these conditions have been found to be those where good communications had existed between the spouses before the onset of the illness and where the family included older children who could cope with expanded roles (Kristjanson & Ashcroft 1994).

THE FAMILY CAREGIVER

Family caregivers often experience significant difficulties associated with managing the patient's physical care and these difficulties can intensify as the patient's condition worsens. This, coupled with the distress from watching the physical and sometimes mental deterioration of their loved one, whilst having to cope with the ongoing day-to-day household, social and financial matters, can make caregiving at home extremely challenging. Indeed, research findings consistently highlight the physical and emotional demands that caregiving families face and also reveal significant unmet needs for support (Hull 1990).

Home caregiving often extends over fairly long periods of time with all of the implications that this can have for carer strain. It has been found that the duration of time between stopping active treatment and death was more than three times longer in those patients who were being cared for at home than was the case for those who died in hospital (Parkes 1988). Also, symptom control was reported to be less effective and the degree of family strain was significantly higher when dying patients were cared for at home (Parkes 1988).

The 78-year-old woman quoted below was caring for her 80-year-old husband. It offers insight into the demands that some caregiving relatives can face.

Tom started complaining of pains in his stomach ... he couldn't get to the commode in time and he messed himself and he was crying ... I told him not to worry and I managed to get him into the bath. When he was in the bath he was rubbing my face and saying 'This shouldn't be happening – you shouldn't be having to do this for me.' That happened a lot on that Sunday (colic and faecal incontinence) but I couldn't get through to my doctor. His phone just kept ringing, ringing, ringing. I thought 'This is just terrible ...'

Societal expectations that female relatives will function as primary care-givers are confirmed in a study by Nugent (1988) who found that 73% of dying patients at home were being cared for solely by female relatives with a further 5% having a female relative significantly involved in providing care (Nugent 1988). Of particular interest is the large number of female caregivers who have to meet the competing demands of their home and children whilst caring for ageing parents and often also whilst holding down a job. These women can experience significant stress and emotional conflict as they try to respond to the myriad and often conflicting demands that are placed upon them. Although these female carers can bear a considerable burden, and often experience health problems attributable to the stress of caring, their support needs largely go unrecognised. Indeed, little attention has been directed at establishing just how such relatives cope with the demands placed upon them (Nugent 1988).

Around 50% of family carers live alone with their dying loved one and nurses need to be sensitive to their needs for support. Caregivers can become very isolated and their needs include having the presence of supportive people around them. It has been found that valuable social support can come from friends and family but health professionals, such as nurses, can also provide crucial support, not just by delivering care but by offering affirmation, advice and support to family carers. Nurses can also assist relatives to gain timely access to a range of services, equipment and resources to support their caring efforts. Caregivers have also been found to benefit greatly from brief periods of respite or 'time out' from the relentless task of caring (Nugent 1988).

Whilst many relatives do manage to continue to provide care for the patient right up to the time of death, others experience severe difficulties with the demands of caring. In the absence of adequate support in the community, the complex array of stresses that can be experienced by family caregivers can lead them to relinquish the carer's role and to seek hospital admission for the patient. Research evidence confirms that unrelieved carer strain and problems in achieving adequate symptom control are the two most frequently cited reasons for hospital admission in the last days of the patient's life (Hull 1990).

Relatives' subsequent grief reactions may be influenced by a range of factors, such as the duration of the illness, the effectiveness of symptom control in the period leading up to the patient's death and the location of the death (Klagsbrun 1994, Kristjanson 1989). Reducing the potential for future regret by offering support to the family in the difficult period follow-ing hospital admission should be a priority if chronic guilt and unresolved grief are to be avoided. Nurses need to be acutely sensitive to the relatives' feelings as many will be experiencing profound sadness and regret when they find they can no longer care for their relative at home.

The following quotes offer examples of the conflicting emotions that relatives can experience about the admission.

> *I feel in a way relieved that she's in here but in a way I feel guilty too. Because I was the one that was always with her and I still miss her … [struggling for control] But I feel as if some of the worry has been taken off me. It was all getting a wee bit too much for me. But I do feel guilty.*

> *I've felt guilty about my dad being in here and I'm obviously sad. Guilty because, well, we're not able to look after him in the way that he needs. So there is a lot of guilt there … you know?*

■ REFLECTIVE PRACTICE 8.2   Relatives as caregivers

Points to ponder:

• Is the current reliance on unpaid female caregivers sustainable in our society?
• What factors might influence future provision of family carers?

EXPERIENCES OF HOSPITAL CARE

Ward climate and facilities

In the author's recent research, relatives of dying patients were critical about the poor provision of basic amenities that hospitals provide for relatives' comfort and privacy. These deficiencies were particularly evident when the family had to stay overnight in the wards. Some of the discomforts mentioned by the relatives included having sat at the bedside on an upright chair all through the night, having been required to go down five flights of stairs to reach a public toilet, having all communications with staff whilst standing in the open corridor and having no private space to go to when they were distressed. The need for access to a private area for relatives to receive information from staff and for brief periods of respite from the emotionally charged environment of the bedside was a very strong feature in the phase one data. However, despite some very critical comments about the facilities in hospitals, the relatives were very emphatic that, in their judgements, the nurses were not to blame for the poor provision.

One elderly woman offered an account of how she received her husband's prognosis from the consultant whilst they both stood in the corridor with people walking all around them. The quote is offered here as it so vividly illustrates the distress that can result from communications where sensitivity is lacking.

> *There's nowhere where you can be alone for a minute or two. I mean, what would that doctor have done if I had fallen at his feet in the corridor or burst into floods of tears? I just flew for my daughter and we had a wee cup of tea in the staff canteen. But even there you had no privacy. She was crying … and I was crying and we'd nowhere to go …*

Initiating contact with staff

Relatives visiting dying patients in hospital often experience difficulties in knowing which nurses they should approach and, indeed, when it might be best to make an approach. Relatives consistently report that they feel very hesitant about disturbing busy nurses. It is a very common perception of relatives that if they were to interrupt staff then some other very ill patient might be deprived of care. Relatives are also very anxious not to be judged as being 'a nuisance' and will go out of their way to avoid incurring the staff's disapproval. Consequently, as they sit in hospital wards, the relatives become adept at picking up cues from the staff. They note that some nurses seem to be open and friendly and are willing to make eye contact and smile, and this makes it easier for relatives to make an approach. Conversely, when they perceive that staff are adopting a more distant stance, rarely smiling at them or making eye contact, relatives are more hesitant about making an approach to staff (McIntyre 1996). The relatives' perceptiveness in this regard is clearly evident in the following quote.

> You get a kind of feel for which nurses are going to be the most forthcoming. There are some that you would approach more readily than others ... it really depends on their attitude. If you feel that their attitude is good and that they're quite happy to talk to you, then that's the one you'll seek out. The attitude of the nursing staff is really important.

Access to information

Relatives of dying patients consistently and repeatedly describe their needs for information about the patient's care and progress and their need to have this information regularly updated (Hull 1992, Kristjanson & Sloan 1991, Lugton 1989, McIntyre 1996). The literature confirms that relatives appreciate information being offered to them rather than them having to actively seek it out. The family also appreciate having continuity of information and they value having regular contact with the same member of staff.

Relatives' information needs are not entirely straightforward. For example, whilst on some days relatives seem to want to receive very detailed information, at other times (perhaps when their own emotional strength is at a lower ebb) they will only seek out basic details about the patient's comfort. This suggests that relatives might benefit from being offered some control over the timing, pace and volume of information exchange. This would allow the relatives to accommodate their fluctuating capacity to confront the reality of their situation (McIntyre 1996). The following quote underscores the shifting information needs of the family.

> Sometimes you don't want to hear. I suppose it's just that sometimes ...
> there are some days when you want to hear and other days when you feel that you just can't take too much detail.

■ REFLECTIVE PRACTICE 8.3   Communication with relatives

Explore the potential for practice development within your own clinical area

- Set up an informal discussion group with clinical colleagues
- Evaluate current practice in relation to communication and information-giving with relatives of patients with advanced illness
- Search the literature for five or more recent research articles and three or more text books that focus on communication practice in terminal illness
- Report and critically evaluate the evidence from the literature and discuss as a team whether changes in practice might be required

Relatives' stress

Within every stressful encounter there will be a range of potentially stress-inducing factors from within the situation, within the environment and within the individual that will operate in a transactional manner, each affecting the other (Wrubel et al 1981). These aspects of the stress experience can readily be related to the experiences of families who have a dying relative in hospital.

Factors within the situation

Although the experience of each person who is facing the loss of a loved one will be unique, relatives in this situation have been found to report common feelings of vulnerability, loss of control and stress (McIntyre 1996). In particular, when the illness has had a long duration, perhaps spanning months or even years, and when the progression of the illness has been fluctuating and unpredictable in character, relatives' coping resources can be seriously undermined. Furthermore, the all-pervading nature of the relatives' stress, in that every aspect of their existence is dominated by their loved one's illness, can erode the coping capacity of relatives. This is graphically revealed in the following exemplar.

> It's a terrible time. I think I could have coped with it better if she'd had a heart attack and died. I'd have been sorry and grieving, but I think this is the very worst thing that could ever happen. It's really awful. Because we know that all this is for nothing. In the end it's all going to be for nothing.

The stress that relatives experience is intensified when they feel unsure about what to expect and their needs for information are not met. It is perhaps worthy of note that of the situational factors described above, the relatives' need for information represents one factor that is amenable to manipulation by nurses.

Factors within the environment

The hospital environment can have a potentially intimidating effect on relatives. Findings from the author's study indicate that nursing interventions that are aimed at making the ward seem less threatening and more welcoming and comfortable can significantly enhance relatives' coping resources.

The research findings also confirm that the relatives' stress is reduced when they can be with their dying, loved one in a quiet, private setting and when the attending family is given access to facilities for rest and refreshment (McIntyre 1996). Conversely, as the quote below reveals, the stress is intensified when the environment is not appropriate to the family's needs.

When he was moved to a room of his own it was the best thing. He was more comfortable and happier. And we were more comfortable too. We could sit there with some privacy. There were children coming into the ward, which was disturbing too. Don't misunderstand me – they have to have their families up to see them. But the way we were feeling, we just wanted to be alone.

Other factors relevant to the ward environment relate to the emotional climate in the ward and, in particular, to relationships between relatives and nurses. Data from the author's own study revealed that when changes occurred so that closer and more relaxed relationships were established between nurses and relatives this yielded reciprocal coping benefits for both. These findings are supported by Nugent (1988) who asserts that supportive social relationships are central to most coping activity and that coping effectiveness tends to be very highly dependent on the establishment of supportive relationships with others (Nugent 1988).

Factors within the individual

Whilst it is acknowledged that perceptions of stress and coping responses will be influenced by personality factors and by specific coping styles, it is not within the scope of this chapter to examine these individual characteristics in any detail. However, it is important that nurses recognise the ways in which personal factors, such as age, physical frailty or economic hardship, may contribute to the stress experienced by the dying patient's relatives. Many relatives will themselves be elderly and, in common with their counterparts in the general population, they are likely to be experiencing a range of health difficulties.

As the following quote confirms, the added stress caused by the impending death and the discomfort of sitting at the bedside, often for days on end, can add to the relatives' general vulnerability.

I have angina and recently I have had to take more tablets than usual and I find I have to sleep propped up. I just feel so drained at times. Really drained. I find that I have to rest in the mornings. You just have to try to pace yourself.

Being in the relatives' role is clearly hard, demanding work. If asked how they are feeling, most relatives will describe feeling 'exhausted', 'worn out' or 'drained'. They are likely to be sleeping little and badly, and most will be tending to get by on snacks rather than eating normally. The following exemplar offers a clear illustration of the strain that relatives commonly experience.

I am absolutely physically exhausted as well as emotionally. Last night I felt that I had come to a pitch where if I didn't put my head down I would just fall down. Other nights my mind is so active that I find great difficulty in sleeping.

Relatives commonly describe their concentration and memory as very poor and many also report feeling irritable and depressed with all of the implications this might have for relationships, both within the family and between relatives and staff. As might be expected, the impact of a terminal illness on family relationships can be variable. Whilst some families will be drawn closer together by the stress they are facing, making relationships stronger than ever, in other families the emotionally charged situation of a terminal illness can cause conflicts to surface, adding to the family's general distress (McIntyre 1996).

■ **CASE HISTORY 8.1   Family, role and gender issues in palliative care**

Jim and Hannah have been married for 17 years and are both aged 40. They have a 15-year-old son, Peter, a 12-year-old daughter, Amy, and a 5-year-old son, Sam.

Three years ago Hannah was diagnosed as having breast cancer and is now nearing the terminal stages of her illness.

Jim's parents live some 60 miles away and are both well. Hannah's father lives nearby but her mother died of breast cancer, at age 50.

■ **REFLECTIVE PRACTICE 8.4   Family, role and gender issues: analysis and discussion**

In relation to case history 8.1, consider some of the potential issues that may arise in relation to:

• Hannah's self-concept and social and gender role expression
• The impact on different members of the family in the lead up to Hannah's death and the period following it
• The resources that might be utilised to support this family

Socioeconomic factors

Financial strain is frequently experienced by families facing a progressive illness. Costs involved in travelling, often for long distances, to and from hospital, and loss of earnings on the part of the patient and/or relative, can all add to the stress that relatives experience. Regrettably it is not common practice for health professionals to sensitively assess for possible economic hardship in families and, as relatives consistently place their own needs well behind those of the patient, unless discreet enquiries are made, needs in this area tend to go unmet. The following quote highlights a not uncommon situation where a family budget has become strained owing to the illness.

I've been unemployed ever since she took ill … and what with fares to the hospital and buying stuff to bring in … It fairly runs away with the money.

Attitudes to the forthcoming death will inevitably be coloured by a range of societal, religious and cultural factors and, in particular, by the habitual patterns of communication that operate within the family unit. As social and spiritual issues are addressed elsewhere in this book, attention will now be directed at some of the issues that underpin communication in families who are coping with a terminal illness.

■ REFLECTIVE PRACTICE 8.5   Relatives' stress

Reflect on your own professional practice and consider whether enquiries are normally made into the general health and well-being of relatives of ill patients.

Patterns of family communication

Social mores will profoundly affect the communication patterns that surround death and dying and, as a result, in most societies the dying process tends to be supported by unwritten rules which govern the ways that death should be managed and confronted. Patterns of communication within the context of terminal care often reveal a complex web of coping strategies being used by those who are caught up in the situation. A pivotal issue, which will profoundly influence the nature of communications, would seem to be whether, and by whom, the forthcoming death is acknowledged and accepted.

It is now more than 30 years since Glaser & Strauss first described the ways in which communications operate between dying people, their families and those involved in their care (Glaser & Strauss 1965). They described a range of awareness contexts by placing these along a continuum to represent degrees of awareness and acknowledgement of forthcoming death.

The state of 'closed awareness' lies at one end of the awareness continuum. In this situation there is no acknowledgement, by any of the parties involved, of the fatal prognosis. At the opposite end of the continuum is 'open awareness' where there is honest and open dialogue about the impending death. Between these positions lie the intermediate states of 'suspicion awareness' where the family and caregivers are aware of the prognosis and the patient harbours unconfirmed suspicions, and 'mutual pretence' where all parties are aware of the prognosis but all tacitly elect to pretend otherwise (Glaser & Strauss 1965). The following quote from a woman whose husband is dying offers a clear example of mutual pretence.

> He [husband] doesn't say a lot … At least he's not telling me a lot. The doctor has told me all that's happening but he'll not say anything to upset me.

This whole area of awareness, pretence, truth telling and collusion raises a number of difficult ethical issues for health care professionals.

Collusion, denial and hope

In a Gallup survey published in 1990, 94% of those polled indicated that they would want to be told the truth about any serious illness which they had (Hodson 1990). Despite this finding, a conspiracy of silence frequently surrounds disclosure of a fatal prognosis. This would seem to be based on assumptions that if dying patients were to be told the truth they would simply 'turn their faces to the wall'. Using this assumption as their justification, health professionals and relatives often collude with each other to conceal the truth of the prognosis from the patient (Seale 1993).

Despite recent moves towards more open disclosure of prognosis, it is still fairly common for relatives to be given the diagnosis first and for the patient not to be told at all (Seale 1993). The uncomfortable situation where relatives know the full prognosis but the patient is left in ignorance has been described as the slippery slope to moral quandary (Shea & Kendrick 1995). Whilst relatives undoubtedly act from a beneficent perspective when they withhold the truth of the prognosis from the patient, collusion of this type raises a number of fundamental ethical issues. Indeed, it has been argued that such deception, however benevolent, denies patients due respect and may also deprive them of the opportunity to take their proper leave of family and friends (Bakhurst 1992).

However, as is usual with ethical dilemmas, there is another side to this highly sensitive debate. Whilst the literature convincingly underscores the value of open, honest communication during terminal illness, the suggestion that 'open awareness' is universally preferred can be challenged. For example, the habitual communication patterns that operate within some families might make open disclosure wholly inappropriate. In families whose usual style of interactions do not normally include exploring deep emotions, their coping success might depend upon their decision to avoid open discussion of the prognosis. Indeed, forcing the truth on those who do not want it could be just as inexcusable as proscribing honest discussion (Seale 1991).

Nevertheless, care must be taken that we do not underestimate people's inner resources. Moreover, whilst avoiding deceit will always remain a basic moral canon, it should also be acknowledged that when health professionals are breaking bad news 'the truth need not be breached with a fist of steel but it can, rather, be embraced by a velvet glove' (Shea & Kendrick 1995). Whilst the ways in which families with a dying relative cope with terminal illness are still poorly understood, the author's own research reveals that relatives' main coping responses include seeking out information from staff, seeking support from family and friends and employing a range of psychological defences, which include denial and, allied to this, the preservation of hope (McIntyre 1996).

Within the context of terminal illness, denial can involve avoiding thinking about or discussing the fatal prognosis, or indeed simply refusing to believe it. The use of denial as a coping strategy is closely allied to the need to preserve hope, even in the face of certain death. During a progressive and fatal illness, those closest to the patient can repeatedly be thrown into chaos as the illness moves from stage to stage. Whilst denial is commonly viewed as a pathological response it is important that health professionals recognise that denial can operate as an important and valuable buffer against stress. Indeed, by blunting the full force of the truth, denial can allow situations to be viewed more positively, thus lowering anxiety and distress, aiding decision-making and assisting day-to-day functioning.

According to Russell (1993) denial can offer protection from the threat of disintegration that might came with the complete loss of hope (Russell 1993). In the author's research, denial was found to operate at different levels and was often employed with considerable insight. The following quote illustrates the tenuous, yet vital, protection that denial can offer as relatives juggle the demands of the patient's illness and the ongoing concerns of everyday life.

> I can go for days without getting upset and then maybe all of a sudden all I do is bubble [cry]. At times I feel it's just not penetrating what's happening to her and then all of a sudden just the daftest wee thing brings it all back into focus...

Within the context of terminal illness, denial can therefore represent a rational and vital buffer against hopelessness (Russell 1993). Hope can operate as a significant coping resource within a close relationship and has dynamic and reciprocal properties in that evidence of hope in one person has a role in maintaining a sense of hopefulness in the other (Herth 1990, 1993).

Nurses can help support and sustain hope in relatives, and therefore also in dying patients, by maintaining a caring presence with the family, by ensuring that optimal standards of comfort and care are provided for the patient, by providing regular information for relatives and by making adequate provision for the relatives' physical and emotional comfort (Herth 1993, McIntyre 1996). Crucially, nurses need to convey a sense of their availability to the family so that a supportive relationship can be formed between the staff and relatives.

■ **REFLECTIVE PRACTICE 8.6 Reflecting on hope**

Consult one or more of the articles cited below, or seek out recent publications that explore the concept of hope, and read the material and reflect upon the implications that any insights gained might have for your own practice.

Herth K 1993 Hope in the family caregiver of terminally ill people. Journal of Advanced Nursing 18: 538–548

Russell G 1993 The role of denial in clinical practice. Journal of Advanced Nursing 18: 938–940

Scanlon C 1989 Creating a vision of hope; the challenge of palliative care. Oncology Nurses Forum 16: 189–283

Shea T, Kendrick K 1995 With velvet gloves: the ethics of collusion. Palliative Care Today 4: 9–10

Relatives' support needs

The literature is consistent in finding that relatives' greatest support comes from seeing the patient well cared for with symptoms being adequately controlled (Hull 1990, Klagsbrun 1994, Kristjanson & Ashcroft 1994, McIntyre 1996). When pressed to express their own support needs, relatives consistently report that they place a high value on being made to feel welcome in the ward and in having unrestricted access to the patient. Also high in their priorities is to regularly receive up-to-date information about the patient's condition and care. As discussed above, when staff take time to talk to the family and to listen to their concerns, this is much commented upon and appreciated. Also, in the potentially alienating environment of hospital, relatives seem to need reassurance that the special status of their dying, loved one will be recognised. When relatives see the staff showing friendship towards the patient they feel comforted. In such an emotional climate, if the relatives have to leave the patient's bedside for a spell they are reassured that there will be someone there who really cares about their relative until they return (McIntyre 1996). The importance to the family of this bond being established with the staff is poignantly confirmed in the following quote.

Knowing there are people there and not just for their medical expertise, but for their comfort as well. They are so friendly to my mum and to the whole family. That it is really excellent. It's made such a big difference. It's comforting to me too.

By way of summary, the factors found to reduce the stress experienced by relatives are listed in Box 8.1. The factors found to increase the stress experienced by relatives are listed in Box 8.2.

■ **BOX 8.1**

Relatives' stress is reduced by:
- Seeing the patient comfortable with symptoms relieved
- Getting regular updates from nurses and doctors
- Carers who know and are known to the patient and their family
- Having the patient's 'special status' recognised by staff
- A caring manner and relaxed friendship of staff
- Having a private place to rest that is very close to the patient
- The bed space being protected from noise and bustle
- Support of family and close friends
- Access to social worker and pastoral support

■ **BOX 8.2**

Relatives' stress is increased by:
- Seeing their relative suffer pain or distress
- Not knowing what to expect (or when)
- Busy wards, loud televisions, noisy children 'running wild'
- Lack of privacy and basic amenities for comfort
- A change in care setting close to the end
- Staff who act distantly and formally to the family
- Feeling that the patient has been denied respect or has been 'written off'

This brief overview has sought to offer a representative sample of the views and feelings expressed by relatives who have a dying family member in the hope that we may gain some insight into their experiences and needs. The nature of the relatives' situation is such that, regrettably, we cannot substantially relieve the pain and grief which the family are suffering. However, by the way we practice we can support relatives in practical and caring ways, and we can also seek to ensure that no avoidable distress is caused whilst the family are in our care.

Relatives' expectations are modest and nurses have considerable potential to relieve certain aspects of their distress. Relatives in the author's study consistently and frequently expressed the value that they placed on staff who will ensure the patients' physical comfort and who are willing to 'be there' with the family during this difficult time. One elderly relative sums up what she needs from nurses in a few words.

Just show that you care. That you see the patient as a person.

CHANGING PRACTICE BY RESEARCH

As discussed above, following phase one of the study the staff nurses attended a 2-day workshop where the research findings were used to develop standards for improved family care and support in the nurses' own wards.

A quality assurance framework was selected for implementing change as it was judged likely that the nurses would already be familiar with standard setting. The standard setting approach also meant that the intervention could be developed by those directly responsible for implementing the changes in practice. This 'bottom up' approach is known to be important for developing feelings of ownership and commitment to a change initiative, thus increasing its potential for success (Harvey 1994, Kitson 1993). Finally, standard setting encourages reflection on practice and also promotes ongoing evaluations of nursing care (Methot et al 1992).

Having heard and discussed the phase one findings, the staff nurses identified key issues that needed to be addressed in their own wards. Box 8.3 presents the list that was collectively drawn up by the nurses during the workshop.

■ BOX 8.3

Areas needing to be addressed in the standards

- Access of relatives to comfortable, private accommodation
- Access of relatives to a named nurse who has knowledge of the patient's prognosis and treatment and relatives' understanding and acceptance
- Access of relatives to other members of the care team
- Interprofessional communication and record keeping
- Family support and information around the time of death
- Access of relatives to spiritual support and to support agencies

The workshop facilitators then delivered a broadly theoretical overview of quality assurance and of standard setting using the Dynamic Standard Setting System (DySSy) approach (Harvey 1994). During the remainder of the workshop the nurses developed the first draft of their standards, working in two groups, each supported by a facilitator.

The final half day of the workshop was devoted to addressing the nurses' own specific concerns. Both groups elected to focus, first, on difficulties that nurses experience when interacting with dying patients and their families and, second, on measures to manage the stress that nurses experience with this aspect of their practice.

STAFF NURSES AS CHANGE AGENTS

During the intervention period, the staff nurses became very actively involved with their ward colleagues, managers and other professionals within the multidisciplinary team in their efforts to bring about the required changes in their wards. Considerable energy was invested in securing improvements in facilities for relatives' comfort and privacy. To this end the staff nurses were involved in extensive liaison with a range of personnel who included builders, estate managers and various charities. In some wards a relatives' room was acquired, where no such facility had previously existed, whilst in some other wards efforts were directed at upgrading the existing provision.

Initiatives to improve communication were implemented in most wards. The most notable change in practice was in the active steps that nursing staff took: first, to initiate contact with relatives, second, to identify themselves by name to relatives and thereafter to maintain regular contact with the family. Initiatives to improve interprofessional communication were also launched in four of the wards. These mainly took the form of including nurses in interviews with relatives when bad news was being broken or when new information was being given to the family.

ANALYSIS OF CHANGE

In the author's study the crucial driving force for change came from the staff nurses who, in their change agent capacity, represented the 'leverage point' that provided the momentum for change. Changes were found to be most evident in those wards where the staff nurse/change agents were experienced, charismatic, opinion leaders who were able to carry their ward teams along with them. Conversely, less confident and less affiliative nurses seemed to experience difficulty in driving the changes forward. The influence of the change agent's personality on the success of a change initiative, and the benefits of providing support for the change agents as they work to implement change, have been widely reported in the literature (Stevenson 1990, Swansburg 1993, Titchen & Binnie 1993, Wright 1989).

The planned change approach used in this study enabled the staff in the wards to design, implement and evaluate their own change strategy and although the magnitude of change was not uniform, positive changes were recorded in all but one of the study wards.

SUMMARY AND CONCLUSIONS

Findings from phase one of the study confirmed that when relatives of dying patients remain in the ward for long periods of time, staff can face a range of difficulties as they seek to accommodate and relate to the family. In the emotionally charged situation of terminal illness, relationships between nurses and relatives can be somewhat uneasy and conflict ridden.

Barriers were found to exist at the very point of contact between relatives and staff and there was clear evidence of the discomfort that both relatives and nurses experience when approaching each other. It was also revealed that relatives commonly felt inhibited about approaching nurses. Indeed, a concern that was almost unanimously expressed was that relatives did not want to be seen as a 'nuisance' by disturbing busy nurses. Relatives also reported not knowing whom they should approach, and when, and consequently relatives commonly experienced unmet needs for information and support.

The nurses' phase one data also revealed that the nurses' discomfort about approaching relatives stemmed from several sources. The nurses' perceptions of the high expectations that relatives had of them had an intimidating effect and the anticipation of failure that this generated often caused the nurses to avoid approaching relatives. Nurses felt further constrained by lack of privacy when communicating with distressed relatives, by lack of knowledge about the relatives' current awareness of the patient's prognosis and by lack of confidence in their own communication skills. The findings confirmed that nurses experience significant stress when dealing with relatives and that they also had significant unmet needs for support.

The effect of the intervention was to dismantle some of these barriers and to do so in quite simple but fundamental ways.

When the relatives' feelings and experiences were illuminated through the phase one data and were presented to the nurses, this had a truly galvanising effect. The feedback of the phase one data, and the experiential workshop that followed, caused the nurses to re-evaluate their communication skills and to reassess their potential to change aspects of the environment of care and their own practice. These perceptual shifts enabled the nurses to reappraise the threat that caring for relatives presented. As a result of these reappraisals, new coping possibilities emerged and the nurses' perceived comfort in their role increased.

From this new world view, the nurses' approach strategies to relatives changed, nurse–relative dialogue flourished and relationships with the patient's relatives were established. Data from **both** relatives and nurses confirm that this resulted in a reduction in the nurses' use of distancing and avoidance tactics and in a reciprocal reduction in stress reported by both relatives and nurses. It is possible that the nurses had previously held unrealistically high expectations of themselves and they could now see that providing support for the dying patient's family was within their professional expertise and coping capacity.

*Over the months a lot of the staff are finding it easier to approach relatives.
You try to build up a relationship so that the relatives feel more at ease
approaching you. In turn we all feel better about approaching them.*

A shift had occurred in many wards to a more holistic and family-oriented
approach to care. From this new perspective, the dying patient's family
became intrinsic to, rather than adjuncts of, the care. More spontaneous
interactions between nurses and relatives were established and a concern
for, and involvement in, family support developed.

Nurses had seemingly lowered their guard and had moved in closer to
establish an emotional connection with the family. This was substantially
confirmed in the relatives' accounts where relatives commonly described
the ward atmosphere as friendly and relaxed. The reciprocal benefits of
these altered relationships, and of the improved facilities in the wards,
offered a compelling message in the research findings. Indeed, the most
striking insight to emerge from the study was the extent to which reciprocal
benefits could accrue when support strategies were implemented. This was
most powerfully revealed where nurses' approach strategies to the family
changed and where provision of facilities for relatives was improved.

The crucial importance of providing comfort at the bedside, and of offering a private area where relatives could rest and where they could receive
information and support from staff, was evident in the findings. Such a
facility not only supports the relatives during what is an emotionally intense
experience, but also acts as a potent coping resource for nurses. When
nurses were able to offer relatives these amenities they reported a reduction
in their own subjective experience of stress which, in turn, resulted in
reduced use of distancing behaviour and in enhanced communication.
A private room for communicating with the family therefore represents
a **crucial** coping resource for both relatives and staff and has significant
potential for enhancing the quality of care during terminal illness. Furthermore, when these crucial areas of communication and facilities were
improved, and nurses felt able to deliver high-quality care, the positive
feedback that this generated provided the impetus needed to implement
further improvements in practice.

The following quote confirms that the warmer relationships that were
established between nurses and relatives appeared to yield reciprocal benefits.

*It's nice for them to be able to relate to you and in a strange way you get
something back from that. In those circumstances it's not that stressful.
You are there for them and giving them a part of you, which is nice.*

Another compelling message in the data relates to the dynamic characteristics of denial and hope. Indeed, denial, often regarded as a rather negative concept, was found to operate as an important coping strategy, which
most relatives will employ in fluctuating measure and often with considerable insight in the time leading up to the death of their loved one.

It is crucial for nurses to recognise that for the patient and close family to
openly acknowledge the imminence of death a profound shift in emotional
orientation within a relationship may be required, which can be of such

magnitude and significance that for some it will represent a step quite beyond contemplation. For such families, whilst there may be tacit acknowledgement of the reality of death, pretence will continue to the end. This need that some families have to preserve hope of recovery right to the end is poignantly illustrated in the following quote.

I don't know how to put it … but just don't let her give up hope. I want her to have a wee bit of hope.

In families where open disclosure of the prognosis is preferred, it is still likely that a point will be reached in the cancer journey when all hope of recovery is finally dismantled and the forthcoming death is confronted fully and openly by the patient and family. Nurses need to be acutely sensitive to the shifting needs of the grieving patient and family with all of the implications that this has for their needs for privacy, support and comfort, in whatever form this may represent for that particular family.

The findings from this research confirm the transactional nature of the stress that is experienced both by relatives of dying patients and by the nurses who provide terminal care in hospitals. It has been established that whilst the source of that stress was not directly amenable to amelioration, it is possible to support and augment the coping resources, both of relatives and nurses, by modifying the physical environment and by enhancing the emotional climate of care.

Benner & Wrubel (1989, p. 62) offer a particularly apt closure to this chapter.

Nurses do not cure stress but they can help people to survive it by establishing a healing relationship and by helping them to mobilise their emotional and spiritual resources.

REFERENCES

Aranda S 1995 Conducting research with the dying: ethical considerations and experience. International Journal of Palliative Nursing 1: 41–47

Bakhurst D 1992 Debate – on lying and deceiving. Journal of Medical Ethics 18: 63–66

Benner P, Wrubel J 1989 The primacy of caring: stress and coping in health and illness. Addison Wesley, California

Cartwright A 1991a Balance of care for the dying between hospital and community; perceptions of general practitioners, community nurses and relatives. British Journal of General Practice 41: 271–274

Cartwright A 1991b Changes in life and care in the year before death 1969–1987. Journal of Public Health Medicine 13: 81–87

Clarke J 1991 Moral dilemmas in nursing research. Nursing Practice 4: 22–25

Eve A, Jackson A 1994 Palliative care services – where are we now? Palliative Care Today 3: 22–23

Ford G 1994 Definition and prospects. Palliative Care Today 3: 21

Glaser B, Strauss A 1965 Awareness of dying. Aldine, Chicago

Harvey G 1994 DYSSY, tutorial package. National Institute for Nursing, Oxford

Herth K 1990 Fostering hope in terminally ill people. Journal of Advanced Nursing 15: 1250–1259

Herth K 1993 Hope in the family caregiver of terminally ill people. Journal of Advanced Nursing 18: 538–548

Higginson I 1993 Palliative care; a review of past changes and future trends. Journal of Public Health Medicine 15: 3–8

Hodson P 1990 Whose death is it anyway? The Observer 11th March 1990. In: Hunt G 1991 The truth about terminal cancer. Nursing 4: 9–11

Hull M 1992 Coping strategies of family caregivers in hospice homecare. Oncology Nursing Forum 19: 1179–1187

Hull M M 1990 Sources of stress for hospice caregiving families. Hospice Journal 6: 29–54

Janes J 1992 Facing that final journey. Nursing Standard 7: 52–53

Kitson A 1993 Accountability for quality. Nursing Standard 8: 4–6

Klagsbrun S 1994 Patient, family, and staff suffering. Journal of Palliative Care 10: 14–17

Kristjanson L J 1989 Quality of terminal care: salient indicators identified by families. Journal of Palliative Care 5: 21–30

Kristjanson L, Ashcroft T 1994 The family's cancer journey: a literature review. Cancer Nursing 17: 1–17

Kristjanson L J, Sloan J A 1991 Determinants of the grief experience of survivors: two empirical studies. Journal of Palliative Care 7: 51–56

Lugton J 1989 Relatives – communicating in the hospice. Nursing Times 85: 28–30

McIntyre R 1996 Nursing support for relatives of dying cancer patients in hospital: improving standards by research. Unpublished PhD Thesis, Department of Nursing and Community Health, Glasgow Caledonian University, Glasgow

Methot D, Caesar J, Duquette A M 1992 Empowering staff nurses through quality assurance. Journal of Nursing Care Quality 6: 9–14

Nugent L S 1988 The social support requirements of family caregivers of terminal cancer patients. Canadian Journal of Nursing Research 20: 45–58

Parkes C M 1988 Not always: special issue: controversies in palliative care: a thematic issue. Journal of Palliative Care 4: 50–52

Raudonis B 1992 Ethical considerations in qualitative research with hospice patients. Qualitative Health Research 2: 238–249

Registrar General for Scotland 1994 Populations Statistics Branch Report. General Register Office for Scotland, Edinburgh

Russell G 1993 The role of denial in clinical practice. Journal of Advanced Nursing 18: 938–940

Scanlon C 1989 Creating a vision of hope: the challenge of palliative care. Oncology Nursing Forum 16: 189–283

Scottish Partnership Agency for Palliative and Cancer Care 1995 Directory of palliative care services in Scotland 1995. Scottish Partnership Agency for Palliative and Cancer Care in conjunction with the Health Education Board for Scotland, Edinburgh

Seale C 1991 Communication and awareness about death – a study of a random sample of dying people. Social Science & Medicine 32: 943–952

Seale C 1993 Changes in death and dying: the past 25 years. Critical Public Health 4: 4–11

Shea T, Kendrick K 1995 With velvet gloves: the ethics of collusion. Palliative Care Today 4: 9–10

Stevenson D 1990 The energy crisis of change. Nursing Practice 4: 15–17

Sudnow D 1967 Passing on: the social organisation of dying. Prentice Hall, New York

Swansburg R C 1993 Introductory management and clinical leadership for clinical nurses. James and Bartlett Publishers, Boston

Thompson I E, Melia K M, Boyd K M 1993 Nursing ethics. Churchill Livingstone, Edinburgh

Titchen A, Binnie A 1993 Research partnerships; collaborative action research in nursing. Journal of Advanced Nursing 18: 858–865

WHO 1990 Cancer pain relief and palliative care. Technical report, Series No. 804. World Health Organization Expert Committee, Geneva

Wright S 1989 Changing nursing practice. Edward Arnold, London

Wrubel J, Benner P, Lazarus R S 1981 Social competence from the perspective of stress and coping. In: Wine J, Smye M (eds) Social competence. The Guilford Press, New York, pp 61–99

Loss, grief and bereavement

9

Margaret Kindlen   Val Smith   Margaret Smith

Bereavement is the state of having lost someone through death and is a complex process involving psychological, social and biological processes. [Osterweiss et al 1984]

INTRODUCTION

Nurses working in palliative care have a direct exposure to loss in many different contexts. They expect that their patients will die. In addition they appreciate the need to support family members up to, and immediately following, the death of a patient. What is perhaps not so clear is the nurse's role in supporting those relatives through bereavement. The WHO (1990), in its definition of palliative care, states that families should be helped to cope during their relatives' illness and in bereavement. Where then does the nurse's responsibility begin and end?

It is not our intention, in this chapter, to create bereavement counsellors. We will explore ways in which nurses can help the bereaved relatives of patients to whom they have provided palliative care, in whatever context they work. We will examine the research that has led the way in providing information about how individuals respond in different circumstances. Some limitations in the current literature will be highlighted. To date, research has seemingly not addressed what bereaved individuals want from society at the time immediately before and following the death of a friend or relative. Against this background we will integrate the notion of bereavement support with that of health promotion in an attempt to offer guidance on how nurses can optimise the support offered in organisation and community settings.

LEARNING OUTCOMES

The chapter draws from the authors' combined interest in the process of bereavement and from personal, clinical and teaching experience in palliative care. It will fulfil requirements for PREP in the categories of reducing risk, care enhancement and patient, family, client and colleague support. By the end of this chapter the reader will have:

- Explored the concept of bereavement
- Examined a broad range of research into bereavement
- Identified risk factors for individuals during the grieving process
- Considered ways that nurses can facilitate individuals through the process of grief

WHO ARE THE BEREAVED?

Bereavement and other forms of loss

Similar responses to bereavement are seen in other forms of loss experienced through life. Some authors believe that maturational and situational losses, such as loss of childhood innocence, favoured objects, growing older and life crisis events, prepare individuals for major losses such as bereavement.

■ **REFLECTIVE PRACTICE 9.1   Your life map**

A good way of looking at your experience of loss is to use a life map. To do this:

- On a piece of paper draw a straight line to represent your age in years
- Mark on the line significant events that have happened throughout your life
- On the left side of the line indicate with a 'T' those events that have been particularly traumatic for you to deal with. On the right hand side mark with 'E' those events that have been enjoyable
- Finally, mark with a circle on the line those events that have (although painful) helped you 'grow' and mark with a box those events (although enjoyable at the time) that have restricted your life and about which you have regrets

Look at the line and count how many events involved some kind of loss.

This exercise helps to identify how many of life's experiences can have both losses and gains, and that many different types of losses occur. For example, leaving home and starting nurse education is a gain of independence and a new start to life; at the same time it is a loss in the sense of moving from home and a loss or change in some friendships and ways of being looked after by parents.

You may wish to ask a colleague or a friend to do this activity. This will help you to compare your perception of life events with someone else's and provide an opportunity for you to perhaps discuss coping strategies in positive and negative circumstances.

This activity may also provide a starting point if ever you need to think of a way to start to begin a small group teaching session.

Reactions to a bereavement will vary according to an individual's previous experience of loss, e.g. redundancy, possessions, his ability to deal with loss and exposure to death. Accordingly, Faulkner (1995) stresses that we should not make assumptions about the magnitude of a loss.

Bereavement affects everyone at some time in life. It is an experience that cannot be avoided. An important issue for nurses to understand is how people are able to cope with this usually stressful event. Lindemann (1944) presented grief as a normal process and stated that only the more complicated bereavements should be considered as pathological. Averill & Nunley (1988) continued the debate, suggesting that the meaning which society gives to loss affects its interpretation and people's orientation to the bereaved state. Engel (1961), in contrast, suggested that grief should be considered as a disease and that this would legitimise medical interest and research.

Many factors influence how people respond to bereavement. Different cultures and societies approach death and grieving differently. Although there is significant continuity between different cultural approaches to bereavement, there can be a marked variation, so that different cultures will probably require alternative types of help or support (Neuberger 1987). Very little research has been carried out with regard to cross-cultural differences or to investigate whether these variations are caused more by genetic predisposition than by cultural influences (Osterweiss et al 1984). The cultural influence of western society appears to discourage people from talking about their experience of grief and expects them to 'return to normal' as soon as possible (Gorer 1965). This chapter will concentrate on bereavement in western society within a predominantly Christian context.

Research indicates that there is an increased mortality and morbidity following bereavement, with an increase in accidents, cardiovascular disease, infectious diseases and suicide. In addition, an increase in smoking, alcohol consumption and the use of tranquillisers and hypnotics is evident (Osterweiss et al 1984). There are also social and economic consequences for the bereaved as they struggle to adjust to their altered lifestyle (Lopata 1979, Marris 1958). This recognised morbidity may be only the tip of the iceberg. People's lifestyles are often affected for many years following the death of someone close. It is still unclear whether this morbidity applies to all sections of the population or solely to those who have particular difficulty with their bereavement. There are, however, some people who do appear to have an increased risk of problems with their bereavement (Parkes 1986, Raphael 1977, Vachon et al 1982a).

Effects of bereavement

Most significant losses occur within the family context. Each family has its own style of coping and this influences how the family unit deals with crisis situations. For example, some families are open in their style of communication, whereas other families use a more closed framework (Bowen 1978). The functional role of individual members of the family is also an important influence in how each family member deals with the loss (Berger 1988). Bereavement is not, however, limited to family relationships. Partners (whether heterosexual or homosexual), friends and colleagues have all had different and special relationships with the person who has died. In addition, remember that children's experiences of death and coping with loss will also have an effect on their response in later life (Lopata 1979, Osterweiss et al 1984, Raphael 1984, Schowalter 1975). Although this is noted, much of the research available concentrates on bereavement in the adult.

The attention given to grief in different individuals varies. Some people find that a profound bereavement for them is trivialised by family and friends. This can sometimes be the case when the person who has died is elderly and infirm. Bereavement in those with cognitive difficulties is also poorly understood. Finally, in the context of bereavement, the death of a pet is not always accepted as a significant loss, yet for the individuals concerned this may be the most upsetting and hardest loss ever experienced.

■ REFLECTIVE PRACTICE 9.2   Review of life map

Look back to your life map and select one event that involved loss. Alternatively, you might like to think of a time when you lost something of importance – your car keys, perhaps.

- Remember what or how you felt at the time
- List the different feelings and emotions
- What did you do after finding out about the loss?

Read the section below about manifestations of grief. Return to your list and compare the thoughts, physical feelings, emotions and actions with those identified in a normal response to grief. This will demonstrate that although similar responses are experienced in consequence to life events, the intensity of the feelings differ, depending upon the importance or significance of the event.

Bereavement support

Benner (1984, p. 47) suggests that:

> *A person can receive help without asking for it and can ask for it without being able to receive it. Even 'help' sometimes does not help; some individuals with strong need for personal control may not be able to acknowledge that they need help or even that they are being helped.*

Although directed towards exploring expert practice in nursing, Benner's words can be applied in bereavement. She presents the theme of 'helping' in eight competencies. The term 'helpful' encompasses a wide range of interventions and behaviours that may be seen by the bereaved relative as of benefit to them. We therefore suggest that Benner's concept of 'helping', with some adaptation, can be subsumed into the nurse's role when supporting individuals through grief (see Box 9.1). We will see below how this helping model compares favourably with Worden's tasks of mourning. In these models of grief there is no suggestion that the relationship with the dead person should be relinquished. Walters (1996) also challenges the idea of bereavement being a journey towards having a life without the deceased. The purpose of grief he writes 'is to construct a durable biography that enables the living to integrate the memory of the dead into their ongoing lives – the grief process being about having conversations with others who knew the deceased'.

■ **BOX 9.1**

The helping role (adapted from Benner 1984)

1. Creating a climate for establishing commitment for healing
2. Providing comfort measures and preserving personhood in the face of pain and extreme breakdown
3. Being with a relative
4. Maximising the relative's participation and control in his future
5. Providing comfort and communication through touch
6. Providing emotional and informational support
7. Guiding the person through emotional and developmental change – providing new options, closing off old ones
8. Teaching mediating – using goals therapeutically

MANIFESTATIONS OF GRIEF

Marris (1986) writes:

> *The need to grieve almost certainly derives from fundamental aspects of our being, however social forms may modify its expression. Yet grieving, unlike other generic human behaviours, does not at first sight appear to be useful to the bereaved. Since it characteristically discourages him or her from at once replacing the lost relationship, it can even seem harmful. What then is its function? Grieving, I argue, is a process of psychological reintegration, impelled by contradictory desires at once to search for the recovery of the lost relationship and to escape from painful reminds of loss.*

Different authors have defined grief in different ways. Lindemann (1944), a pioneer in the field, provided a reference point for defining normal and morbid forms of grief. His work, however, was with specific groups, such as bereaved disaster victims and their close relatives following the Coconut Grove fire.

For example, from 101 interviews with recently bereaved individuals, he identified many common factors. Much of Lindemann's research was with psychoneurotic patients who experienced bereavement during the course of their treatment. Although his sample populations cannot be considered typical, he provided a milestone from which subsequent research has been developed.

Worden (1991) identifies categories of physical sensations, health concerns, thoughts, behaviours and feelings, including:

- Hollowness, tightness of stomach, chest, shoulders and throat
- Sensitivity to noise
- A sense of depersonalisation and a feeling of unreality
- Breathlessness and deep sighing
- Muscular weakness
- Fatigue, lack of energy
- Dryness of mouth

The psychological manifestations include a feeling of shock or numbness, helplessness, yearning, anxiety and guilt. A preoccupation with the past is quite usual, as are hallucinations or the sense of the presence of the deceased. The intensity of these emotions is often quite startling with the bereaved never having experienced such strong feelings before. The behaviour of the bereaved person may also undergo changes with the onset of absentmindedness, social withdrawal, crying and difficulty with decision-making. It is from these manifestations of grief that the various authors have developed their theories.

Theoretical frameworks

Bowlby's (1980) theories of attachment and loss developed from his studies of children separated from their mothers. Bowlby (1980) suggests that making attachments are for security and safety, and that this is normal behaviour for both children and adults. When the attachment figure disappears, or is threatened, an intense feeling of anxiety and threat occurs. These intense feelings are generated in the surviving family when a loved one dies. After some modifications to his ideas, Bowlby (1980) and later Parkes (1986) suggested that there are four stages in the grieving process (Table 9.1).

Although the various authors have described the process of grief in different ways, the manifestations of grief already identified are mentioned in their writing to a greater or lesser degree. All would agree that grief does not progress in an orderly manner but that the bereaved person

Table 9.1 Stages in the grief process	
Bowlby (1980)	**Parkes (1986)**
Numbness	Shock and alarm
Yearning and searching	Searching
Disorganisation and despair	Anger and guilt
Reorganisation	Gaining a new identity

oscillates between the various stages of mourning – sometimes getting 'stuck' at a particular point – and need extra time or help before they are able to move on.

Parkes (1986) further addresses the issue of loss and grief within the context of psychosocial transitions. He suggests that loss and grief are components of life changes that require the individual to revise her view of the world. Other psychosocial transitions, for example, may include redundancy, divorce and the loss of a limb. These events will produce similar manifestations of grief to those found in bereavement. He contends that psychosocial transitions have three main characteristics. They:

- Require people to make major revisions of their assumptions about the world
- Are lasting in their implications, rather than transient
- Happen over a relatively short period of time

He suggests that bereavement can therefore be seen within the overall context of life's psychosocial transitions.

Carter (1989) reviewed theories of bereavement in an interesting ethnographic study. She interviewed a sample of 30 adults who were bereaved between 3 and 23 years previously. They were asked to give an account of their bereavement and this was compared with the theories of bereavement. Although similarities were identified, some significant differences were evident. Some of these differences may be a result of differing perceptions of a given situation by health care professionals as compared with those of bereaved relatives.

Grief resolution occurs, according to Parkes (1986), when the bereaved person is able to find a new identity after their life situation has been changed by death. When, for example, the widow is able to see herself as a widow and not as her dead husband's wife, she has accepted the absence of her husband and the new role she has to undertake. This concurs with Worden (1991) who suggests that resolutions occur when the bereaved person is able to emotionally accept that their loved one is dead and move on in a positive way with a new life. Bowlby (1980), on the other hand, suggests that for some, mourning continues and the bereaved relative never fully recovers their former state of health and well-being. This is supported by one widow who explains, 'you don't get over it; you get used to it' [Parkes & Weiss 1983, p. 155].

One view is that for the majority, bereavement is resolved after about 2 years following the death (Penson 1990, Vachon et al 1982b, Worden 1991). This does not mean, however, that the bereaved has let go of all attachments with the deceased but rather has 'emotionally relocated the deceased and moved on with life'. Stroebe et al (1993) draw attention to the importance of the ongoing relationship with the deceased. They suggest that the place this relationship has with the bereaved is part of the adaptation to the loss. People are changed by bereavement, and the process of grief allows the development of a changed but ongoing relationship with the person who has died (Klass et al 1996).

Lindemann (1944), Bowlby (1980) and Parkes (1986) describe grief in stages, as a rather passive process that happens to the person, whereas Worden (1991), by identifying tasks of mourning, puts more emphasis on the role of the individual in coming to terms with their own personal loss. As a development of stage theory, Worden defined that four major tasks of mourning are to:

- Accept the reality of the loss
- Work through the pain of grief
- Adjust to an environment in which the deceased is missing
- Emotionally relocate the deceased and move on with life

Worden considered that these tasks must be accomplished for equilibrium to be re-established and the process of mourning to be completed.

■ REFLECTIVE PRACTICE 9.3   Tasks of mourning

Compare the tasks of mourning described by Worden (1991) with the competencies required in a helping role (adapted from Benner (1984) in Table 9.1).

- The competencies within the helping role are required by the nurse to assist the bereaved person with each of the tasks suggested by Worden (1991). How would you rate these competencies in yourself and what plans can you make to validate and improve them?
- Enquire about appropriate skills-based communication courses. When you next attend a personal development interview negotiate with your manager for an opportunity to attend a course

---

Uncomplicated/complicated grief

Uncomplicated grief is characterised by all of the feelings and emotions described above. Eventually, periods of normality occur and become increasingly longer. When there are complications, different patterns emerge. These are collectively known as complicated grief (Worden 1991).

- Chronic grief, when mourning is of excessive duration with the person unable to return to normal living.
- Delayed grief, when normal grief is inhibited or postponed only to return with greater intensity at a future loss.
- Exaggerated grief, when the person becomes totally overwhelmed and may develop severe depression or become dependent on alcohol or other drugs.
- Masked grief. Some grief reactions can be masked, for example, when the bereaved individual exhibits physical symptoms similar to those that had been experienced by the deceased.

Interestingly, Parkes & Weiss (1983) comment that in their experience, chronic grief is the most common problem. They also suggest that the widely held view that early distress following bereavement is essential for normal grieving, is not supported by the available research.

PREDICTORS OF GRIEF

Different studies have identified a number of factors that can be used to predict the outcome of bereavement on an individual (Parkes 1995). Although they do not necessarily provide an accurate prediction of risk, the following factors will either help or hinder the grieving process and can be used to guide a health carer when assessing families:

- Relationship between the bereaved and the deceased
- Circumstances surrounding the death
- Life and physical fitness of the bereaved
- The bereaved person's personality
- Social factors
- The dead person's age
- The family circumstances and situation

Parkes (1993) strongly advocates the assessment of risk factors in those who will be most affected by the patient's death. This should be possible in palliative care, given the type of relationship that is encouraged between professionals, patients and informal carers. Parkes (1993) advocates the use of genograms to map out relationships, previous bereavements and other major losses, such as divorce. A genogram, says Parkes (1993, p. 667), 'is more useful in palliative care than a stethoscope'.

Genogram

A genogram is a map that identifies family relationships in a coded format. The starting point is one family member. Symbols identify male and female family members and a series of horizontal and vertical lines represent links within and between generations (Fig. 9.1).

The genogram shown in Figure 9.1 represents three generations of a family. You should note the familial trend in breast cancer from Susan through to Elizabeth. Should Elizabeth's cancer progress to a palliative care situation then this genogram would indicate that special attention needs to be given to Joan who has experienced multiple bereavements.

■ REFLECTIVE PRACTICE 9.4 Construct a genogram

If you have not used genograms in your practice, take time now to construct one. You could use your own extended family as an example or, alternatively, choose a patient that you are currently looking after. A useful reference is Dobson (1989).

Children's perception of death, for example, will be influenced by their stage in development. Communication between different family members and with the child is important. The work of children's bereavement support groups, such as Winston's Wish in Gloucester (Stokes et al 1995),

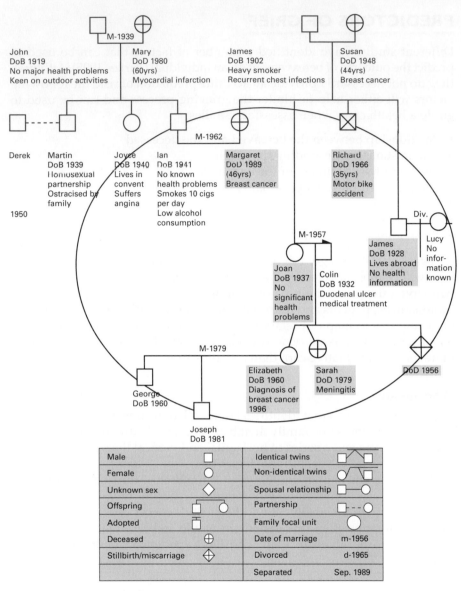

Fig. 9.1 Example of a genogram.

has raised awareness of the special needs of children who are grieving. Glazer & Clark (1997) explored the need for parenting classes as part of a hospice bereavement programme. They concluded that it was important to normalise the parenting process for children who were grieving. Parents were provided with opportunities to deepen their relationships with their children, to understand and to respect the individual nature of grief work with a child.

Factors influencing bereavement outcome

Research has indicated that many of the factors considered to be 'high risk' in the adjustment to a significant loss can be identified at the time of bereavement and may be used to help in predicting a good or poor outcome for the bereaved person (Parkes 1975, Vachon et al 1982a, Worden 1991). Not all authors, however, agree with these identified risk factors (Osterweiss et al 1984). Retrospective studies, while able to include a larger population, rely on the recollections of the bereaved person and risk introducing a bias to the findings. Robertson et al (1997) discuss collecting data during the grieving process. There are competing beliefs. It has been argued that collecting data from vulnerable people who are less able to make decisions is an intrusion of privacy to the point of being an infringement of rights. The counter argument is that people benefit from being able to talk about their feelings. There is a wider ethical debate to be considered here in relation to gaining informed consent from vulnerable people and also the issue of professionals acting as gatekeepers and preventing opportunities for willing subjects to participate in studies of this kind.

In their Harvard bereavement project, Parkes & Weiss (1983), identified some predictive variables for bereavement outcome. The sample, however, was from younger widows and widowers and, as such, may not be comparable with other groups of the bereaved. Vachon et al (1982b) studied a sample of widows with a wider age range (22–69 years). This sample excluded relatives of patients who died in the emergency room, those who were certified dead on arrival and those lost to follow-up. The study claims further factors indicative of high risk. This is yet another study that could be criticised for under-representing the bereaved population. It could be argued that the excluded groups of bereaved relatives have the potential for higher than normal distress associated with bereavement.

Bowling & Cartwright's (1982) study of elderly widows found several factors that indicated a high risk of poor bereavement outcome. The limitation in this study was the timing of the data collection – between 4 and 6 months following death – which, as already suggested, is long before grief resolution can be expected to be complete.

Suicide

According to Breibart & Passik (1993), patients with cancer are more at risk of committing suicide than the general population. Moreover, this is likely to occur in the advanced stages of disease and is associated with suffering caused by pain, poor prognosis and a sense of hopelessness, disinhibition and feelings of helplessness. There is evidence that bereaved relatives of those who have committed suicide have very difficult times during grief. Gallaher-Thompson et al (1993) conducted a study with the hypotheses that reactions to suicidal deaths were more extreme and longer lasting than natural deaths. They compared a group of bereaved spouses, following a natural death, with a group of spouses following a suicidal death. A group of non-bereaved was used as a control. Variables were matched as closely as possible. Interestingly, at 8 weeks following bereavement there were virtually no differences between the bereaved groups in the range and intensity of responses. However, in the longer term symptoms of depression and anxiety persisted for longer periods in the suicide survivor group and grief resolved at a much slower rate than in the natural death survivor group. The authors attribute the non-significant difference factor in early bereavement to the acute phase of mourning, which is intense, regardless of the mode of death.

■ **REFLECTIVE PRACTICE 9.5   Bereavement through suicide**

Find out what professional support is available locally for people who have been bereaved by suicide. If this is an area of inexperience for you, arrange to speak to a professional who has expertise in this specific area of bereavement.

You may find it helpful to read biographies of those who have experienced this type of loss. It may also be useful to compare the experiences of bereavement by natural death and bereavement by suicide.

Examples of biographies giving insight into the death of a spouse, either subsequent to death by natural events or through suicide are:

- 'A grief observed', by Lewis (1966) in which the author recounts his experience following the death of his wife who had cancer
- 'She never said goodbye' by Dykstra (1989). This gives an account of a widower's grief following the suicide of his wife who felt unable to continue living with the consequences of a diagnosis of Alzheimer's disease
- 'A special scar' by Wertheimer (1991) provides insight into the feelings and experiences of people bereaved by suicide

---

Social networks

Maddison & Walker (1967, p. 1058) examined the widow's interaction with the environment as seen by the widow herself during the bereavement crisis. Widows who perceived their environment and social networks as unhelpful had a poorer bereavement outcome and identified more unsatisfied needs than the group who did not perceive their environment as particularly unhelpful. Maddison & Walker (1967) identified this crisis period as the first 3 months after the husband's death.

Other factors may also prove to be significant in bereavement outcome. Hinds (1992) found, for example, that family members identified several sources of distress including loneliness, uncertainty about the future, disruption of lifestyle and helplessness. This suggests that the overall environment is a factor that needs consideration in the period before death. Bowen (1978) considers that the family unit is significant and suggests that those relatives who are able to express their emotions freely subsequently cope more effectively with loss. Stedeford's (1981) experience concurs with this. She reports that 'the couple or family who talk together, and who are able to take leave of each other, seem to cope with bereavement better' [Stedeford 1981, p. 787].

Personality

There may be a correlation between expression of emotion and personality traits to explain why individuals fall into either the high- or low-risk groups with regard to their bereavement outcome (Murgatroyd & Wolfe 1982, Vachon et al 1982a). Vachon et al (1982a, p. 787) point out that

It is easy to hypothesise an individual who is psychologically distressed because of a pronounced lack of support from her social network: It is equally easy to hypothesise the individual who, because of her continued psychological distress, has exhausted network resources and so is unsupported.

Here, the suggestion is that the underlying personality of the person may give a strong indication of their ability to adjust to bereavement. Vachon et al's (1982a) study involving 'low-risk' widows provided evidence to suggest that personality factors had a significant and protective role in this group of women.

Vulnerability versus personality

Caplan's (1981) research claims that psychological stress increases the individual's vulnerability and that those specific aspects of the individual's functioning that are weakened by the effect of the stress are complemented by social and professional networks of support.

These ideas are much in line with several general theories of stress and crisis intervention (Bailey & Clarke 1989, Murgatroyd & Wolfe 1982, Sutherland & Cooper 1990) and also fit in with Parkes' (1972) theories of psychosocial transitions mentioned above. Bereavement therefore not only produces manifestations of grief, but also may produce a crisis in the individual's life that requires many different coping strategies.

People with learning disabilities

The principles of dealing with loss in individuals with learning disabilities are very close to the heart of palliative care. Professionals in palliative care often get to know families well and are in a position to assess risk factors and the need for bereavement counselling. People with learning disabilities reach adult life, live in the community and, more frequently than 20 years ago, outlive parents. It is likely that nurses will meet patients in palliative care who have sons or daughters with some degree of learning disabilities. It is now more widely accepted that the experience of bereavement for people with learning difficulties follows much the same pattern as observed in the general population (Oswin 1981). The same is true for elderly people with cognitive impairment, as in Alzheimer's disease. However, Strachan (1981), in his study with a group of residents in long-term institutional care, reported that few of the residents maintained contact with relatives during the terminal illness. Ward staff often did not discuss the death because they thought the resident would not understand or that they would be unnecessarily upset. An earlier study by Emerson (1977) pointed out that where patients with learning disabilities were reported to be showing a sudden change in behaviour, manifested in aggression or withdrawal, 50% of such patients had suffered a recent bereavement. Kitching, in 1987, pointed out that grief is often a delayed process for people with learning disabilities. They may not immediately understand the full implications of the loss but come to feel the impact of the separation later.

Tuffrey-Wijne (1997) points out that people with learning disabilities have their own particular gifts and life experiences that help them to cope with bereavement, provided that they are well supported. In the same way as any other person working through the grief process, there is, for them, an opportunity for growth.

High-risk factors

It must be remembered that predictors of probable outcome only provide an indication of those who may have difficulty with their bereavement and do not give any definite answers (Parkes 1986). In addition, as already stated, most of these studies are based on a defined section of the population, namely widows and widowers, and therefore these predictors may not apply to other groups, for example, adult children, parents or siblings. Although a variety of different methodologies have been used to identify risk factors, there is sufficient evidence to suggest that certain factors can be identified to indicate those who are at high risk of having difficulty with their bereavement (Sanders 1988).

ANTICIPATORY GRIEF

There are conflicting beliefs about the role of anticipatory grieving. Some suggest that advanced warning can be of benefit whilst others indicate no difference (Bowling & Cartwright 1982, Sweeting & Gilhooly 1990, Welch 1982).

Anticipatory grief was first discussed by Lindemann (1944) when he identified the manifestations of grief in the relatives of those (e.g. soldiers going to war) who potentially could die. Welch (1982) describes anticipatory grief in the relatives of cancer patients as a process 'characterised by cyclical periods of mental anguish and feelings of loss'. Such feelings begin when the initial diagnosis of a malignancy is heard and express the expectation of the loss of a significant relationship and social role through the impending death of a loved one.

The stages that people exhibit in the adjustment to the forthcoming death of a loved one can be compared to the stages of grief as described by Bowlby (1980), Lindemann (1944) and Parkes (1986), in their work on bereavement, and Kubler Ross (1970), in her work with dying patients.

Anticipatory grief has been described by other authors as a component of coping, the process starting with diagnosis and continuing until well after death (Hampe 1975, Weismann 1979). Many of the studies of anticipatory grief have been with the parents of dying children and these appear to be remarkably consistent in the stages of grief that they identify

(Sweeting & Gilhooly 1990). Predeath grief has also been found in studies with adult patients. What is not clear is if this anticipation has any effect on the postdeath grieving process. Parkes & Weiss (1983), in their Harvard study, examined the grieving process in widows and widowers who were under the age of 45 years. They found that those with less than 2 weeks' warning of the impending death had more difficulty in their adjustment following the death than those who had a longer warning. It could be argued that anticipation was helping their grieving. Alternatively, the interpretation could be that sudden deaths generate more traumatic responses. Allan & Hall (1988) suggest that too much anticipation can produce additional problems involving severe psychological and physiological stress combined with an economic price from patients and the family. Bowling & Cartwright (1982) found the length of illness preceding the death had no influence on the bereaved relatives' subsequent adjustment.

NEEDS OF RELATIVES

Several studies over the last 20 years have identified important needs that relatives have during the terminal phase of an illness or dying. In Hampe's (1975) study the following list of needs emerged from spouses of dying patients:

- Being with the dying person for as long, and whenever, they wished
- Help in caring for physical needs
- Assurance of the comfort of the patient
- Being kept informed about care plans and about impending death
- Being able to express emotion with others, and having comfort and support from relatives and friends
- Having acceptance, support and comfort from health care staff

Whilst similar needs have been identified in other studies, Freihofer & Felton (1976) and Hull (1991) found that relatives did not welcome the encouragement, received from nurses, for them to express their emotions and to cry. Hull (1991) suggests that the desire to express emotion may depend on whether the particular family wanted to share their feelings at that time. Freihofer & Felton (1976) point out the significant implications of relatives' preference for most nursing to be directed towards support, comfort and prevention of suffering of terminally ill persons rather than towards the family. Similarly, Weismann (1979) writes that helping a patient to have a 'good death' helps the relatives in their bereavement. Bass & Bowen (1990) found that family caregivers who had difficulty during the terminal stages of the illness reported more difficulty later with their bereavement. By being aware of the needs of relatives, the health care team can plan interventions that can then improve their care (Dracup & Breu 1978). This period of time before death is increasingly recognised as having an influence on the postbereavement period. Bereavement care therefore needs to be considered within the whole context of the dying patient's final illness.

■ REFLECTIVE PRACTICE 9.6   Relatives' involvement in patient care

In the previous section there is discussion about the needs of relatives and the benefits of their participation in patient care. Is this an observation you have made?

Nurses in the community work with relatives to provide care in the last stages of life. If you work in hospital, a palliative care unit or in a nursing home, take time here to consider the group of relatives that are currently visiting patients or residents in your care.

Arrange to have a discussion with your colleagues to establish the benefits and difficulties encountered by staff and by relatives when families participate in both physical and psychological care of patients. When discussing this think about barriers that staff may put forward to create difficulties for relatives.

LIMITATIONS IN BEREAVEMENT RESEARCH

Bereavement is a multifactorial and complex issue. Many studies have been directed towards identifying risk factors and have achieved some success. Assessing the effectiveness of interventions has been more problematic. Conflicting results indicate the complexity of the subject. Structured quantitative methods have been favoured. Little research has considered how needs change over time. This highlights that a specific type of support offered at one stage in the mourning process might not be suitable at another stage. Because the variety of bereavement programmes offered rarely conform exactly to previous research studies, it is difficult to say with any certainty if the same positive results are being achieved. The literature suggests that many organisations develop their bereavement programmes on an *ad hoc* basis with minimal evaluation of their effectiveness.

Most of the studies cited have been carried out with widows and, to a lesser extent, widowers. It therefore may not be possible to extrapolate this data to other groups. Little is known about the effect of grief on parents, adult children and siblings, although some studies have concentrated on special types of losses (Osterweiss et al 1984).

One aspect of research that has not been pursued to any extent is families' perception of what they find helpful or unhelpful. Some semistructured interviews and questionnaires have identified areas that the bereaved have found to be either helpful or unhelpful (Bowling & Cartwright 1982, Maddison & Walker 1967, Vande-Creek 1988). These studies were of a semistructured nature and may not have allowed the participants to raise issues of significance to them.

BEREAVEMENT CARE

One of the authors conducted a small study to examine the bereavement support offered by a group of hospices in Scotland (V Smith, unpublished work, 1993). Data collected from three hospices indicated that although a wide variety of services were available, there was little uniformity between the hospices. Little attempt was made to assess the effectiveness of the support offered, or to question why people declined the support that was available. In the conclusion to the report, the following questions were raised:

- Were the relatives' needs being met?
- Was the support offered suitable?
- If the support was unsuitable, why was this the case?

Bereavement has been found to cause an increased risk of deterioration in both physical and mental health (Osterweiss et al 1984, Parkes 1986). The aim of any bereavement support service is to prevent, when possible, the detrimental consequences of bereavement. Lattanzi (1988) reminds us that 'we cannot take away people's pain but can offer to stand with them in some critical moments, giving them time and a human message that will encourage them to continue into the future'. He further suggests that to be effective, bereavement support services should have clear and achievable goals. For example they should:

- Provide information about the normal
- Enable grieving individuals to review and reflect upon their loss
- Assess individual coping ability, stress levels and available support
- Encourage bereaved individuals to use existing support systems or to create additional sources of support

A hospice, familiar to one of the authors, invested both considerable time and resources into establishing a bereavement service. All staff are offered training on loss and grief. Following training sessions staff are interviewed to assess their readiness to join the bereavement team. In keeping with Parkes' (1993) recommendation, staff in this hospice view bereavement care as an integral part of the overall support for patients and their 'family' group from time of first contact. Families are assessed informally and, where appropriate, a prebereavement care plan is implemented. This involves a member of the team being designated as the family key worker who befriends the family and continues to offer support following the bereavement. Support is tailored to meet the preferences of the bereaved persons and ranges from a telephone call or letter of invitation to group sessions held at the hospice. One-to-one support is available and bereaved individuals are encouraged to make contact with their key worker if and when a listening ear is needed. A monthly review includes an opportunity of supervision for the key worker, together with an evaluation of client progress.

Another example of a bereavement service offered by a hospice is a more formal one, comprising a two-member home care nursing team and a social worker. Four to 8 weeks after bereavement, relatives and friends are invited to attend group sessions on a fortnightly basis. An invitation is given to join a group for a maximum of six sessions, at any time during the first year of bereavement. One-to-one support is available for those who find group sessions unhelpful. Individual cases are reviewed through the hospice's weekly, multidisciplinary team meeting.

Some hospitals operate schemes that involve independent bereavement counsellors, social workers, clinical psychologists or the local mental health services. Community nurses and palliative care specialist nurses include early bereavement support for families as a recognised component of service they provide. Although this may be time-limited, it generally provides an opportunity to assess how different family members are coping.

Evaluation of bereavement support services has been mostly confined to those provided by hospices. Lattanzi-Litch (1989) examined the services offered by 266 hospices. Only 6.5% of the bereaved were referred to outside agencies. The success of hospice-delivered services is open to debate. Parkes (1980) reports that people who choose to participate in many of these services appear to find them helpful. Wilkes (1993) found that the commonest method of evaluation of bereavement services was the take-up of the service and the feedback from clients. Others believe that there is no definite research evidence to support their value (Osterweiss et al 1984).

Assessment of risk

Stroebe et al (1988) note that the important strength of any service provision is the assessment which drives it. The 'at risk' questionnaire developed by Parkes & Weiss (1983) has been extensively used at St Christopher's Hospice, London. It formed the basis of Parkes' (1981) evaluation study of the hospice bereavement service. This involved identifying those individuals most at risk of experiencing difficulty with their bereavement. In the Lattanzi-Litch (1989) study, 77% of hospices used a bereavement assessment tool. Those that did identify high-risk individuals, however, did not necessarily target their resources towards those individuals. Walshe (1997), from her review of assessment of grief, makes recommendations for provision of education about grief assessment, more careful timing for assessment and more careful selection of assessment tools.

■ REFLECTIVE PRACTICE 9.7   Continuity of support

Earlier in the chapter you were asked to select two families and to construct genograms to identify those members of a family who might have difficulties in bereavement.

• What provision did you make for the continued support of relatives?
• Would your colleagues agree to compile a protocol for assessing and meeting the needs of bereaved individuals?

A different approach will be needed, depending on where you work. The focus needs to be on referral to the primary care team, and acknowledgement ought to be given to the bereavement process beyond the acute period: this is generally accepted to be the first 2 to 3 months.

Once need has been identified, the type of support offered may vary between individuals. Parkes & Weiss (1983) warn that 'forms of intervention that are appropriate for one type of bereavement may be useless or even harmful in another'. Raphael & Nunn (1988) recommend that a therapeutic assessment be made prior to counselling. This enables a 'profile of bereavement coping and vulnerability' to guide a specific rationale for bereavement intervention.

Professional and social bereavement support

When appropriate support is offered to those at high risk of a complicated bereavement, morbidity is reduced. This was illustrated in Raphael's (1977) study involving 200 widows. Those at risk of post bereavement mortality were randomly allocated to either the intervention or non-intervention group. One-to-one counselling provided for the intervention group had a significant effect in lowering the morbidity when compared with the control group. In a similar study at St Christopher's Hospice, London, Parkes (1981) also found that when support was offered to selected high-risk bereaved families, they showed a significant improvement in health outcome when compared with a control group receiving no support. Other studies have shown less clear results and this may be attributed to the fact that the subjects in the studies conducted by Raphael (1977) and Parkes (1981) were restricted to high-risk individuals only.

Maddison (1968), in his study of widows, identified several factors that were consistently helpful or unhelpful for the poor bereavement outcome group. These included:

- Lack of permissive support
- Blocking the expression of their emotion
- Opposition of their wish to review the past and talk of their husbands
- Encouragement to take up new interests and even romantic relationships

This study demonstrates that adjustment depends, at least in part, on the survivor's perception of the environment. It makes no claims about the quantity of support provided or about the accuracy of the widows' perceptions. It must, however, be acknowledged that behaviour described as unhelpful during the first 3 months of bereavement may not be perceived so 12 months later.

In a structured telephone interview, widows and widowers reported to Vande-Creek (1988) that family, friends and neighbours were more helpful than professionals following the death of their spouses. Cartwright et al (1973) similarly found family and friends were identified as most supportive by a sample of elderly, bereaved widows. Both of these studies were carried out retrospectively, several months following the death, and therefore relied on the widow or widower's recollection of what occurred. These studies focus on the early phase of bereavement and therefore do not take into account the complete grief process. Parkes & Weiss (1983) also found that family support was important but suggested that the period of time the support was available was more significant than the number of people involved. This echoes the importance of informal support promoted in Chapter 4 of this book.

Group therapy or group sessions are provided by some organisations. Although the effectiveness of this has not been systematically tested, it is suggested that there is some improvement in those in groups with a high risk of poor bereavement outcome (Parkes 1980, Vachon & Stylianos 1988).

Volunteer and self-help programmes

Self-help groups are associations of people who come together for the specific purpose of sharing the same problem or life situation in order to benefit from mutual aid. Such groups are available to offer support to the bereaved and are often initiated by bereaved individuals and are directed towards people who have experienced a similar loss. Examples are CRUSE, Sudden Infant Death Support (SIDS) and Compassionate Friends. CRUSE is probably the most well-known voluntary bereavement organisation in the UK. It offers a combination of professional and volunteer support, including self-help groups.

Widows-to-widows programmes were first introduced by Silverman (1970) following his study with newly bereaved widows. Widows contacted each other to offer friendship and support. In some cases, contact was sustained for several years, developing into a lasting friendship. This has become a model for many subsequent self-help programmes. Prior to this study, doctors largely provided grief counselling, thus associating those requiring assistance with grief with 'mental illness'. In the initial period of bereavement, family, friends, clergy and funeral directors have a presence in offering support. Later, in the phase which Silverman calls 'recoil', many of those people have withdrawn by the time the impact of loss most affects the widow. Silverman & Silverman (1975) concluded that the most appropriate time to introduce interventions for bereaved individuals is about 6 weeks following the death. Many programmes are now available throughout the USA. Some are similar and others have evolved from the one developed by Silverman (Osterweiss et al 1984).

A systematic comparative study of self-help by Vachon et al (1980) showed a significantly improved adaptation to bereavement in the intervention group as compared with the control group. The intervention was initially in the form of personal contact by another widow who had fully adjusted following her bereavement. Later, the 'new' widow was introduced to an appropriate self-help group that was supervised by trained facilitators. Parkes (1980) reported that where there are trained facilitators leading groups the outcome is better.

One limitation of self-help groups is the appeal that most have to middle-income widowed people rather than to the lower income groups, who tend to be more at risk. Self-help groups are one aspect of bereavement support.

Support prior to bereavement

There is some evidence to suggest that support prior to bereavement has a place in reducing morbidity in the post-bereavement period. Less deterioration was reported in the health of relatives of patients who had been in the palliative care unit compared with relatives of patients from general wards. In the palliative care unit, family support was provided during the terminal stages of the illness and following the death of the patient. This was not the case in the general wards, where no specific support was offered to the family (Cameron & Parkes 1983, Ransford & Smith 1991). One criticism of these studies, however, is that the sample may have been biased because of the previous selection of patients who were transferred to the palliative care unit. Vachon (1988), in her literature review of counselling and psychotherapy in palliative/hospice care, suggests that there is little evidence in the form of documented evaluation to support the effectiveness of services. She urges that careful documentation of the evaluation of the psychological aspects of hospice care should be given serious consideration. Pottinger's (1991) study highlighted that the hospices which offered services to meet emotional needs of the bereaved were the most sought after by relatives. She did, however, offer a note of caution with regard to the expectations of support services, stating that although hospice staff can lessen the anxieties of the moment, the support offered may be not adequate to sustain the bereaved person in the longer term.

The time of death

The actual time of death is a particularly important stage in the bereavement process. Little research is available to discover what occurs at this time but it is a time that may have an impact on the relative's subsequent ability to cope. Cathcart (1988), for example, suggests that viewing the body is beneficial for the majority of close relatives. Useful information has been developed about how to cope with the bereaved relative at the time of death (Burgess 1992, Cathcart 1989, Clarke 1993). These are mostly guidelines and have been written from personal experience and anecdotal evidence. Some work has been carried out studying death in the accident and emergency department and the provision of support offered to bereaved relatives (Ashdown 1985, Burgess 1992). Tye (1993), in a self-administered, structured questionnaire, reviewed the nurses' perception of the needs of suddenly bereaved relatives. Although the nurses appeared to have an overall awareness of need, there were differences in their perceptions of helpfulness as compared with relatives in previous studies. Findlay & Dallimore (1991), in a study of bereaved parents in the accident and emergency department, found that 46% considered they had been dealt with unsympathetically and in some cases their overall needs had not been met. The literature suggests that improvements are being made into the care of bereaved relatives at the time of death (Burgess 1992), but more research is needed to determine what is happening in many situations and if relatives' needs are being met.

PERSONNEL INVOLVED IN BEREAVEMENT SUPPORT

A variety of personnel are involved in bereavement support – often a combination of professionals and volunteers (Parkes 1980). Lattanzi-Litch (1989) found that in 48% of hospices that employed a bereavement co-ordinator, the post holder was from a social work, nursing or clerical background and generally the ratio of volunteers to staff was four to one. In a study by Wilkes (1993) social workers, nurses and volunteers were found to be the key people offering support, with mention also of trained counsellors, psychologists and doctors in a few units.

Whereas Parkes (1981) recommends that training for volunteers is important in the provision of bereavement services, Silverman (1970) maintains that in the widow-to-widow programmes, professional training will alter the type of support provided. He suggests that volunteers assume professional values rather than the qualities of a befriender. In Lattanzi-Litch's (1989) study, despite the fact that 92% of hospices offered training to bereavement volunteers, little uniformity was found in the programmes. The training period varied from 2 to 40 hours. Wilkes (1993) made similar findings, with some units providing little or no training at all. This needs to be considered in the context of Parkes' (1981) suggestion that, following training, it takes volunteer counsellors about 1 year to become proficient.

CONSTRAINTS TO BEREAVEMENT SUPPORT

Although a range of bereavement support is offered by different organisations, Lattanzi-Litch (1989) and Wilkes (1993) identified a shortage of resources being linked with the difficulties for further development of bereavement services.

The conclusion from the literature review undertaken here suggests that the provision of a service for everyone who is bereaved would be extremely costly. Evidence shows that such a service would be of little benefit in reducing morbidity, except to some extent in the high-risk groups. Indeed, for some in the low-risk groups, intervention may even be harmful (Parkes & Weiss 1983, Vachon & Stylianos 1988). Most importantly, many people probably do not want or need help to deal with their emotions. Family and friends can provide sufficient support. It is questionable that self-selection for bereavement intervention is appropriate because those individuals at most risk of difficulties with their bereavement may not recognise the need or feel able to seek help (Vachon et al 1980).

■ REFLECTIVE PRACTICE 9.8   Bereavement support

The data presented above refers to Lattanzi-Litch's (1989) study where the funding for health care is different from the UK.

- To what extent however, do the factors identified above compare with your situation?
- What could be done to overcome any obstacles?

In 1991 an SHHD (Scottish Home and Health Department) report, 'Everybody's death should matter to somebody', prompted action from the SHHD. Task forces were initiated in all Health Board areas in Scotland to examine ways of supporting dying patients and their relatives. A subsequent SHHD report, 'Arrangements for the care of the dying and bereaved', was published in March 1997. This details the response from different Health Boards and is recommended to you for further reading.

For most people, bereavement is a normal process and therefore an emphasis on intervention could medicalise this normal process. Evaluation of bereavement service offered is important in the current climate of quality assurance and audit. To date, no studies appear to have been carried out to consider the costs and benefits of bereavement support.

Important factors in a bereavement support service

Overall, it appears that bereavement support is of use to some people in certain circumstances. The following factors are important in the provision of bereavement services.

- Assessment of need is a key element
- A close social network is the most appropriate way to give support immediately following the bereavement
- The support of family and friends should be sufficient for people who experience normal reactions to the loss
- One-to-one support from someone who has experience of bereavement may be useful several weeks after the bereavement
- Support groups are more appropriate several months after the bereavement
- Formal programmes in the early stages of bereavement may be helpful for high-risk groups
- Psychotherapeutic interventions may be warranted for those who display particular difficulties

THE NURSING ROLE

Against a background of research, which has apparently failed to examine what bereaved individuals consider to be helpful both around the time of death and in the immediate post-death period, we are faced with the task of offering a framework to nurses to help with this very task.

The UK is a death-denying society that risks medicalising the normal processes of dying and bereavement. Grief is thought of as a process to get through as quickly and as quietly as possible. Faulkner (1995) points out that difficulties arise because society's expectations about the perceived loss can sometimes be at odds with the individual's perspective. Many rituals around this significant time, for family and friends, have disappeared, leaving a bereaved individual isolated and often confused about the feelings they have. Some people experience more difficulties than others, but with support the bereaved individual can survive the death and adjust to a new life. Nurses need to recognise this and be prepared to help individuals (before and after bereavement, and in different contexts) for as long as support is required. To achieve this nurses also need to appreciate that individuals will respond or react differently. They need to:

- Understand what grieving means for individuals
- Recognise when people are grieving
- Be prepared to spend time with people who are grieving

- Identify factors that may give rise to a problematic bereavement
- Recognise the strengths and limitations in their skills and advise patients about other agencies appropriate to an individual's assessed needs

Bereavement and health

Health has been described as not so much a definition as a way of life, or a pursuit of well-being (Jackson 1989). Simnett (1995) describes 'health promotion' as an umbrella term for a range of activities. The two funda- mental aims are:

- To improve health and well-being
- To empower people and communities to take charge of aspects of their lives that affect their health

So, what is the relationship between health promotion and bereavement care and palliative care? Health is a political issue as are mortality statistics. Increased morbidity and mortality are related to bereavement. It therefore seems logical to consider the care of bereaved individuals in the context of health promotion. The hospice movement since inception has promoted the idea of living with progressive disease and with maintaining independence, if not in physical, certainly in psychological terms. Whilst recognising that the emotional and physical debility imposed by bereavement creates a temporary deviation from well-being, there can be no doubt that the out- come is for return to health and, for some, to improved health.

It is not the remit of this chapter to consider health promotion in a broader concept but it is perhaps worth mentioning that society's attitude towards death may have a significant influence on bereavement outcome. So long as death is seen as a totally negative experience, to be avoided at all costs and pushed into the background, the process of grief will be seen as something to fear and avoid. If death can have a more central place in society, perhaps the process of grief can be better understood and accepted. This would allow the bereaved to have some time and space to move at their own pace and in their own way through their grief. It is in this broader context of health and bereavement that health promotion has a valuable place.

PRINCIPLES OF NURSING INTERVENTIONS FOR DEALING WITH LOSS

Care of the bereaved must start before bereavement and will result in the prevention of psychiatric and physical disorders (Parkes 1993). This means being honest with families and informing them of situations as, when and before they happen. Parkes (1993) recommends that there should be regular discussions of family problems in which the multidisciplinary team present their findings and assessments of the families. This guarantees that the family remains the focus of care. It encourages the multidisciplinary team to develop the interest, knowledge and skills to ensure high-level, expert care (Parkes 1993). Important principles that underpin nursing intervention will be discussed here. In particular we will draw together the needs of relatives, as identified by Hampe (1975), the competencies that Benner (1984) identified in the helping role of the nurse and the tasks that Worden (1991) suggests that the bereaved individual needs to work through during the process of bereavement.

■ **BOX 9.2**

A model of helping

Relatives of dying patients need to be:

- With the dying person for as long, and whenever, they wish
- Helped to care for physical needs
- Assured of the comfort of the patient
- Kept informed about care plans and impending death
- Able to express emotion with others, and have comfort and support from relatives and friends
- Offered acceptance, support and comfort from health care staff

Resolution of bereavement requires that an individual:

- Accepts the reality of the loss
- Works through the pain of grief
- Adjusts to an environment in which the deceased is missing
- Emotionally relocates the deceased and moves on with life

Nurses involved in 'helping' require to be competent in:

- Creating a climate for establishing healing, marshalling any appropriate agency to help at different points along the journey to rehabilitation
- Providing comfort measures and preserving person-hood in the face of pain and extreme breakdown
- Being with a relative
- Maximising the relative's participation and control in his future
- Providing comfort and communication through touch
- Providing emotional and informational support
- Guiding the person through emotional and developmental change – providing new options, closing off old ones
- Teaching and mediating – using goals therapeutically

Using a model of helping to achieve the tasks of mourning

People need permission to experience the magnitude of their loss and to explore their own mechanisms of coping. Worden's (1991) tasks of bereavement present a framework to enable people to work through the various stages of mourning. Alongside the grieving individual, nurses have an important role in assessing 'at-risk' criteria and in offering support through effective helping skills before and following bereavement.

■ **CASE HISTORY 9.1** **Grace and Janet**

Grace was 86 years old and had lived with the effects of Alzheimer's disease for 10 years. She had spent the last 2 years in a nursing home during which time her physical health and cognitive abilities had deteriorated. Her daughter Janet, a nurse, had maintained a close, loving relationship with her mother. As a result of successive transient ischaemic episodes, Grace was aphasic. Despite this there was a very special bond and an exceptional non-verbal communication rapport between mother and daughter.

Nursing home staff systematically adjusted their input to accommodate the needs of Janet, who continued a high level of input into her mother's care. This involved complementing her mother's attempts to fulfil activities of daily living. Throughout the 2 years that Grace had been in the nursing home, nurses facilitated continuity of care between her frequent visits home and the nursing home. Janet held on to the aim to grant her mother's wish to die at home. Nursing home, GP and community staff were all prepared to accommodate this wish, provided that appropriate circumstances existed.

One day following her return from home, nursing staff became concerned about Grace who was febrile and listless. Her daughter visited, prepared as usual to feed Grace her evening meal. Instead, Janet gave her a drink and settled her mother early for the night. A further deterioration happened overnight and prompted staff to alert Janet to the imminent death of her mother.

Staff were in agreement to relinquish as much of Grace's care as possible according to Janet's wishes. Other family members were contacted. Janet's niece, Lucy, was recognised as her main support. During the following few days until Grace's death, Janet spent many hours attending to her mother's needs, taking respite when other family members visited. Janet negotiated with nursing staff and the GP for suitable analgesia and anxiety-relieving medication for her mother. Staff of the nursing home took on the role of visitors to Grace and provided relief and support to Janet. Kim, Grace's former dog, stayed alongside and provided much needed comfort during the day and night. Grace died peacefully one evening in the presence of Janet, Lucy, Karen (Lucy's 6-year-old daughter) and Kim (the dog).

As Grace died, Lucy's 6-year-old daughter was watching a favourite television programme and was oblivious to the events in the room. An almost tangible feeling of peace prevailed; Karen turned away from the television and after one or two glances towards her great grandmother approached her in her usual fashion, kissed her 'gran' and said good night.

After a few minutes of private grief shared with Lucy, Janet informed the nursing home staff that her mother had died.

This scenario describes the experience of a daughter. Her needs are similar to those identified in Hampe's study. Also evident in the nursing home staff are the competencies that Benner identified in her helping role described above in this chapter.

■ **CASE HISTORY 9.2 Anne**

Anne arrived at the health centre and asked to see the practice nurse. With some embarrassment she told the practice nurse that her dog had died. Her dog had been a constant companion and without him she felt that she could not cope. Further exploration revealed a number of traumatic losses over a period of 5 years. Her father had died 3 years ago, following a lengthy progressive deterioration of multiple sclerosis. Anne had been her mother's mainstay during that time. This had not been realised by primary care staff when Anne herself had undergone chemotherapy following the diagnosis of breast cancer 18 months previously. Nor was it known that Anne's mother had died suddenly 6 months ago. The impact of Anne's grief had placed an enormous strain on a relationship resulting in her fiancée ending their engagement. Anne's dog had been killed in a road accident the day prior to her visit to the health centre.

This woman is currently working through Worden's second task of mourning. The fact that she has sought help indicates a need to express her grief. There are multiple losses here and she will be responding to all of them in different ways. It needs to be remembered that each new loss triggers memories and any unfinished business in previous losses. The nature and intensity of the relationships in previous 'loss situations' needs to be considered along with the nature and intensity of the relationship with the dog. One can speculate about a huge mixture of feelings here. It is quite usual for people to say, 'I don't know how I am going to live without …' and for some to say, 'I want to be with …'

■ **REFLECTIVE PRACTICE 9.9 Helping the bereaved**

In the above scenario there are a number of compounding factors – distressing deaths of parents, a diagnosis of a potentially fatal illness and the rejection of her fiancée.

• How should the practice nurse proceed?

SUMMARY

The study of bereavement is vast and to cover all aspects is beyond the scope of one chapter. There has, however, been a conscious effort on behalf of the authors to facilitate the application of research to the clinical situation. The introductions of the two case histories at the end of this chapter demonstrate such an integration of theory and practice. Both case histories are descriptions of real situations with names and some of the circumstances changed to protect anonymity.

It has been our intention to bring to the attention of readers, no matter the clinical context of work, that:

- Bereavement affects all of us at some time in our life
- It is usually a normal, healthy process
- It is possible to identify factors that might render a person vulnerable during a bereavement
- There are identifiable skills, within the nurses' role, which can be used to assist people before, during and following the death of a significant person
- Every nurse has a role to play in assisting people through a normal bereavement.
- Some bereavements prove to be more complicated and require referral for specialist help

REFERENCES

Allan J D, Hall B A 1988 Between diagnosis and death: the case for studying grief before death. Archives of Psychiatric Nursing 2: 30–34

Ashdown M 1985 Sudden death. Nursing Mirror 161: 22–24

Averill J R, Nunley E P 1988 Grief as an emotion and as a disease: a social constructivist perspective. Journal of Social Issues 44: 79–95

Bailey R, Clarke M 1989 Stress and coping in nursing. Chapman Hall, London

Bass M D, Bowen K 1990 The transition from caregiving to bereavement: the relationship of care related strain and adjustment to death. Gerontologist 30: 35–42

Benner P 1984 From novice to expert. Addison Wesley, New York

Berger R 1988 Learning to survive and cope with human loss. Social Work Today April 24: 14–17

Bowen M 1978 Family therapy in clinical practice. Jason Aronson, New York

Bowlby J 1980 Attachment and loss, Vol. 3. Loss sadness and depression. Penguin, London

Bowling A, Cartwright A 1982 Life after death: study of elderly widows. Tavistock, London

Breibart W, Passik S 1993 Psychiatric aspects of palliative care. In: Doyle D, Hanks G, Macdonald N (eds) Oxford Textbook of Palliative Medicine. Oxford Medical Press, Oxford, pp 244–256

Burgess K 1992 Supporting bereaved relatives in A and E. Nursing Standard 6: 36–39

Cameron J, Parkes C M 1983 Terminal care: evaluation of effects on surviving family of care before and after bereavement. Postgraduate Medical Journal 59: 73–78

Caplan G 1981 Mastery of stress: psychosocial aspects. The American Journal of Psychiatry 138: 413–420

Carter S L 1989 Themes of grief. Nursing Research 386: 345–358

Cartwright A, Hockey L, Anderson J C L 1973 Life before death. Routledge & Kegan Paul, London

Cathcart F 1988 Seeing the body after death. British Medical Journal 297: 997–998

Cathcart F 1989 Coping with distress. Nursing Times 85: 33–35

Clarke J 1993 The day after a death. Nursing Times 89: 46–47

Dobson S 1989 Genograms and ecomaps. Nursing Times 85: 54–56

Dracup K A, Breu D S 1978 Using nursing research findings to meet the needs of grieving spouses. Nursing Research 27: 212–213

Dykstra R 1989 She never said goodbye. Highland Books, Suffolk

Emerson P 1977 Covert grief reactions in mentally retarded adults. Mental Retard 6c: 46–47

Engel G L 1961 Is grief a disease? Psychosomatic Medicine 23: 18–22

Faulkner A 1995 Working with bereaved people. Churchill Livingstone, Edinburgh

Findlay I, Dallimore D 1991 Your child is dead. British Medical Journal 302: 1524–1525

Freihofer P, Felton G 1976 Nursing behaviours in bereavement: an exploratory study. Nursing Research 25: 332–337

Gallagher-Thompson D et al 1993 The impact of spousal bereavement on older widows and widowers. In Stroebe M, Stroebe W, Hansson R O. Handbook of bereavement, Cambridge University Press, Cambridge

Glazer H R, Clark M D 1997 Parenting classes as part of a hospice bereavement program. Hospice Journal 12: 22–40

Gorer G 1965 Death, grief and mourning in contemporary Britain. Tavistock, London

Hampe S O 1975 The needs of the grieving spouse in a hospital setting. Nursing Research 24: 113–120

Hinds C 1992 Suffering: a relatively unexplored phenomenon among family care givers on non institutionalised patients with cancer. Journal of Advanced Nursing 17: 918–925

Hull M M 1991 Hospice nurses caring support for 'caregiving families'. Cancer Nursing 14: 63–70

Jackson M O 1989 Paths towards a clearing: radical empiricism and ethnography inquiry. Indiana University Press, Bloominton

Kitching N 1987 Helping people with mental handicap: a case study with discussion. Journal of the British Institute of Mental Handicap 15: 60–63

Klass D, Silverman P, Nickman S (eds) 1996 Continuing bonds: new understandings of grief. Taylor and Francis, Bristol

Kubler Ross E 1970 On death and dying. Tavistock, London

Lattanzi-Litch M 1988 The voice of clinical and personal experience. Journal of Palliative Care 4: 81–83

Lattanzi-Litch M 1989 Bereavement services: practices and problems. Hospice Journal 5: 1–28

Lewis C S 1966 A grief observed. Faber, London

Lindemann E 1944 Symptomatology and management of acute grief. American Journal of Psychiatry 101: 141–148

Lopata H Z 1979 Women as widows. Elsevier, New York

Maddison D 1968 The relevance of conjugal bereavement. Psychiatry 41: 223–233

Maddison D, Walker W L 1967 Factors affecting the outcome of conjugal bereavement. British Journal of Medial Psychology 113: 1057–1067

Marris P 1958 Widows and their families. Routledge & Kegan Paul, London

Marris P 1986 Loss and change, 2nd edn. Routledge & Kegan Paul, London

Murgatroyd S, Wolfe R 1982 Coping with crisis. Open University Press, Milton Keynes

Neuberger J 1987 Caring for dying of different faiths. Lisa Sainsbury Foundation, London

Osterweiss M, Solomon F, Green M (eds) 1984 Bereavement: reactions, consequences and care. National Academy Press, Washington DC

Oswin M 1981 Bereavement and mentally handicapped people: a discussion paper. Kings Fund Centre, London

Parkes C M 1972 Bereavement studies of grief in adult life. Tavistock, London

Parkes C M 1975 Determinants of outcome following bereavement Omega 6: 303–323

Parkes C M 1980 Bereavement counselling: does it work? British Medical Journal 5th July: 3–6

Parkes C M 1981 Evaluation of a bereavement service. Journal of Preventative Psychiatry 1: 179–188

Parkes C M 1986 Bereavement. Penguin, London

Parkes C M 1993 Bereavement. In Doyle D, Hanks G, Macdonald N (eds) Oxford textbook of palliative medicine. Oxford Medical Press, Oxford

Parkes C M, Weiss R S 1983 Recovery from bereavement. Basic Books, New York

Penson J 1990 Bereavement: a guide for nurses. Harper Row, London

Pottinger A M 1991 Grieving relatives: perceptions of their needs and adjustment in a continuing care unit. Palliative Medicine 5: 117–121

Ransford H E, Smith M L 1991 Grief resolution among the bereaved in hospice and hospital wards. Social Science and Medicine 32: 295–304

Raphael B 1977 Preventative intervention with the recently bereaved. Archives of General Psychiatry 34: 1450–1454

Raphael B 1984 Anatomy of bereavement. Basic Books, New York

Raphael B, Nunn K 1988 Counselling the bereaved. Journal of Social Issues 44: 191–206

Roberston B J, Jay J, Welche S 1997 Can data collection during the grieving process be justifiable? British Journal of Nursing 6: 759–764

Sanders C M 1988 Risk factors in bereavement outcome. Journal of Social Issues 44: 97–112

Schowalter J E 1975 In: Schoenberg B (ed) Bereavement: its psychosocial aspects. Columbia University Press, New York

Silverman P R 1970 The widow as a caregiver in a program of prevention with other widows. Mental Hygiene 54: 540–547

Silverman P R, Silverman S M 1975 In: Schoenberg B (ed) Bereavement: its psychological aspects. Columbia University Press, New York

Simnett I 1995 Managing health promotion: developing healthy organisations and communities. Wiley & Sons, London

Stedeford A 1981 Couples facing death: unsatisfactory communication. British Medical Journal 283: 1098–1110

Stokes J, Wyer S, Crossley D 1997 The challenge of evaluating a child bereavement programme. Palliative Medicine 11: 179–190

Strachan R 1981 Reaction to bereavement: a study of a group of mentally handicapped hospital residents. Journal of British Institute of the Mentally Handicapped 9: 20–21

Stroebe M, Stroebe W, Domittner A 1988 Individual and situational differences in recovery from bereavement: a risk group identified. Journal of Social Issues 44: 143–158

Stroebe M, Gergen M, Gergen K, Stroebe W 1993 Broken hearts of broken bonds. American Psychologist 47: 1205–1212

Sutherland V J, Cooper C L 1990 Understanding stress: a psychological perspective for health professionals. Chapman & Hall, London

Sweeting H, Gilhooly M 1990 Anticipatory grief: a review. Social Science and Medicine 30: 1073–1080

Tuffrey-Wijne I 1997 Bereavement in people with learning disabilities. European Journal of Palliative Care 4: 170–173

Tye C 1993 Qualified nurses' perspectives of the needs of suddenly bereaved family members in the accident and emergency department. Journal of Advanced Nursing 18: 948–956

Vachon M L S, Lyall W A L, Rogers J, Freedman-Letofskky J, Freeman S J J 1980 A controlled study of self help intervention for widows. American Journal of Psychiatry 137: 1380–1384

Vachon M L S, Sheldon A R, Lancee W J, Lyall W A L, Rogers J, Freeman S J J 1982a Correlates of enduring distress in bereavement; social network, life situation and personality. Psychological Medicine 12: 783–788

Vachon M L S, Sheldon A R, Lancee W J, Lyall W A L, Roger J, Freeman S J J 1982b Predictors and correlates of adaptation to conjugal bereavement. American Journal of Psychiatry 139: 998–1002

Vachon M L S, Stylianos K L 1988 The role of social support in bereavement. Journal of Social Issues 44: 175–190

VandeCreek L 1988 Sources of support in conjugal bereavement. Hospice Journal 4: 81–92

Walshe C 1997 Whom to help: an exploration of the assessment of grief. International Journal of Palliative Nursing 3: 132–137

Walters T 1996 A new model for grief: bereavement and biography. Mortality 1: 7–25

Weismann A D 1979 Coping with cancer. McGraw Hill Book Company, New York

Welch D 1982 Anticipatory grief: reactions in family members of adult patients. Issues in Mental Health Nursing 4: 149–158

Wertheimer A 1991 A special scar. Routledge, London

Wilkes E 1993 Characteristics of hospice bereavement services. Journal of Cancer Care 2: 183–189

Worden W 1991 Grief counselling and grief therapy: a handbook for the mental health practitioner. Routledge, London

WHO 1990 Cancer pain relief and palliative care. Technical Report series 804, World Health Organization, Geneva

USEFUL ADDRESSES

CRUSE
126 Sheen Road
Richmond
Surrey TW9 1UR
0181 940 4818 (administration)
0181 332 7227 (CRUSE bereavement line)

The Compassionate Friends
53 North Street
Bristol BS3 1EN
01272 539639

London Association of Bereavement Services
365 Holloway Road
London N7 6PN
0171 700 8134

Ethical issues

10

Sally Lawton   Dorothy Cyster

ETHICS AND PALLIATIVE CARE

The purpose of this chapter is to discuss some of the everyday ethical issues that may arise in palliative care nursing. Through the description of three case histories, various ethical principles and theories will be explored, giving the reader an opportunity to apply theoretical, ethical frameworks to particular situations.

It is anticipated that this chapter will enable the development of the knowledge, skills and attitudes that are required in ethical decision-making. However, the chapter does not intend to provide the reader with easy solutions to ethical problems faced by nurses in palliative care settings. In fact, it may raise more questions than answers. The study of ethics encourages us to look at a particular problem from all angles before making a considered decision. As there are often no straightforward answers, this decision-making process may leave you rather unsettled and confused, but in the process you will have considered a range of possible solutions.

LEARNING OUTCOMES

We consider that this chapter addresses the PREP categories of care enhancement and patient, client and colleague support. By the time that you have read this chapter, you should be able to:

- Define the term 'ethics' and its relevance to palliative care
- Identify ethical issues that arise in palliative care settings
- Develop your problem-solving skills to enhance nursing care

DEFINING ETHICS IN PALLIATIVE NURSING

It may be difficult to offer a definition of ethics in palliative nursing settings that accurately reflects its relationship to everyday nursing practice. A dictionary definition of ethics may link it to the study of morals, but, for many of us, 'morality' is not an issue that is thought about on a daily basis. A further definition of morals states that it is a distinction between right and wrong, the power of distinguishing between right and wrong and the requirements to which right action must conform (Allen 1990). This suggests that to understand morals and ethics, the person has to have some knowledge of a decision-making process as well as knowing what may be right or wrong in any given situation. As there are so many interpretations of what is 'right' or 'wrong', one of the difficulties in the study of ethics is appreciating the range of views that individuals may hold.

Just as a definition of ethics may be difficult, ethical and moral problems may also be hard to define. Aroskar (1989) suggests that an ethical problem is more than an issue of making a difficult choice. It is defined as 'those problems in professional practice in which there is a conflict about the morally right action to take or in which the duties and obligations of health care professionals are unclear'.

When questions such as 'What should I do now?' start to be asked, perhaps it is a sign of an ethical problem, as noted by Omery (1991). An ethical problem could lead to a choice having to be made between two equally unsatisfactory alternatives. Each alternative would involve sacrificing a principle.

Ethical problems are often problems of communication. They are created and solved by communication. In such circumstances, there is room for reasonable disagreement. Duncan's (1992) study confirmed this view when ethical problems were investigated. Interprofessional communication was one of the key issues raised that was identified by the sample. Furthermore, Rodney (1989) identified the feeling of senselessness in nurses when faced with decisions that had been made without any consultation of the team or interaction with relatives of patients. This reflects the lack of influence that the nurse may have within a team and the need for increased teamwork. As it may be the nurse who spends the greatest amount of time with a patient, decision-making without involving the nurse may mean that an important contribution is missed. Also, divisions may appear within the team about the particular role that each member may play. This is evident in the literature on ethics and also with the division made between medical and nursing ethics. This division seems to have occurred largely for historical reasons, stemming from the USA in the 1980s when nurses were attempting to gain professional status and a greater degree of autonomy from the medical profession. It was stated that nursing had its own professional ethical code. However, this division is unnecessary and unhelpful as ethical issues, like care issues, cut across disciplines. Health care workers increasingly depend on team work. Shared care means shared responsibility and shared moral values. Scott (1995) and Seedhouse (1988) have advocated the need to focus on the ethics of caring within health work rather than continuing such differences. 'Shared care presumably means shared responsibility for care and this should encompass shared morals, as well as clinical responsibility [Scott 1995].' If the patient is the central focus of care, then the ethics of caring can be promoted. This is particularly relevant in the nursing of patients who are reaching the end of their lives. At an everyday level, the nurse working with patients in palliative care settings may be more aware of the different focus of care that regards death as a normal life event. However, there may still be many decisions that have to be faced, which prove to be problematic; some examples of ethical problems are shown in Box 10.1.

■ **BOX 10.1**

Examples of ethical problems
- Divided loyalties, e.g. 'whistle-blowing'
- Conflicts of interest, e.g. participation in research
- Conspiracies – interprofessional rivalry where the patient is not involved in the decision-making process

---

Writers such as Allmark (1992) and Seedhouse (1988) have argued that health care (and therefore nursing) is an ethical concern in itself because of the continual interaction with fellow humans.

In the rapidly changing health care environment, the process of decision-making may be increasingly complex, adding to the pressures that nurses and other health care workers face daily. In addition, the growing awareness of ethico-legal issues suggest a need for decisions to be based on sound reason in order to (potentially) be justified at a later date. Patients and clients are more aware of their 'rights' and are encouraged to be autonomous. This has been exemplified in the 1990s with the development of government initiatives, such as the Patient's Charter. This document sets out expected levels of service, how to access such services and where to obtain information. This is not a new phenomenon in palliative care. The 'Dying person's bill of rights' (anon) addressed such issues, highlighting the need for respect, individuality and truthfulness in the final stages of an illness.

ETHICS IN PALLIATIVE NURSING

Patients in palliative care settings may be particularly vulnerable to decisions about their future care. In such situations, the nurse may find that the decision-making process does not fully involve the patient. Through the development of the moral imagination, the nurse develops an ability to empathise with patients; this therefore improves communication skills, which is essential in palliative care settings, and may help the patient and her family make an informed decision about her care at a difficult time. We suggest that there are many issues to consider, but we are focusing on advocacy and autonomy, caring, respect, justice as fairness and trust.

Advocacy and autonomy

Patient advocacy would be difficult to achieve if the nurse had no ability to rationalise problems and settings with the patient. Having knowledge of ethical decision-making would enable the nurse to develop respect for the individual's choices, especially if they differ from the nurse's or other health carers' personal views. In the three case histories that are presented in this chapter, the issue of patient advocacy is a central feature. In general discussion, the role of nurses (amongst others) as patient advocates is often raised without question. However, the concept of advocacy begs further investigation.

The nurse may act in a supportive role and as an advocate for the patient as they reach their own level of autonomy. Kendrick (1994) also noted that advocacy should 'reflect the patient's interpretation of his or her own best interests'.

The challenge in this is that, at times, patients may choose to do things their way, making choices that reflect different values from those held by the nurse. This highlights the notion of autonomy. Beauchamp & Childress (1983) define an autonomous person as someone who 'determines his or her course of action in accordance with a chosen plan by himself'. This reflects the right of the patient to choose how to live.

However, Penn (1994) has commented on the fact that some patients may not want to become autonomous, especially in life-threatening situations. This provision of autonomy may add to the stress already faced by the individual.

Consider, for a moment, the 'rights' of a person in choosing where they would like to die. The patient may wish to die at home, but the relatives may be distressed at such a thought. This is unsurprising in today's society where the health care system has become the main care agency at the beginning and the end of most people's lives. What is the role of the nurse in this situation? If it is one of advocacy, then whose advocate should she be? If she is purely the patient's advocate, can resources be guaranteed and justified for the support that the family might need?

The nurse may feel that the situation at home is not suitable for the patient's needs, but if the patient wants to stay at home, can the nurse deny this? In another situation, the carers may want to keep the patient at home without realising the implications and the demands that this may place on them. Is a nurse able to give enough information about the likely progress of an illness without terrifying the relatives? In such situations, the illness may become the focus of the whole life of the family, causing additional stress and tension among other family members. Again, it has to be questioned how a decision, respecting the views of all concerned, can be made in such situations.

■ REFLECTIVE PRACTICE 10.1   The nurse as an advocate

Write down three examples of when you have acted or would act as a patient's advocate in a palliative care setting.

The developing role of the nurse places issues of accountability and responsibility for actions on the individual practitioner. Such developments have been endorsed in UKCC documents such as the 'Scope of professional practice' (1994), 'Guidelines for professional practice' (1996) and the 'Post registration education programme' (1990). One of the outcomes of these professional developments means that we can no longer 'pass the buck' to our medical colleagues and leave them to grapple with the problem to find a solution. However, this may be an uncomfortable development for some nurses who may have felt less responsible for decision-making.

Caring

The central focus of ethical decision-making and its links to caring further confirms the need to develop some understanding of the central links between ethics and caring. This is supported by Wells (1988) who wrote:

> *Just as nurses have a responsibility to offer appropriate and meaningful care to the sick, so also is it incumbent upon them to protect human rights and those values which help make them. Not to recognise that sick people have inalienable rights is ultimately to deny those rights to ourselves.*

In everyday language, this may be referred to as 'doing as you would be done by'. While this seems fairly straightforward in theory, what does it actually mean in practice?

■ REFLECTIVE PRACTICE 10.2   Caring

What does the maxim 'do as you would be done by' mean to you as a person and in your professional role within palliative care settings?

If you have thought about issues such as being treated fairly, being shown respect and dignity as an individual and not being excluded from care because of your age, gender, religious or cultural background, and being kept fully informed about issues that relate to you, then you are identifying ethical principles. We will now discuss these principles in more detail.

ETHICAL PRINCIPLES

Writers such as Beauchamp & Childress (1983) would classify the concepts mentioned above as ethical principles as follows:

- Respect for person
- Justice as fairness
- Doing good when acting in the best interests of the patient (beneficence) and not doing harm (non-maleficence)

Such principles are the foundation of nursing and personal moral guidelines. In this context, then, caring for others also means caring for ourselves and acknowledging the importance of ethical principles and theory. Indeed, if the UKCC (1992) 'Code of professional conduct' is studied, such ethical principles guide its clauses. However, as Chadwick & Todd (1992) note, the Code cannot make a decision in an individual situation. This supports the idea of developing knowledge about ethical frameworks.

Role conflicts can occur as the nurse can have a number of roles in life, for example, manager and citizen as well as nurse. If considered in more depth, these principles address a wide range of issues. For example, respect for persons would include autonomy, dignity, being non-judgemental, keeping a person fully informed, obtaining full informed consent, advocacy and truth-telling. Doing good and not doing harm would apply in issues such as obtaining informed consent for treatment or research, truth-telling and the protection of a person from harm.

Respect

At a simple level, respect for persons includes considering the labels that are used to describe people. How do you think respect is altered if a patient is called by her condition, rather than by her name. To hear a nurse say 'We've got an obstruction coming into the ward' sounds more like a traffic hold-up rather than a person in great pain with a life-threatening condition. If we consider how quickly patients adopt a passive role when they are admitted to hospital, the sense of self may well be lost in the process, especially if they are in great pain, in distress or experiencing great fear.

Issues that should *not* interfere with the caring dimension include how likeable the patient is and how responsible the nurse feels that the patient is for his condition. This culpability was raised as an ethical issue by Omery (1991). In this study, the patients were seen as being responsible for their illnesses, which made the nurses question whether they were deserving of care. This would contravene the ethical principles outlined above with specific regard to respect of the individual.

Respect and caring are vital elements of the role of the health care worker in palliative care settings. Such elements reflect the central role of the patient. As McGee (1994) said 'nursing care without respect dehumanises people, but it could be argued that respect is difficult to define, although it is a term regularly used. We see it as valuing the view of an individual. This is contrary to the superficial knowledge about people that we sometimes hold and consequently base our judgements on.

Another aspect of respect is maintaining confidentiality. In the community setting, it can be easy to be drawn into conversation unwittingly about a patient. Your arrival at a house may be seen by a few people and sometimes you find a neighbour waiting by the car to 'have a wee word' with you. While most of this is done for genuine reason and concern, it can place the nurse in a difficult position when trying to avoid the discussion of confidential issues.

In addition, it also has implications for the keeping of accurate records in the home and hospital setting as you have to consider who might be reading them. Similarly, in the hospital setting, confidential information is often exchanged behind curtains, which are not soundproof.

In other situations, the patient may be labelled as a 'victim' of a particular condition and, rather than be respected, be pitied. Within such a high technologically based health care system, dying, it could be argued, is the ultimate sign of failure. If the system is focused on cure and survival, then having to face issues of mortality are bound to place additional stress on the providers of care, the family and the patient. In addition, patients who are not responding to treatment may be made to feel guilty by staff whose aims of treatment are curative.

Justice as fairness

Justice as fairness would incorporate equity in accessing care in the health context as well as considering the quality of a person's life. In this definition, justice encompasses equal respect for a person's rights as well as being aware of legal implications. There is a link between the notion of respect for the individual and trying to promote the quality of a patient's life. Within the health care system, the quality of life may be assessed in a systematic way using a tool such as the quality adjusted life years scale (QALYS). This may then determine whether a particular treatment will be used, based on the likely outcome, and may be used to distribute rationed care. However, it has to be questioned whether the advance of the consumerist and technological society has meant that there is an expectation that no-one should die and that everyone, no matter how ill, should have the 'right' to treatment and life. It almost appears as if the general public have never been aware of the finite nature of resources in the NHS or that such developments in health care treatment are relatively recent.

Jeffrey (1993) has argued that the use of QALYS is questionable in advanced palliative care because QALYS measures physical health alone. How the person determines their quality of life also includes psychological, social and spiritual factors. Who is in the best position to decide a patient's quality of life within a system of finite resources? Is it possible to maintain the ethical principle of justice, meaning equal access to any resources in such a system?

Perhaps this challenge to the purely physical basis of care rationing was shown in the recent publicity given to the Child B case in the autumn of 1995. This child, who had a complicated form of leukaemia, was denied treatment by a health authority. Her father took the case to the High Court in an effort to overturn the decision that, he argued, was made on economic, rather than clinical grounds.

In the event, an anonymous benefactor paid the £75 000 for her treatment in a private hospital. The publicity grew when he went to court again, in October 1995, to enable her identity to be made known. Through the media, this child spoke about her fight against her illness and the battle for survival. She died in May 1996, again with much publicity. This aptly summarises the public notion about the 'fight' against illness, and particularly cancer, which is often described as a battle. Does this reinforce the notions of death being a sign of failure? What effect may this attitude have on a patient who feels too weary to 'fight' and what is the role of the nurse in such situations? This particular case also highlights the feeling within the general public and the media that the health care system has a duty to provide treatment.

Trust

Nursing theorists, such as Watson (1989), have written about the importance of developing a helping relationship that is based on trust. If a patient loses trust in the nurse or the health care system, then it could be argued that he may become more vulnerable as he will not know when someone is being honest with him. This notion of trust is closely linked to respect. We would argue that trust and respect have to be developed over time and are relevant, especially when nursing patients in the final stages of an illness. If that trust is broken, then it may be impossible to regain it.

■ REFLECTIVE PRACTICE 10.3   Palliative care services

Do you know what palliative care services are available locally and nationally for patients? If not, seek out the nearest palliative care service and find out what might be available should a patient with advanced disease, in your care, require more help than can be provided by your professional team.

ETHICAL THEORY

The ethical principles outlined above may be interpreted in ethical theory through a number of different approaches. The first approach is known as 'deontology', which can be defined as the notion of duty or doing what is right. When considering the ethical principle of truth-telling, for example, deontologists would view truth as important, regardless of the situation. They would argue that it is important to always tell the truth. Through the consideration of ethics in contemporary nursing, the traditional view of the nurse, always acting out of a sense of duty, may be challenged. In the history of nursing, there are many close links with the notions of duty, obedience and the place of the nurse firmly in the control of non-nurses. In early nurse education programmes, the role of the nurse was closely linked to the Victorian expectation of the role of women. This could be recognised as a deontological approach to nursing.

The other major ethical approach is known as 'consequentialism'. This is interpreted as considering the outcome of an action, rather than the action itself. In the example of truth-telling, the consequentialist would tell the truth if the consequences would not be more damaging than the truth that was to be told. A person who is in a state of denial may find such 'truth' difficult to accept and therefore the nurse would have to carefully consider the effect of telling the truth in such a situation. As we work through each of the examples, we will highlight the different approaches that both deontologists and consequentialists would suggest.

ETHICAL FRAMEWORKS

As shown in this chapter, ethical issues may present themselves as daily problems in palliative nursing situations. In this section, attention is given to three ethical frameworks that may assist in the thought processes that nurses experience when confronted with such situations. The use of such problem-solving approaches focuses on the central place of ethics in daily nursing practice. As Greipp (1992, p. 734) noted:

Ethical decisions should be an integral component of all practice, not just those monumental decisions involving life and death, donors and transplants.

Crigger (1994) has argued that the existing ethical theories are based on masculine notions and she has argued for the inclusion of the feminist notion of caring, which combines the deontological and consequentialist theories in decision-making. The first step in such a combined approach is to use intuition. This occurs when a situation is noted and has known ethical principles applied to it. If there is no conflict, then a resolution can be determined. However, if there is still some uncertainty, then a process of critical thinking begins. The features of the situation are examined, the opening thoughts being 'should something be done in this situation?' The final test of the theory in this framework is to apply it to other potential situations, which may include others and the individual. Perhaps this framework is the one that is used by many people who are making decisions regularly without using a predetermined framework. Such is the nature of nursing work that time to 'mull a situation over' is often not available.

Three ethical frameworks will now be identified and applied in turn to palliative care settings through three Case histories. The frameworks are:

- Seedhouse's ethical grid
- Greipp's framework
- Niebuhr's response ethics

Seedhouse's ethical grid

The first Case history illustrates an ethical problem, within the hospital setting, concerning a person called Sophie. It highlights issues of patient autonomy, informed consent and respect for a person. Seedhouse's ethical grid (1988) is used to analyse it.

This framework is composed of a four-layer grid, which enables differing solutions to ethical problems to be worked through in a logical manner (Fig. 10.1).

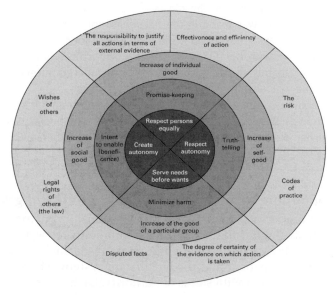

Fig. 10.1 Seedhouse's ethical grid.

The four layers are:

- The central layer, which addresses the purpose and is the most important box. Seedhouse advises that at least one box from this layer is used in all deliberations made in the context of health work. This layer provides the core rationale – the 'central conditions' necessary for health (Seedhouse 1988)
- The second layer, which refers to deontological principles
- The third layer, which refers to consequentialist ethical principles
- The final, outside layer, which refers to external forces influencing care

Each of the boxes within the four layers is independent and detachable, yet all the boxes have strong relationships with one another. The grid can be seen in different ways, for example, as a spiral or as a two- or three-dimensional object. The four distinct layers of the grid are shown in order to illustrate that at least four different sets of elements make up comprehensive ethical deliberation. Seedhouse's ethical grid is illustrated in Case History 10.1.

■ CASE HISTORY 10.1   Sophie

Sophie, a 72-year-old woman, was admitted to her local District General Hospital in a state of collapse. The decision to have emergency surgery to repair a suspected perforated bowel was taken although Sophie thought that she told the admitting nurse and doctor that she wished to be left to die. Despite this, she was rushed to the operating theatre. During the surgery, an inoperable rectal cancer was discovered and a palliative colostomy was fashioned. Following her transfer to the surgical unit she made a steady recovery and learned to care for the colostomy.

Three years previously, a diagnosis of a squamous cell carcinoma of the floor of Sophie's mouth had been made and this tumour had metastasised into the lymph nodes in her neck. Although she had been given the option of surgery at that time, she decided that she did not want to undergo such mutilating surgery. This decision was made in the full realisation that her life would be shortened by not having the surgery. She had spent a long time discussing this potential outcome with her GP so felt that an informed decision had been taken. However, in this situation, the decision to undergo surgery had been taken while she was unable to express her wishes clearly.

On her recovery, Sophie felt anger that she had not been left to die as she had wished or, as she expressed it, that she had been helped to survive. Two weeks after her discharge home from hospital, Sophie took a fatal overdose of morphine elixir.

Analysis of Sophie's story using Seedhouse's ethical grid

There are a number of key issues in this Case history, namely, personal autonomy, doubts about the 'right' action to take in respect of treatment and/or the withdrawal of treatment, information sharing, and a conflict of interests between a patient and the health care system. The solution rests with our conscience, not with status or authority. Each layer of the grid will now be explored.

The central layer In Sophie's case, her decision regarding initial surgery was respected; however, when emergency surgery was required on the second occasion, her autonomy as an individual was not respected. One could argue that it could not be respected as it would have led to harm, only to herself. In some instances, the autonomy of a patient has to be questioned if her decision will lead to harm to other people, which was not an issue in Sophie's case. Seedhouse (1988) states that personal autonomy refers to 'a person's capacity to choose freely for himself, and to be able to direct his own life'. Autonomy is, however, restricted by other factors, such as the law, social tradition, other people's autonomy and the prevailing circumstances of a person's life. Personal autonomy depends upon the physical ability, knowledge and understanding of the choice and option.

Seedhouse (1988) acknowledges that the idea of respecting autonomy is bedevilled with controversy but reminds us that 'many large medical ethical problems hinge upon this principle'.

In Sophie's case, as in many other palliative care situations, people dying still have a right to treatment or a right to decline treatment if they wish. As we have seen, problems arise when they are unable to express their wishes. In this situation, one can only take the best course of action for that person to minimise their suffering and try to act as they would have wished. Relatives and close friends can be a helpful guide in this respect, providing insight into what the patient would have intended. In the box 'serving needs before wants' we are considering the needs of all and 'justice as fairness' is concerned with the treatment of all persons with equal respect.

The second inner layer From a deontological point of view, staff in this situation might have felt that it was their duty to preserve life at all costs and to ensure that the remaining time left for Sophie was of as good a quality as it could possibly be.

The surgeon, it could be argued, acted out of beneficence to do good and prevent harm coming to Sophie. However, the psychological aspects of this need to be examined. Seedhouse (1988) states that truthfulness is an important principle of conduct by health care workers. Sophie had been told the truth, but owing to the sudden deterioration of her condition, communication had temporarily broken down. The issue of promise-keeping as a central duty to maintain professional trust is an issue in this case. Has the patient been fully informed? Can she make an informed choice? To minimise harm may entail inflicting 'harm' for the sake of beneficence. In this case, it was the surgery. Was treatment necessary – a fundamental need or not? If the ethical principle of doing good and not doing harm is applied, then it could be argued that the health care team acted out of a sense of duty to the patient.

The third layer Which group or individual would benefit most in this situation? The surgeon's intentions were to promote the individual good of Sophie, but this also had an unfortunate outcome for her. Perhaps this shows the different interpretations of her well-being and quality of life. Within this layer, the needs of the family and staff would also be considered as a particular group of people. In Sophie's case, she had no close family or friends, so the staff could focus their attention on her. The appropriateness of the surgery may have met the needs of the staff, who did not want to see her suffer, but it is questionable whether Sophie felt the same way. For Sophie, it is her happiness that is paramount. She had already refused curative surgery as, in her opinion, it would have been mutilating. She knew the consequences of that action. Was it unethical to go against them? Could further consultation with knowledgeable colleagues have cancelled the surgery?

Does the 'happiness' of the staff have any bearing, in this instance, as they would account for the greater number of people. On her discharge home, Sophie had made a decision to end her life. However, the staff may feel that they acted in the best interests of the patient, in the given circumstances, by performing surgery. This shows that decisions have to be taken rapidly in an emergency situation. In this situation, if the full facts had been known, the decision-making process would have been very difficult for all staff involved. Following an incident such as this, all staff may be left feeling guilty and even inadequate. Debriefing sessions with staff can be beneficial in such situations to permit the expression of feelings and views as well as rectifying any misconceptions. It can also be used to consider future action in similar situations and be a way of thanking staff for their efforts.

The outer layer The factors here influence the decision about the actions taken because of legal requirements and professional codes of conduct. Seedhouse (1988) advocates that one of these boxes should be used on all occasions to justify the actions in terms of the external evidence. In the box that mentions the degree of certainty of the evidence on which action is taken, the health care team were presented with an acutely ill person needing treatment. It may have been hard to justify *not* operating in such a situation. However, this would need to be balanced against the wishes of Sophie.

Discussion

The suicide of a patient, then, may be regarded as a failure by the staff because of a feeling that the care was not good enough. Is this applicable in Sophie's case? If we reflect upon the UKCC 'Code of professional conduct' (1992) in this situation, what guidance can clauses 1, 2, 5 and 7 offer the nurse?

• Clause 1. Act always in such a manner as to promote and safeguard the interests and well-being of patients and clients.

• Clause 2. Ensure that no action or omission on your part, or within your sphere of responsibility, is detrimental to the interests, conditions or safety of patients and clients.

• Clause 5. Work in an open and co-operative manner with patients, clients and their families, foster their independence and recognise and respect their involvement in the planning and delivery of care.

• Clause 7. Recognise and respect the uniqueness and dignity of each patient and client, and respond to their need for care, irrespective of their ethnic origin, religious beliefs, personal attributes, the nature of their health problems or any other factor.

The philosophy of the modern hospice movement emphasises the importance of the quality of life, rather than the quantity of life. As Saunders (1993) wrote:

> *... you matter because you are you. You matter to the last moment of your life and we will do all we can, not only to help you die peacefully, but to live with you until you die.*

In this case, Sophie had decided that she did not consider her life to have sufficient quality to continue living. She was in full possession of her mental faculties and had made a rational decision about her future. It was *her* life. Likewise, it could be argued that she had the right to choose to end her life. The hospice movement advocates that with good palliative care and support, patients should not have cause to feel suicidal, but there will always be those who feel that they can no longer battle on with the effects of their disease. If the health care team are confident that the best palliative care has been offered, then it would seem necessary to respect a patient's decision to reject it. The nurse cannot take responsibility for the decision of a patient, although it is extremely difficult not to intervene and do what we think is best for the patient. This is why there is a need in the educational process to consider personal as well as professional ethics.

The notion of religion may also intervene in such moments because some people hold the view that it is a sin to take one's own life as life itself is in the gift of a Supreme Being who has the power to give and take life. For the individual contemplating suicide, this may instil feelings of guilt at the very thought of suicide. This is exemplified in the Christian religion where there is importance attached to the meaning of suffering and that the process of dying might involve suffering. Many of the original hospices that were set up had, and some still have, a religious foundation, and therefore their hospice philosophy reflects such a religious ethic.

Staff who are caring for patients, such as Sophie, will have to consider and reflect on their own religious beliefs, or lack of them, in such situations. In nursing, students are taught not to be judgemental and not to allow personal views and beliefs to influence decision-making. However, the individual nurse has to recognise when such a conflict may arise. Within palliative care nursing this can prove to be difficult when intense feelings and beliefs can obscure objectivity.

■ REFLECTIVE PRACTICE 10.4   Sophie

Reflect on Sophie's story. Should the notion of duty (the deontological approach) have more importance than the consequences of acting or not acting in a particular situation?

Greipp's model of ethical decision-making

The second case history illustrates the notions of respect, advocacy and justice as fairness, doing good and not doing harm, and trust. It will be analysed using Greipp's framework (Fig. 10.2).

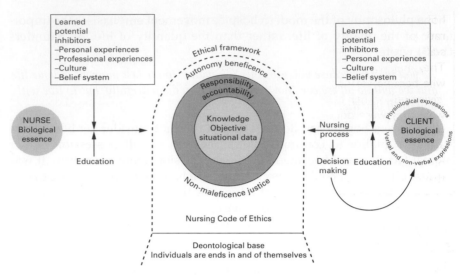

Fig. 10.2 Greipp's model of ethical decision-making. Printed with permission of Blackwell Science Ltd., from Greipp M (1992) Greipp's model of ethical decision-making. Journal of Advanced Nursing 17: 735.

The ethical framework described by Greipp (1992) was developed to raise awareness of the complex demands of today's health care system in which social, legal and economic factors affect health care decisions. The model places ethical principles centrally, with nursing influences and client influences on either side. It stresses the importance of existing knowledge, culture and education on the central ethical principles and the influence of our personal beliefs on our professional practice. Learned potential inhibitors have been identified by Greipp who acknowledges the importance of education in counteracting these personal feelings, as in Case History 10.2.

■ **CASE HISTORY 10.2   Tom**

Tom was a 59-year-old man who had taken early retirement from his work. Two years previously, a malignant melanoma was excised from his arm and he had made a good recovery. Recently, he had become very tired, breathless and anaemic. Investigations revealed that pleural metastases had developed. A course of palliative radiotherapy followed to alleviate his symptoms but, despite this, his condition deteriorated and he was admitted to an acute medical ward. As he was dehydrated, an intravenous infusion was started. Owing to his deteriorating condition, it was suggested that he could be cared for more appropriately in the nearby hospice where he would obtain the peace and privacy that he needed. Although Tom was in favour of such a move, his family were unhappy about the prospect of moving him. They had not fully appreciated the severity of his illness and, to them, the hospice meant death. Following a meeting with one of the medical team from the hospice who explained the function of the hospice to them, Tom was transferred to the hospice with the intravenous infusion still running. His condition was deteriorating daily and he was becoming increasingly breathless. After a few days, the staff at the hospice felt that the infusion was not serving any useful purpose. They met with the family to explain the proposed plan for its removal. Tom's wife became very angry and upset, accusing the hospice of poor care and of 'giving up' on her husband too soon. She felt that 'at least the hospital knew what they were doing as they saw that he needed fluids and nourishment'. 'If you take it down, he will die,' she said. It took the hospice staff a long time to gently explain that the intravenous infusion was no longer an appropriate part of his care and she finally agreed to its removal. Tom died peacefully later on that night with his family beside him.

Analysis of Tom's story using Greipp's model of ethical decision-making

The nurse is concerned with the care of Tom and wishes to offer him the best care possible. In her professional judgement, this may mean withdrawing the intravenous infusion, keeping him comfortable and keeping the relatives fully informed about his condition. The nurse has learned to do this from her previous experience and education. Perhaps she also considers how she or one of her family should be treated in a similar situation. The influence of her cultural and religious background may make this situation easier or more difficult to deal with. If she has worked extensively in a 'curing' environment, she may feel that Tom's impending death is a failure of the system. Such feelings may also affect the other members of the health care team who are looking after Tom.

The central ethical principles in this situation are determined as the right to treatment, respect and autonomy. It could be argued that Tom is no longer able to be autonomous because of his illness. In this instance, the family have a crucial role to play as they want to be involved in treatment decisions. We know that Tom has expressed his wishes about his care, but the nurse has to strike a balance between respecting his wishes and those of the family. The potential conflict seems to be between the differing interpretations of the ethical principles of beneficence (doing good) and non-maleficence (doing harm). The family may also be feeling a sense of injustice that Tom is not having 'proper' treatment or access to a wide range of treatments.

Discussion

This incident highlights the issue of hydration, which is a common ethical problem in hospital and hospice settings. The move from curative to palliative treatment can be a painful one for the patient, family and staff as they come to terms with the future. Nutrition is a basic human need and relatives may mention that a lack of nourishment will lead to a patient's death. As in the example above, when there appears to be a decision to withdraw intravenous fluids, then relatives may interpret this as a sign of incompetence and the hastening of death by staff. There is a natural desire to feed a loved one, as nourishment is associated with love and grati-fication. From the perspective of the hospice, and Tom himself, this may be so, but the relatives may have a totally different perspective. Lamerton (1990) writes that 'drip-feeding into veins merely lengthens the process of dying'. Twycross & Lack (1990) in their discussion of the management of cachexia in the dying patient said 'because of the greatly increased metabolic rate, aggressive dietary supplementation is of little value in reversing cachexia'. Twycross & Lichter (1993) discuss the issue of appropriate treat-ment for a patient close to death.

> Measures such as cardiac resuscitation, artificial respiration, intravenous infusion, nasogastric tubes and antibiotics are all primarily supportive measures for use in acute-on-chronic illnesses, to assist a patient through the initial period towards recovery of health. To use such measures in patients who are clearly close to death and have no expectation of a return to health is inappropriate and is therefore bad medicine – we have no right or duty, legal or ethical, to prescribe a lingering death. Therapeutic interventions that can best be described as prolonging the distress of the dying are both futile and inappropriate.

Twycross & Lichter (1993) support the argument by saying that, in certain circumstances, dehydration may well be beneficial and hydration detrimental, reducing incontinence, coughing and congestion, choking and drowning sensations. There is a belief that dehydration in a terminally ill patient is distressing. In other circumstances it certainly is, but when all the systems are shutting down it may not be so distressing (Malone 1994). Over-hydration can be unethical in itself as the patient may drown as the body becomes unable to cope with the additional circulating fluid. This would be a most distressing death for a patient and those caring for them and raises the concern about inflicting unnecessary suffering on a patient and the notion of doing good and not doing harm.

Twycross & Lichter (1993) also raise the point of the importance of making the terminal phase of an illness as normal as possible and this may include removing unnecessary equipment. They note that it becomes more difficult to be close to the individual if faced with a multitude of tubing and, in addition, the focus of care may be directed towards the equipment, rather than the person.

In this situation then there appears to be evidence to support the decision-making process although, as noted by Sutcliffe (1994), there is no conclusive evidence of the effects of dehydration. However, the effects of such decisions on the relatives have to be considered in view of their feelings about the need for nourishment.

Ethical problems were researched by Davidson et al in 1990 when nurses in eight different countries were asked about the action that they would take in a hypothetical situation regarding the feeding of a patient against their will.

Although the decisions reached by the nurses were different, the study found that addressing the problem was difficult for the nurses. Such a finding implies that although the context and culture of the nurses was different and they had different interpretations about the terms used, the actual resolution of the situation was in itself problematic.

For Tom's family, the intravenous infusion was an indication of life, of continuing treatment and hope. When its removal was discussed, this made them face the reality of his situation and they were not ready for such an event. The progression of the illness was more rapid than they realised. This shows that the line between the emotional needs of the family and the patient's comfort, wishes and desires is a fine one, especially if the patient is unconscious (Brooker 1992). This poses the ethical problem in this situation – whose needs are we meeting: those of the patient, the family or the staff? If the patient is conscious, then she will have feelings about fluid intake and respect has to be taken of such wishes. However, if the patient is unable to offer an opinion about this issue, who should act as his advocate?

Brooker (1992) would urge the health care team to consider that intravenous fluids should not be started to ease the conscience of staff or relatives. In addition, the introduction of such treatment should neither add to the distress nor detract from the reality of the patient's impending death.

The important feature of the care of the relatives in Tom's case is the reassurance that Tom has not been abandoned and that because he is dying he has not been offered less treatment. It would be unethical to cause the patient unnecessary suffering merely to appease the relatives. Whatever you do, or fail to do, someone suffers. Therefore it is advisable, whenever possible, to prevent this situation in advance by giving attention to the components of the ethical decision-making process.

■ REFLECTIVE PRACTICE 10.5   Tom

In our discussion of Sophie's suicide story we referred to the relevant clauses in the UKCC 'Code of professional conduct'. In Tom's case what guidance is there in the code for you?

If the ethical principle of justice as fairness is applied in this situation, then did Tom obtain equal access to treatment?

Niebuhr's response ethics

The final Case history is set in the community and highlights the ethical problem that a nurse may face in relation to information giving. It will be analysed using Niebuhr's response ethics.

The use of intuition in an ethical framework is also seen in response ethics, which was developed by Niebuhr in the 1960s (Tschudin 1994). This framework asks the reader to work through a problem by answering a series of questions. It would also seem an appropriate framework to apply in a group setting as well as being used by the nurse working in isolation.

- What is happening here? (Based on your gut reaction)
- What would happen if …? (Certain actions were taken)
- After careful consideration, what is the fitting answer?
- What has been the result of this action?

■ CASE HISTORY 10.3   Meg

Meg was a retired music teacher who lived with her sister, Dora, in the old family home. Following an acute illness Dora died, which devastated Meg.

A few months later, Meg was diagnosed as having a breast carcinoma, which had metastasised. In consultation with Meg's niece, the GP had decided that it would be too upsetting for Meg to know about her diagnosis so soon after Dora's death.

Although the district nurse had been visiting Meg occasionally since Dora's death, she was previously unaware of Meg's recent illness. When she called at the house, later that day, Meg appeared to be in considerable pain, reporting that her abdomen felt 'full-up' and distended. She asked the district nurse what could be wrong.

This presented the district nurse with a problem. Should she be honest with Meg with whom she had already built up a relationship or should she maintain the 'conspiracy of silence'?

Analysis of Meg's story using Niebuhr's response ethics

Niebuhr's response ethics are used to analyse this situation. The first question to ask is '**What is happening here**?' It appears that the nurse has been asked not to disclose information to Meg as it may be too distressing. The difficulty is that the nurse has developed a trusting relationship with Meg and feels disloyal *not* telling the truth. Meg is going to need nursing care and as the nurse respects Meg, it is hard for her to remain silent.

With the problem identified, the second phase of this framework asks the question '**What would happen if** the nurse told Meg the truth?' Is there a possibility that such information would harm Meg? The potential for the distress it may cause might prevent her from making rational decisions. In addition, it might then cause problems with her niece and her GP who also have close links with her.

However, this question can also be reframed as '**What would happen if** the nurse did not tell Meg the truth?' Would this situation affect the relationship and therefore the care that has developed between nurse and patient? How would Meg be able to trust any future information given by any other health professional? Is this an example of a very paternalistic attitude, which denies Meg the opportunity to make her own decisions in a fully informed way?

The third question in Niebuhr's framework invites the nurse to consider both options and make a decision.

■ REFLECTIVE PRACTICE 10.6   Meg

Reflecting on Meg's story, what would you do?

Discussion

Meg's story shows the problem that the nurse may face. If we return to the two approaches to ethics, outlined briefly, i.e. deontology and consequentialism, then the ethical problem can be seen.

If the deontological approach is adopted within the information-giving category, then a nurse may decide that a patient should always be told the truth about a condition. This shows that she feels he has a duty to inform patients in every situation because this is the morally correct thing to do. If the nurse feels that she has a duty to tell the truth, he may feel that it is not right to withhold information.

Alternatively, if he feels that the patient may be harmed by such disclosure of information, from the consequentialist point of view she may feel that it would be better not to tell her. However, this does not solve the problem, because ethical problems in daily practice do not always give the person time to consider varying ethical theories. In this situation, the patient, Meg, is looking at you, a nurse whom she knows, waiting for an answer. If you tell her a lie now, then the bond of trust will be broken between you, making future care difficult.

Meg's story, described above, shows the type of situation that nurses face on a daily basis and could be found in any nursing context. As mentioned above, this district nurse found herself asking 'What should I do?' and reflects one of the primary concerns of this chapter – the notion of respect for the patient as an individual in their own right, and for yourself as a nurse.

■ REFLECTIVE PRACTICE 10.7   Informed consent

How can the nurse promote the notion of informed consent in situations like Meg's?

ETHICAL FRAMEWORKS SYNTHESISED

The similarities between the ethical frameworks outlined above seem to be the importance of intuition and the context of the situation. The adoption of reflection in conjunction with an ethical framework may enable such intuitive skills to develop as well as assisting with reflection on previous experiences. In the three Case histories presented in this chapter, we have used three ethical frameworks to illustrate how they may relate to clinical practice. These Case histories also reinforce the notion that ethical concerns are far from being the preserve of headline-grabbing situations. The nurse working with patients and relatives in any palliative care environment may have to face situations where they have to make a decision under difficult circumstances. We have chosen to focus upon issues of informed consent and advocacy, trust, respect, teamwork and self-awareness. In other situations that the nurse faces on a daily basis, there are issues of resources to deal with. The biggest challenge of all is the individual nature of the situation that the nurse finds herself in at the time.

SUMMARY

We have aimed to discuss some everyday issues, within palliative care, in relation to ethical theory. The Case histories reinforce the stress that may develop in the nurse who faces ethical problems in daily practice. Through-out this chapter, we have linked professional and personal ethics and would stress the need for self-awareness.

Davis & Oberle (1990) have developed a model of supportive care that places great emphasis on the self-integrity of the nurse. In ongoing situations that involve complex decision-making, the nurse has to have some way of maintaining her own self-esteem. Nursing dying people may cause stress, and this stress may begin during nurse education, as exemplified in the account of a student nurse feeling that better care could have been given to a dying patient (Elliott 1994). This stress may be heightened, especially when the care that is needed is not matched by available resources. Gallagher & Boyd (1991) have suggested that some nurses see ethical education as a necessary component in nurse preparation.

Nurses may find themselves in a conflict of roles based on the potential clash between their personal values and the socialisation process into nursing. According to Kelly (1992) such conflicts 'are most likely related to the disparity that exists between the ideals of nursing and the everyday struggle to get through the workload that takes place in the real world of hospital nursing practice'.

This view is also found in the later work of Davis & Oberle (1995) who argue that such stress is demonstrated by disillusionment and burnout. In the community, hospice or hospital setting, it seems vital for the nurse to be able to share feelings with colleagues and reflect on the care that has been delivered in a supportive way. It could be argued that having education in ethics may enhance such a supportive atmosphere. The understanding gained through ethical frameworks may be of value to this process.

A major concern in palliative care settings is the vulnerability of the patient who is in the final stages of an illness. The fear of pain and dying, as well as the fear of death, may add to the burden of the process of decision-making. In addition, there may be some uncertainty and confusion about the options for future care. An explanation of the closeness of ethical principles to the nursing of dying patients may offer a more realistic approach to the study of ethics and ethical problems. It has been noted that nurses face ethical situations on a daily basis, but these situations only become problems when no clear solution can be found. To this end, Case histories from three differing contexts of care have shown that such daily concerns face nurses working in the hospital, hospice and community sectors.

Furthermore, the value of considering ethical issues in some detail may assist in adopting a framework for problem solving in situations where there appears to be no easy answer.

This important link between ethics and caring has to be the central focus of any decisions made in ethical situations. However, this may not make situations any easier to resolve and highlights the presence of ethical problems when there is the potential for harm, regardless of which approach is taken. This situation is made more difficult because of the nurse's wish to care for patients.

■ REFLECTIVE PRACTICE 10.8   Practice development

We leave you to consider the following question:

How does your knowledge of ethics enable you to reflect on and develop your practice?

REFERENCES

Allen R (ed) 1990 The Concise Oxford Dictionary of Current English. Clarendon Press, Oxford

Allmark P 1992 The ethical enterprise of nursing. Journal of Advanced Nursing 17: 16–20

Aroskar M 1989 Community health nurses: their most significant ethical decision-making problems. Nursing Clinics of North America 24: 967–975

Beauchamp T, Childress J 1983 Principles of biomedical ethics, 2nd edn. Oxford University Press, Oxford

Brooker S 1992 Dehydration before death. Nursing Times 88: 59–62

Chadwick R, Todd W 1992 Ethics and nursing practice. Macmillan, Basingstoke

Crigger N 1994 Universal prescriptivism: traditional moral decision-making theory revisited. Journal of Advanced Nursing 20: 538–543

Davidson B, Laan R V, Davis A et al 1990 Ethical reasoning associated with the feeding of terminally ill elderly cancer patients: an international perspective. Cancer Nursing 13: 286–292

Davis B, Oberle K 1990 Dimensions of the supportive role of the nurse in palliative care. Oncology Nursing Forum 17: 87–94

Davis B, Oberle K 1995 An exploration of nursing disillusionment. The Canadian Journal of Nursing Research 25: 67–76

Duncan S 1992 Ethical challenge in community health nursing. Journal of Advanced Nursing 17: 1035–1041

Elliot T 1994 Euthanasia and the nurse. Nursing Standard 10: 55

Gallagher U, Boyd K (ed) 1991 Teaching and learning nursing ethics. Scutari Press, Harrow

Greipp M 1992 Greipp's model of ethical decision-making. Journal of Advanced Nursing 17: 734–738

Jeffrey D 1993 There is nothing more I can do. Patten Press, Cornwall

Kelly B 1992 Professional ethics as perceived by American nursing undergraduates. Journal of Advanced Nursing 17: 10–15

Kendrick K 1994 An advocate for whom – doctor or patient? How far can a nurse be a patient's advocate? Professional Nurse 9: 826–829

Lamerton R 1990 Care of the dying. Penguin, London

Malone N 1994 Hydration in the terminally ill patient. Nursing Standard 8: 29–32

McGee P 1994 The concept of respect in nursing. British Journal of Nursing 3: 681–684

Omery A 1991 Culpability and pain management/control in peripheral vascular disease using the ethics of principles and care. Critical Care Nursing Clinics of North America 3: 551–558

Penn K 1994 Patient advocacy in palliative care. British Journal of Nursing 5: 40–42

Rodney P 1989 Towards ethical decision-making in nursing practice prolongation of life. Canadian Journal of Nursing Administration 2: 11–14

Saunders C 1993 Oxford textbook of palliative medicine. Oxford Medical Publishers, Oxford

Scott A 1995 Moral obligation. Nursing Times 91: 50–51

Seedhouse D 1988 Ethics: the heart of health care. John Wiley, Chichester

Sutcliffe J 1994 Terminal dehydration. Nursing Times 90: 60–62

Tschudin V 1994 Deciding ethically. Baillière Tindall, London

Twycross R, Lack S 1990 Therapeutics in terminal cancer. Churchill Livingstone, Edinburgh

Twycross R, Lichter I 1993 The terminal phase. In: Doyle D, Hanks G, Macdonald N (eds) The Oxford textbook of palliative medicine. Oxford Medical Publications, Oxford, p 653

UKCC 1996 Guidelines for professional practice. UKCC, London

UKCC 1992 The code of professional conduct. UKCC, London

UKCC 1994 The scope of professional practice. UKCC, London

UKCC 1990 Report on post registration education and practice. UKCC, London

Watson J 1989 Nursing science and human care: a theory of nursing. Appleton-Century Crofts, Connecticut

Wells R 1988 Ethics, informed consent and confidentiality. In: Tschudin V (ed) Nursing the patient with cancer. Prentice Hall, London, pp 459–474

FURTHER READING

Glover J 1990 Causing death and saving lives. Penguin, London

Randall F, Downie R 1996 Palliative care ethics, a good companion. Oxford Medical Publications, Oxford

Research and audit: demonstrating quality

11

Keith Farrer

Nothing will improve care than acting on existing knowledge. [Sternwald 1995]

INTRODUCTION

The above quote may seem almost redundant in a discussion of research and quality in palliative care. However, the reality is that although the past decade has brought advances in the alleviation of suffering in patients with advanced incurable illnesses, much of this existing knowledge is not applied. Standards of palliative care are variable between different institutions and geographical regions, resulting in an inequitable service for our patients (Clark 1993).

Quality management in palliative care aims to monitor, maintain and improve the care given to our patients. Research is primarily concerned with generating new knowledge and understanding, which also includes evaluating methods of applying this knowledge to practice. This chapter aims to explore methods of quality assessment and research methods that seek to improve the care given to dying patients and their families. Particular attention will be paid to the challenges that exist in demonstrating quality in palliative care.

LEARNING OUTCOMES

PREP requirements will be met in the areas of reducing risk, care enhancement and practice development through:

- Identifying standards, evaluating and changing practice
- Using audit to assess symptom distress and quality of life
- Using research to demonstrate quality and to generate new knowledge

QUALITY ASSURANCE

The interest in quality assurance in palliative care has mushroomed in recent years. The motivation for this interest is similar to that in other areas of health provision and can be broadly outlined in the following three areas.

NHS reforms

In palliative care, the changes in the structure and organisation of the NHS, brought about partly by the White Paper 'Working for patients' (The Secretaries of State for Health 1989), are having a direct impact on the organisation and delivery of care. These reforms have resulted in an internal market (manifested by the purchaser/provider split) and have placed greater emphasis on the views of the consumers of health services. The philosophy embodied in the recent NHS reforms are manifested by concepts of quality and cost. As nursing services provide elements of both general and/or specialist palliative care delivery, they are now being faced with the task of having to enter into contracts based on the relationship between quality of care and cost – put simply, as value for money. Those palliative care units that are independent from the NHS are not immune to these changes. Funding has previously (post-NHS reforms) been provided from a mix of charitable monies and from regional health authorities. However, increasingly, hospices are having to enter into health authority contracts that include mandatory indicators of quality. Also, alarmingly for those units, there is no guarantee of future financial support from health authorities, whilst some are now faced with the difficult task of competing with other units for a seemingly ever-decreasing 'pot of money'.

Consumerism

The past 10 years has seen the emergence of consumerism as a dominant culture in all public sector services (including the NHS). The general public is becoming better educated and more aware of its statutory rights; partly as a result of improved telecommunications and partly owing to a raised awareness of NHS services, during and after recent NHS reorganisations. Patients (or perhaps more appropriately 'customers') have higher expectations and are becoming more critical of the manner in which care is provided.

Professional issues

In relation to palliative care there are two main professional issues that motivate the drive to ensure good quality services for terminally ill patients.

First is the desire of all professions working in palliative care to ensure that patients and families receive the highest possible quality of care – whether this is to be provided in the patients' own home, in specialist units or in hospitals. This motivation is especially acute when one considers that (unlike in some other areas of health care) we only have one chance to 'get it right' for the dying person. Despite this imperative, there is evidence to suggest that inequalities exist in the provision of palliative care, with access to and quality of clinical care varying from region to region (Clark 1993, Higginson 1993a). If palliative care is to continue to evolve as a credible aim of all health care professionals, then these issues need to be resolved through planned quality and research initiatives. Deming's (1988) belief that quality 'doesn't happen by accident' highlights the need for careful planning to ensure consistent quality in palliative care.

Second, ensuring quality of care in nursing is paramount in maintaining the credibility of nursing's contribution to palliative care. Whilst the obligation for nurses to give good quality care to all patients is not under question, there are important reasons to ensure that this is demonstrated and continually monitored. That nurses should be able to demonstrate their valuable input into providing holistic palliative care is linked to the motivations outlined above. However, the recent changes in the structure of the NHS have made it imperative to demonstrate effective and quality nursing care. The reality of a competitive health care market means that nurses must be able to demonstrate the effectiveness of the care given to patients in order to be able to secure continued funding (failure to do this may result, at the very least, in a reduction of funds required to continue existing programmes of care).

Demonstrating and assuring quality of nursing care is only possible through careful quality management programmes, which integrate methods of care evaluation through audit and evaluation research (Koch & Fairly 1993). However, nursing and other health care professions working in palliative care face enormous difficulties with this task. In order to demonstrate these difficulties it is first necessary to discuss the concept of quality and the origins of quality assurance.

DEFINING QUALITY

Before proceeding to discuss quality in relation to palliative care it is first necessary to attempt to portray what is inferred by the term.

The Oxford Dictionary states that quality is:

A degree of excellence; relative nature, or character ...

This definition infers that quality is on a continuum, i.e. it can be poor, good or somewhere in between, and that it is relative to time and resources invested in the concerned product or service. However, the definition does not shed light on the components and processes by which this 'degree of excellence' is achieved.

The European Organisation for Quality Control (EOQC) cites quality as:

The totality of features of a product or service that bears its ability to satisfy given needs.

Again this definition implies that quality may vary, but differs from the previous definition as it explicitly reflects the current ethos of consumerism, i.e. that quality is driven by the needs of the consumer (the 'customer is always right' ethos!). Nevertheless, the definition does not lead us any closer to determining what the features are that satisfy the consumers of health care. The difficulty in pinning down an all-encompassing definition to illuminate quality is not surprising if quality is considered to be a multidimensional concept. Rather than attempting to produce a conclusive statement to define quality, Maxwell (1984) outlines six dimensions to illuminate quality in health care. These include:

- Appropriateness: that the service is what the population needs
- Accessibility: that services are accessible
- Effectiveness: that the service is achieving the intended benefit for both the individual and the population
- Acceptability: that services are provided such as to satisfy the reasonable expectations of patients
- Efficiency: that resources are not wasted on one service to the detriment of another
- Equity: that there is a fair share for the population

Although this framework offers a useful checklist for looking at quality it is somewhat more difficult to apply, i.e. an efficient service may not always be equitable.

THE ORIGINS OF QUALITY ASSURANCE

The origins of quality assurance are in manufacturing industry. In discussing the differences between quality in manufacturing and quality of a service (such as health care), Parasuraman et al (1985) list the following three characteristics as inherent in all areas that provide a service. These are particularly relevant to the following discussions on quality in palliative care and are as follows:

1 Services are intangible: they cannot (in their entirety) be stored, counted and measured like products in manufacturing industry. This poses difficulty in trying to assure and measure quality in palliative care; namely, that it is not possible to do a final quality check, as standard in manufacturing industry.

2 Services have customers with very heterogeneous needs – in palliative care no patient has exactly the same needs. Indeed, patients with similar disease processes may have very different physical problems and emotional needs. The implication of this is: how do providers of care identify the common or core services that will address the needs of each patient, and which components of palliative care demonstrate good quality of care?

3 Services have inseparability – quality is a process that occurs during the delivery of the care and is not just an end-point. The end-points of health care, whether they be the restoration of health or, in palliative care, a dignified and pain-free death, can rarely be attributed to one intervention from one health care profession. In reality, the delivery of health care is an

intertwined and interdependent series of interventions delivered by a team of different health carers. In quality management and evaluation research this poses difficulties when attempting to determine the impact of intervention by one health care worker in the area being examined.

■ REFLECTIVE PRACTICE 11.1   The concept of quality

The concept of quality:

- Conveys a degree of excellence – this is relative to the time and resources invested in it
- Is multidimensional and linked to the individual's and society's expectations and perceptions
- Is more difficult to demonstrate in a service than in the manufacturing industry

Think about this in relation to palliative care.

AUDIT AND QUALITY ASSURANCE IN NURSING

Confusion between audit and quality assurance remains widespread within nursing. Shaw (1989) defines quality assurance as the definition of standards, the measurement of their achievement and mechanisms to improve performance. Similarly, audit in health care is defined as:

A cyclic activity incorporating evaluation of the quality of clinical practice and action taken in response to the results of this evaluation. [DOH 1994, p. 5]

From the above definition it can be seen that both audit and quality assurance are more than just the setting of standards or the measurement of practice. Inherent in both is the commitment to improve quality through action based on the assessment of current practice. In audit the action taken to improve standards is often referred to as 'completing the cycle'. As it is generally agreed that audit forms one component of the wider concept of quality assurance (Black 1990), both terms will be used interchangeably throughout this chapter.

The quality assurance process within nursing is not new. Indeed, Koch (1992) asserted that as, in the 1980s, the majority of published papers on quality in health care were written by nurses, it suggests that nurses were taking the lead in quality initiatives. Much of this early work focused on the framework for quality assurance put forward by Donebedian (1980). This framework breaks down services into the following three separate, but inter-related, components:

- Structure – the physical and organisational aspects of a service, i.e. staffing levels or equipment available
- Process – the manner by which care is delivered. This includes how, for example, nurses interact with patients, or whether guidelines for good practice are followed
- Outcome – what is achieved from the structure and processes of care

In the UK, much of the quality and audit in health care is based on this model. In nursing in the UK, this framework forms the basis for the RCN's quality assurance programme – the 'Dynamic standard setting system' (Kitson 1988). The foundation of this system is that the involvement of staff in the process of setting and monitoring standards, pertaining to the structure and process of care and evaluating the outcomes of these, will result in sustainable improvements in nursing care.

The impact of this system in the UK has been far-reaching – probably every organisation has been involved at one time or another in the process of setting and attempting to evaluate nursing standards. Indeed, the RCN has produced its own standards of care for palliative nursing (RCN 1993). These standards, produced by consensus opinion of expert nurses working within palliative care, relate to issues of patient care, family care and working within the multidisciplinary team.

THE KEY COMPONENTS OF QUALITY ASSURANCE AND AUDIT PROGRAMMES

Identifying standards

The start of most audit and quality assurance programmes necessitates the identification of a standard. This standard needs to be realistically achievable and measurable. As Higginson (1993b) points out, the development of standards can be very time-consuming. In many areas of palliative care practice, the groundwork has been carried out with standards already formulated. Examples include the RCN's 'Standards for palliative care' (RCN 1993), The National Association of Health Authorities (1987) document on 'Care of the dying' and 'Guidelines for good practice and audit measures' (The Royal College of Physicians 1991). Additionally, guidelines and protocols may exist locally, on areas pertaining to palliative care, which can form the basis of standards. Where standards do not exist it is essential to consult with experts in the field.

Setting standards is only the first step in the audit process and in comparison to the following steps is arguably the easiest. The temptation at this stage can be to set a long list of standards relating to a range of different issues. Often the result of this is that the standards lack focus and are difficult to measure. Setting a few measurable standards, which are likely to improve the quality of palliative care, should be the starting point.

Evaluating practice

There are a variety of different approaches to evaluating practice against the predetermined standards, and the choice depends on whether the structure, process or outcome of care is being examined. Also, a distinction between retrospective and prospective audit needs to be made.

- **Retrospective audit** involves examining care after it has been completed, commonly involving examining case notes of patients. Usually, retrospective audit examines structure and process issues. The limitations of this method are that its success is dependent on the quality of the patients' records. It is also a laborious and time-consuming affair, which can be demotivating for those new to participating in audit and quality assurance programmes. Nevertheless, it can provide extremely useful information with the benefit of not directly intruding on patient care. Examples in palliative care may include examining case notes to see whether appropriate laxatives are being prescribed with opiates or whether patients with pain are being assessed regularly using a pain-assessment tool. Often, retrospective audit is combined with other methods in the evaluation of care. Currently I am using such a method, as part of a wider study of the quality of palliative care in the hospital setting, where patients' drug charts are being reviewed to determine if the WHO guidelines on cancer pain management (WHO 1990) are being followed. This is being combined with a patient survey of pain and other symptoms.

• **Prospective audit** entails evaluating care as it is being delivered and is useful for studying process and outcome issues. Methods of prospective evaluation are not dissimilar to research methods in more formal research projects. In auditing outcome of clinical care, a measurement tool is needed and is often administered by questionnaire or in a structured interview. As with quantitative research methods, the tool needs to be demonstrated to be both valid (that it measures what it is intended to measure) and reliable (that it is consistent). Readers who are not familiar with these concepts should refer to specific research texts (i.e. Polit & Hungler 1991). In palliative care, examples of quality assurance programmes and audits that have focused on outcomes have, in the past, been in areas such as symptom control or patient satisfaction (discussed below). However, recently more attention has been given and work carried out to validate other tools that measure the wider aspects of palliative care (see the section below that discusses current palliative care assessment tools).

Changing practice

The process of changing practice to improve quality is the most difficult aspect of quality assurance and is the subject of many articles in the literature (see Malby 1992). Whilst an in-depth discussion of this literature is beyond the scope of this chapter, it is important to highlight the following points.

First, stressed in much of this literature is the importance of staff being involved at 'grass roots level' in any project from the outset. A failure to involve staff from the outset of any quality initiative is, at best, most likely to result in what Koch (1992) describes as the 'lamentable' position of nurses spending time producing standards of which the end result is for these 'to be left in dusty cupboards'.

In a discussion of quality management, Morgan & Murgatroyd (1994) highlight that although the customers and the rank-and-file workers are the most important in the quality process, they need to be underpinned by support from senior management. Ideally, if quality assurance and audit is to result in improved care, then nurses need to feel supported in their endeavours to strive to deliver good care.

Second, audit and quality assurance activity in palliative care must be multidisciplinary. In defining audit, Closs & Cheater (1996) argue that the emphasis must be on multiprofessional involvement because most health care is not the sole responsibility of one discipline. Palliative care is delivered by a team of health care professionals who are characterised by inseparability (as previously discussed), and therefore quality assurance initiatives that are unidisciplinary are unlikely to produce sustained change or demonstrate that the 'quality of care' can be attributed to one particular discipline.

Finally, audit is more likely to succeed and produce change when it has direct relevance to practice and can be incorporated into clinical practice. For example, an audit of symptom control that uses a valid symptom distress scale can equally form part of a nursing assessment. Many of the tools discussed below can be used as both a clinical assessment tool and for outcome measure.

■ REFLECTIVE PRACTICE 11.2   Quality assurance

If quality assurance and audit initiatives are to improve palliative care, the following need to be considered:

- Involve staff from the outset. Invite and involve other disciplines – it may be possible to combine resources or even carry out a combined project on an area of mutual concern
- Involve senior management and keep them informed at every step of the process
  Additionally, Higginson (1993b) offers the following pointers in starting a project:
- Begin small – don't be too ambitious
- Plan – be meticulous in the planning stage. Ill thought out projects will only result in disillusionment
- Meet regularly – in the often hectic pace of clinical areas it will probably be necessary to set a specific time to meet, rather than wait for that elusive, quiet moment

How can you apply these points in your practice?

PROBLEMS AND CRITICISMS OF THE QUALITY ASSURANCE PROGRAMMES IN PALLIATIVE CARE

Quality assurance and audit programmes certainly have their place in improving and demonstrating quality in palliative care. However, there are limitations in their application to health care and, in particular, practical problems related to the discipline of palliative care.

Perhaps the most fundamental criticism of quality assurance techniques is that they assume that important aspects of health care are easily observable and amenable to measurement. Quality assurance methods (in particular, audit) are based on the principles of measurement (Linderman 1976), which involve assigning numbers to objects, events and experiences. Approaches that rely on the measurement of phenomena are referred to as quantitative. Critiques of this approach (of which there are many within nursing and the social sciences) argue that individuals' experiences are complex and not easily measured. Palliative care is characterised by care that is delivered with sensitive attention to the diverse reactions and needs of people coming to terms with life-threatening illnesses and the personal suffering that this often entails. It aims to address the physical, psychological, social and spiritual needs of the dying and their families. The danger of concentrating on areas that are amenable to measurement, such as patients' physical symptoms, is that the areas less easily measured are given less attention in the quest for improving and demonstrating quality of care. It would also be wrong to present palliative care to interested observers as just a set of observable and measurable standards – palliative care is complex and, in its totality, beyond measurement.

USING RESEARCH TO DEMONSTRATE QUALITY IN PALLIATIVE CARE

The difference between audit and research

The distinction between audit and research causes confusion amongst clinical nurses which, according to Closs & Cheater (1996), is hardly surprising given that both researchers and those involved in audit are frequently unclear about the differences.

Closs & Cheater's (1996) discussion of the differences reveal that although the activities are inter-related they differ in several important areas.

The main difference is the purpose of both activities. As defined above, audit is a cyclical activity that is primarily concerned with improving the standards of care given. This differs from research which, as described by MacLeod-Clark & Hockey (1989), is aimed at generating new knowledge through systematic inquiry. In broad terms, the purpose of health care research is to provide generalisable knowledge that will provide a basis for decision-making in clinical practice. Smith (1992, p. 905) succinctly captures the difference between the aims of research and audit by stating:

> *Research is concerned with discovering the right thing to do; audit with ensuring that it is done right.*

Depending on the purpose of the research it can either be:

• **Theory constructing** (qualitative research), where the emphasis is on a process that begins with a set of observations and progresses to develop theories from these observations. This domain of research is termed qualitative, where the goal is to document and interpret the totality of what is being studied from the subjects' viewpoint or frame of reference (Leininger 1985). It does not involve the use of numbers or statistics but commonly identifies themes, patterns or characteristics from the data collection, which are then employed to develop a theory or theories.

• **Theory testing** (quantitative research). This approach differs from that described above in that it starts with a theory and the purpose is to test this through experimental or quasi-experimental methods. Quantitative research attempts to demonstrate and present its findings in terms of numbers and frequencies (Hockey 1991), and the emphasis is on measuring the variables under study rather than attempting to explore and understand individual situations or phenomena.

However, in practice there is often constant interplay between the construction and testing of theories. As it is beyond the remit of this chapter to illustrate these concepts in more depth, readers new to research methodologies are advised to refer to specific research texts for an overview (Cormack 1991, Leininger 1985, Polit & Hungler 1991).

Evaluation research in health care aims to identify (either through the testing of hypotheses or, for example, in qualitative research by describing indicators of good/poor care) what is the best practice. In contrast, clinical audit does not seek to generate new knowledge; however, it is related to research as it uses the evidence acquired through systematic research as the basis for its standards.

Similarities also exist in the methods used in audit and research (quantitative, in particular); in collecting data both may use questionnaires, interviews or reviews of case notes. However, the emphasis on samples (which patients and how many patients should data be collected from) differs. In determining sample sizes, quantitative research employs strict criteria and methods to ensure that the findings are not likely to have occurred by chance and can be generalised to a broader population. In audit, the clinical significance takes priority over statistical significance. In illustrating this, Closs & Cheater (1996) point out that it is possible (and often clinically relevant) to audit a small sample of patients to see if standards are being reached. They argue that for the patient it can be significant if only one in a small sample does not receive the standard of the care expected. In contrast to this is that it is often difficult to judge the significance, in terms of testing a theory, of results obtained from research using small sample sizes of patients.

The process of determining sample sizes in qualitative methods differs significantly from both audit and quantitative research and depends on the methods being used. Broadly, sample sizes in qualitative methods are smaller owing to the in-depth nature of this type of research – a good introduction to qualitative research methods is described by Hunt (1991).

Perhaps, most importantly, audit should never involve disturbance to patients beyond that required for normal clinical management (Maden 1991), whereas clinical research involves patients being interviewed or completing questionnaires (which may be beyond the requirements for the normal management of patients). To ensure that patients are not caused additional distress by participating in research studies, all proposed studies must have the consent of the relevant local ethics committee. However, under the guise of audit, it is not unusual for patients (and families) to be asked to complete satisfaction surveys. As satisfaction surveys may be construed as beyond the expected clinical management of patients, it is advisable to contact your local ethical committee prior to commencing such a project. Although it is difficult to envisage any harm coming to patients who participate in such surveys, it is possible that some questions will highlight, for a patient, a difficult or poor experience during the course of their care and cause some distress.

Aranda (1995) points out that the emotions of dying patients, such as sadness or tearfulness, are often brought to the surface in the process of participating in palliative care research, and do not necessarily equate to harm being done. In support of this, Aranda (1995) argues that by participating in research, patients are given the opportunity to express their feelings during a research interview, which can be a positive and cathartic experience for them. Nevertheless, it is the job of the ethics committee to examine provisions for dealing with such situations and to ensure that the researchers are sufficiently sensitive to the potentially negative consequences for patients participating in studies.

The opening quote of this chapter implies that within palliative care there exists a knowledge base, which if acted on will greatly improve the care given to patients. The challenge of quality assurance and audit activity is to incorporate this knowledge into practice and demonstrate the improvements in the quality of care given to our patients. However, to ignore the role of research in the pursuit of demonstrating the effectiveness of palliative care would wrongly imply our complete understanding of the processes that determine how we apply this knowledge to practice.

The following sections discuss some previous attempts to demonstrate the effectiveness of palliative care and highlight the difficulties of the research methods used. To summarise, the main difference between audit and research is in the purpose of both activities:

- Audit is primarily concerned with improving standards of care
- Research is aimed at generating new knowledge
- Audit and research are interdependent; clinical audit uses the evidence acquired through systematic research as a basis for its standards
- Although the purposes of both activities are different there are some similarities, particularly in relation to data collection
- If through the process of audit or research patients are disturbed beyond what would be normally required for clinical management, ethics approval should be sought

RESEARCH IN PALLIATIVE CARE – PAST TRENDS AND FUTURE DIRECTIONS

Much of the early work in palliative care research sought to highlight the poor care that dying patients were receiving. The information that was collected was both powerful and shocking and indicated that much work was required to begin to meet the needs of the patients (Corner 1996). Such research included, for example, studies that examined the levels of symptom distress in health care institutions (Hinton 1979, Hockley et al 1988, Simpson 1991) and research that sought to examine, in sociological perspectives, issues such as collusion and patients' awareness of dying (Glaser & Strauss 1965). Many of these studies had a far-reaching impact in developing local services for dying patients and helped to shape the emerging specialty of palliative care.

The last decade has seen palliative care services continue to burgeon, whilst also diversifying into other settings, i.e. acute hospitals and day care.

However, this proliferation of hospice/palliative care services has, in part, been unco-ordinated (Clark 1993) and ad-hoc with evidence that despite this rapid expansion of services there are still inequalities in access to services (Seale 1991).

In parallel with the development of palliative care services there has been an explosion of published research studies. This is reflected in the increase in palliative care journals and publications, which is a reflection of the emergence of palliative care as a distinct specialty. In a review and a discussion on the direction of palliative care research, Corner (1996) cites that much of the previous and current research 'appears to be at the descriptive level' and comments that it is difficult to distinguish between what is audit and what is research. Corner (1996) also infers that that much of the evaluation of palliative care services lacks imagination in the research methods used and has local relevance only (rather than generating new knowledge and understanding, which can be generalised to a wider audience).

It seems that, on the whole, the expansion and diversification of palliative care services is not underpinned by 'sound' scientific evaluations of their effectiveness. Reasons for palliative care research seemingly being 'out of step' with the development of services include the following:

• Palliative care services are funded from a variety of sources, including charities and NHS monies. The priority has been to set up services to meet the perceived needs of patients; whereas rigorous studies of the health care needs of patients and evaluations of the impact of these services have been a lower priority.

• Research in the field of palliative care is practically difficult. Evaluation studies of palliative care are plagued by the difficulties of performing research with very ill subjects. These difficulties include: poor response rates to questionnaires (Aranda 1995); difficulties in recruiting a sufficient number of patients who are able to participate in studies; and high attrition rates from studies owing to deterioration in the participants' general health (Aitken 1986).

• There are methodological problems associated with quantitative studies of the outcome of interventions and palliative care services. These mainly centre on choosing what to measure and selecting a valid and reliable measurement tool. This is discussed in more detail in the section below that deals with 'Measurement tools in palliative care'.

• Finally, the dominant view in health care evaluation has centred on measurement. In order to measure something we first need to be able to understand and conceptualise the issue, something that is very difficult to do in some areas of palliative care.

Although the above reflections on the status of palliative care research are critical of the depth and rigor of current research, there are notable exceptions. These exceptions will be discussed in the following categories:

• Quantitative evaluations of palliative care services
• The use of surveys to evaluate palliative care
• The value of qualitative research methods in evaluation research

Quantitative evaluations of palliative care services

Although there have been many studies describing palliative care services and problems that dying patients encounter (Ellershaw et al 1995, Hockley et al 1988), few have been large enough to generate any meaningful conclusions. Corner (1996) suggests that the preoccupation with describing activities and problems, rather than 'actively evaluating existing and new approaches to care' is a reflection of the new and emerging nature of the specialty of palliative care.

Traditionally, health care services have been evaluated by comparing the outcomes of two different services (i.e. a hospice to a hospital oncology unit). Such studies usually involve an established service (the control group) being compared to a new or different method of delivering care (i.e. a hospice). These evaluations have been noticeably absent in palliative care research evaluations.

An exception to this is 'The national hospice study' of in-patient hospice, home hospice and conventional care, which was carried out in America in the late 1980s (Greer et al 1986). The motivation for this study was to determine whether hospice care was effective and, if so, eligible for Medicare (US-state funding). This study measured a variety of outcomes in a sample of over 1700 patients receiving care in either hospice, at home (supported by hospice home care) or in hospital oncology units. The results revealed small significant differences in pain and other symptoms but failed to detect significant differences in overall quality of life, and satisfaction with care – as reported by family members (Greer et al 1986). However, Higginson (1993a) points out that some of the 'sampling inconsistencies' limit the conclusions that we can draw from this study. Specifically, as the study was non-randomised the results may be attributed to differences in the patient populations studied rather than to differences among the care given in the hospital, hospice and community settings.

The only fully randomised study (considered by some to be the gold standard in evaluation research) of a specialist palliative care service was also carried out in the USA. In this study, Kane et al (1984) randomly allocated patients to either hospice or conventional hospital care and, as with the previous study, measured a variety of outcomes. In general the findings are similar to the above study, with increased patient and family satisfaction with care demonstrated in the hospice setting. However, pain and symptom control were not shown to be statistically different between the two settings. This may have been a result, in part, of the fact that the patients randomised to the hospice group were admitted to the hospital when beds were not available – on average, 13.2 days were spent by patients in hospital when they were allocated to the hospice sample! Nevertheless, this and the previous study tentatively show that the quality of care in hospice is as good (and in some aspects better) than hospital care. However, in commenting on these studies, Aitken (1986) argues that other advantages for patients in hospices may not have been sufficiently demonstrated owing to a lack of reliable measurement tools. The criticism of this and other evaluations of palliative care services are related to the limitations of the methods used; namely, that quantitative methods fail to highlight aspects of palliative care that are not amenable to measurement.

The use of surveys to evaluate palliative care

In the UK there has been a proliferation of the use of the survey as a method of evaluating the provision of palliative care, both at national and regional/local level.

Surveys are normally quantitative in nature and can be categorised as descriptive or explanatory (Abramson 1990). Descriptive surveys seek to describe the characteristics or variables under study, whereas explanatory surveys aim to test theory through the use of large samples and data sets.

Surveys into palliative care have mainly been at the descriptive level, with some of these using very large samples to gain a national picture of the care of the dying. A recent survey by Addington-Hall & McCarthy (1995) repeated a survey performed in the UK 20 years previously by Cartwright et al (1973). In both surveys, random samples of bereaved relatives were interviewed using the same structured interview schedule. Addington-Hall & McCarthy (1995) concluded, following analysis of the data obtained from over 2000 relatives, 'that there is some way to go before all dying patients receive high-quality care'. As with the original survey by Cartwright et al (1973), there were many patients with unmet physical, emotional and social needs.

The past decade has seen a proliferation of satisfaction surveys, in both health care evaluations and audit, brought about mainly through the consumer movement seen in wider society. Although the participation of patients in the evaluation of nursing practice should be encouraged, the use of satisfaction surveys are fraught with difficulties. Central to these difficulties is a lack of understanding of the concept of satisfaction. In a discussion of the concept of satisfaction, Lawler (1971) points out that we need to understand this concept before we can explain why certain factors cause it. In palliative care, where a cure of the illness is not possible, we do not know to what extent factors such as anger, expectations of health care and past experiences with health care professionals influence patients' overall satisfaction. Moreover, Fitzpatrick (1984) notes that the consistently high satisfaction found in most health care surveys may not be a true reflection of satisfaction/dissatisfaction, as patients may be reluctant to express criticism for fear of treatment being compromised. Additionally, when palliative care is being provided in busy wards, patients may not wish to be seen to be critical of overburdened staff 'doing their best'. Currently, the lack of research into the concept of satisfaction and the components necessary to produce it in palliative care, make the use of satisfaction surveys of questionable benefit in the evaluation of services.

To conclude, the recent expansion and diversification of palliative care services are not underpinned by sound scientific evidence of their effectiveness in improving patient care. Quantitative research methods have their place in the evaluation of palliative care but are practically difficult and cannot entirely capture the breadth and scope of the specialty. Furthermore, the lack of research into the concept of satisfaction and the components necessary to produce it in palliative care, make the use of satisfaction surveys of questionable benefit in the evaluation of services.

MEASUREMENT TOOLS IN PALLIATIVE CARE

There are many tools that have been designed for assessing the distress and quality of life of people with different illnesses and health deficits. However, this section will deal only with those tools that have been either designed or used in palliative care. In choosing a tool to evaluate any aspect of palliative care it is important that it meets the criteria of being valid, reliable, sensitive to changes over time and appropriate for the purpose that it is being used for (see Box 11.1).

■ **BOX 11.1**

Criteria for measurement tools

Validity. This is the term used to describe whether the tool measures what it is intended to measure (Polit & Hungler 1991). For example, a valid depression measurement tool, for palliative care, needs to differentiate between normal sadness and grief associated with dying and clinically significant depression.

Reliability. This is the term used to describe whether the tool consistently measures the same concept, when applied in different settings by different people. One would expect a reliable tool to yield the same results when measuring the same concept at different times (test–retest reliability) and rated by different users (inter-rater reliability).

Sensitivity. This is concerned with the ability of the measurement tool to detect clinically significant changes over a period of time. Visual analogue scales are considered to be the most sensitive scales, whilst simple verbal descriptive scales are usually less sensitive. Sensitivity is particularly important in clinical audit where the emphasis is to monitor clinical practice over a time period

Appropriateness. Is concerned with the ability of the measure to be used in the intended setting. Is it short enough for ill patients to complete? Is it culturally appropriate (if it was designed in a different country)?

In the reality of clinical practice, particularly in palliative care, there is never going to be a tool that completely satisfies all these criteria and that is suitable across all the different settings in which palliative care is delivered. When attempting to evaluate a palliative care service there is always going to be some conflict between, for example, a valid tool that is sensitive to differences in the area being measured and a tool that is sufficiently short for patients that are very ill.

Although patient participation should be the gold standard in the evaluation of patient care, there is a proportion of patients in our specialty that cannot participate because of illness – some authors have put this figure at 50% (McWhinney et al 1994). The temptation is to accept this and concentrate on patients who are able to complete the necessary questions. However, in doing this we risk not evaluating the care given to the patients who arguably have the greatest palliative care needs. In order to achieve this, some tools have been designed to be completed by proxy (for the patient), by either relatives (commonly, bereaved relatives) or by the professional carers. Although this may be the only method of gaining valuable information about patients with advanced disease, findings obtained in this way should be treated cautiously. Information gained, for example, from bereaved relatives may be affected by both their memory of events and the process of bereavement. Nevertheless, such studies do give us valuable, albeit tentative, information about the care of patients with advanced disease that otherwise would not have been available. Those planning audit or research studies need to consider what tools should be used and by whom they will be completed. If a study aims to assess the care given to all patients in a specialist palliative care unit, a number of tools will be required that allow patients, where possible, to participate and perhaps enable relatives or carers to participate when patients are too ill. Such an approach will add to the richness of the evaluation rather than detracting from the methodological rigor of the study. Table 11.1 presents some of the more common tools used in palliative care evaluation studies.

> ■ **REFLECTIVE PRACTICE 11.3   Quality of life evaluation tools**
>
> Are you familiar with any of the tools described in Table 11.1?
>
> • Select a tool from each section and discuss with your colleagues the possibility of using one of these in your practice.

THE ROLE OF QUALITATIVE RESEARCH IN THE EVALUATION OF PALLIATIVE NURSING

Quantitative research is based on the assumption that the social world is amenable to measurement and that theory can be tested through the application of experimental research designs. Critics (of which there are many in nursing and other social sciences) argue that the emphasis on measurement in quantitative research methods does not lend itself to the human sciences (see Leininger 1985 for a fuller discussion of this area). The increasing recognition of the limitations of quantitative research has seen the emergence of an alternative approach – termed qualitative research. This approach to research evolved at the turn of the 20th century in anthropological and phenomenological circles. Qualitative research has increasingly gained recognition in the health sciences in the last 20 years.

Qualitative research is based on the belief that there is more to 'knowing' than what can be seen or measured and that it is equally important to study an individual's experiences within the context under investigation (Leininger 1985). Its focus is much broader than the often narrow focus of the traditional research methods. It aims to generate theory and knowledge

Table 11.1 Common symptom distress scales, quality of life and specific palliative evaluation tools

Name and author of the tool	Areas measured	Comments
Symptom distress scales		
Rotterdam symptom checklist (De Haes et al 1990)	34 symptoms, including physical and psychosocial problems. Each problem assessed on a Likert scale	The scale was developed in patients with different stages of cancer – either disease-free or undergoing chemotherapy. Although good evidence of validity and reliability exists, its length makes it inappropriate for use with patients who are very ill
Edmonton symptom assessment system (Bruera et al 1991)	Nine physical and psychological symptoms measured on visual analogue scales	This scale has been developed for use in hospice but may equally be of value in a hospital setting. The scale is designed so as the scores are 'charted', making the tool a good ongoing clinical assessment and audit tool. Evidence of validity and reliability is limited to the North American population
Symptom distress scale (Holmes 1989)	10 physical and psychological symptoms measured on a numerical scale	This tool has been developed from McCorkle & Young's (1978) tool in the USA. It has been extensively validated in the UK and is the most commonly used scale in cancer research nursing. Although simple to use, very ill patients may find it difficult
Wisconsin brief pain inventory (Daut et al 1983)	Measures pain and its impact on the psychological and social well-being of the patient on 12 scales. Items are measured on a 0–10 scale	This tool is particularly useful in palliative care as it considers pain as a multifaceted concept. It is well validated with patients with chronic pain. An abbreviated form is currently being used to study the incidence of pain in patients with cancer in different settings across Scotland (Fallon, personal communication, 1997)
Hospital anxiety and depression scale (Zigmond & Snaith 1983)	Two subscales, consisting of 14 items, measuring anxiety and depression	Designed for use in patients with a physical illness. Easy and quick for patients to complete. Some doubt over the validity of the depression subscale in dying patients. Needs further testing

Table 11.1 Common symptom distress scales, quality of life and specific palliative evaluation tools (contd)

Quality of life (QOL) tools

Spitzer quality of life index (Spitzer et al 1981)	Measures five domains of QOL: physical activity, daily living, perception of own health, support from family and friends and outlook on life. Within each of these five areas are three statements, which are scored 0, 1 or 2	Developed specifically as a brief and simple measurement of quality of life. Shown to be valid and reliable in oncology patients. However, little evidence of testing in patients with advanced cancer. Designed to be completed by 'proxy' by the patient's physician, and therefore validity of the results may be questionable
The functional living index (cancer) (Schipper et al 1984)	The instrument contains 22 items covering physical, functional, psychological and social areas. Each of the questions are measured on a seven-point numerical scale	Although quite long, it can be completed by patients in 10 minutes. It was developed and tested in ambulatory oncology patients and therefore its applicability to patients with advanced cancer is questionable
European organisation for research and treatment of cancer – QLQ-C30 (Aaronson et al 1993)	30 questions and a global QOL core covering the physical, functional, psychological and social domains of QOL	Internationally tested, demonstrating good validity and and reliability amongst cancer patients with early and advanced stages of cancer. Shown to be sensitive to changes in QOL over time. Its length may make it difficult for some patients to complete
Global quality of life score	May be administered as a single visual analogue score or a numerical scale (as found in the last question of the above tool)	Most patients would be able to rate their QOL on a single scale. Donnelly & Walsh (1996) report that this is the QOL assessment tool of choice for seriously ill patients. The major disadvantage is that it does not give any information on what component of quality of life (i.e. physical or social) is good or poor
Specific palliative care evaluation tools		
Support team assessment tool (STAS) (Higginson 1993b)	17 items assessing areas of importance to patients with palliative care needs, including: communication, planning affairs and home support	Designed for use by community specialist palliative care services. Widely used and well validated. It relies on being completed by the professional and is therefore

Table 11.1 Common symptom distress scales, quality of life and specific palliative evaluation tools *(contd)*

		only as valid as the person who is able to make accurate judgements on behalf of the patient. Also limited on the assessment of patients' symptoms
Palliative care assessment tool (PACA) (Ellershaw et al 1995)	Measures symptom control (eight core symptoms plus patient-reported symptoms), patients and relative insight, and facilitation of patient placement	Specifically designed to assess the impact of hospital palliative care teams, in the areas measured, over a time period. Initial tests of reliability are good. More work is needed to confirm its validity, particularly in relation to the insight scores which may, in some patients, measure denial rather than lack of insight
Patient evaluated problem score (PEPS) (Rathbone et al 1994)	Patients are asked to list problems 'impairing their quality of life – whether physical, emotional, social or spiritual'. These problems are then rated, by the patients, as mild, moderate or severe	This is a patient-centred approach (rather than a tool) for evaluating patient problems which, when combined with, for instance, a global quality of life score (as described by the author) provides a very useful clinical assessment and audit tool. **(The author has found this method very useful in the hospital. As part of clinical assessment it has been used on the first patient visit and then repeated 1 week later. This provides useful patient-generated information on the team's effectiveness in helping with the most commonly reported problems.)**
Regional study of the care of the dying questionnaire (Addington-Hall & McCarthy 1993, Cartwright et al 1973)	This questionnaire assesses a number of areas of palliative care as reported by bereaved relatives	The current questionnaire was adapted from a previous study by Cartwright et al (1973). The results gained from using this tool should be treated with some caution, as they are dependent on the memory of bereaved families. Nevertheless, this is a very useful tool for evaluating 'by proxy' palliative care services, and the results from the two previous studies by the authors are *available for comparison*

based on the in-depth study of human behaviour in different contexts. The methods and tools common to qualitative research are very different from the previously discussed research methods. Although a full discussion of the methods are beyond the scope of this chapter, the list below outlines some of the more common methods:

- Interviews
- Observation
- Participant observation
- Case studies (Clark 1997)

The aim of qualitative research is to identify, document and interpret the life events under investigation. At no time does the researcher attempt to manipulate or measure the variables being studied. To this end, the focus of qualitative research is led by the area under investigation in contrast to quantitative methods where the researcher has a predetermined agenda to study.

The data, often rich accounts of individuals' experiences in the area being studied, are analysed according to the qualitative approach the researcher adopts. This analysis aims to describe and identify common themes that emerge from the data. Often, researchers will formulate theories based on the relationship between the themes that are found during the course of the study.

The role of qualitative research in evaluating palliative care is to inductively develop theory and deepen our understanding of what constitutes quality and good nursing care of patients receiving palliative care in different settings. Many of the qualitative studies in palliative care give rich accounts of the experiences of patients in the adversity of a life-threatening illness. Some of these have helped to deepen our understanding on what constitutes good quality of care from the patient and family perspectives.

The following two studies, found in the palliative care literature, are good examples of this:

- 'Indicators of quality of palliative care from a family perspective' (Kristjanson 1986). This American study used open-end interviews, with 20 families selected by purposive sampling methods, to describe the indicators that families of the terminally ill perceive to be important in the care of the patient and themselves. The data obtained from the interviews were analysed for recurring themes. The study suggested that a number of factors relating to the behaviour of care givers was important in providing good quality care. These factors included: open communication with the patient and family about diagnosis, good attention to symptom relief and a compassionate attitude to the patient and family.

- 'After diagnosis of cancer: the patient's view of life' (Bliss & Johnson 1995). The authors of this study use critical incidents of good and bad experiences, as reported by patients, to gain an understanding of their needs following diagnosis. The strength of this study is its longitudinal design, in that patients were interviewed twice (following diagnosis and 1 year later). As with the study discussed above, patients valued sensitive communication. Additionally, the provision of support in the community was valued highly by both the patient and the family. Interestingly, the authors report that patients were more likely to remember the good experiences (rather than the poor experiences) after a year.

Both nursing and palliative care has a long track record in the use and development of qualitative research. Early examples of qualitative studies in palliative care, such as Glaser & Strauss's (1965) seminal work on awareness of dying, have helped to shape the modern approach to the care of the dying. If we are to continue to provide a high standard of care to dying patients then further qualitative studies need to be undertaken to enable us to understand, more fully, patients' and families' perceptions of palliative care delivery.

Although Morse (1991, p. 11) commented that the development of qualitative research in nursing is 'accelerating in nursing at breathtaking speed', good qualitative evaluations of the first-hand experiences of patients receiving palliative care are rare. Most qualitative research in palliative care has focused on bereaved relatives and, although by no means unimportant, do not provide us with a deeper understanding of the first-hand experiences of patients. Moreover, many evaluation 'surveys' purport to use qualitative methods, when in fact the focus of such studies (i.e. patient satisfaction surveys) is quantitative, with the odd token open question thrown in. Such approaches to evaluation research do little to add to the credibility of qualitative research and, at worst, reduce its methodology to what Morse (1991, p. 14) describes as 'a free for all'.

Qualitative research methods have much to offer palliative care evaluation research but should not be seen as a soft option (Clark 1997). Qualitative research in itself is difficult to master and requires of the researcher a high degree of self-awareness and reflective skills. This, coupled with the sensitive issues surrounding the care of the dying, makes it important for anyone embarking on this type of research in palliative care to obtain good research techniques and personal supervision.

> ■ **REFLECTIVE PRACTICE 11.4   Qualitative research**
>
> Given that qualitative research methods require a high level of interpersonal and self-awareness skills in the researcher, what implications does this have for supervision?

CONCLUSION

In a review of published palliative care evaluation studies O'Hendley et al (1997) comment:

That although the palliative care movement is widespread, research assessing its effectiveness is limited.

The priority for all professionals working in this specialty must be to start to address this. The risk of failing to evaluate palliative care practices, in a climate of scarce resources, is that funding will be reallocated to other services that have been shown to produce positive outcomes. The lack of evidence of effectiveness in palliative care is not, I believe, the result of antipathy or a lack of desire in nurses to evaluate their practice but is a reflection of the practical and ethical difficulties associated with evaluating palliative care. Although there are no simple answers, the challenge facing nursing and all professionals is to find new and innovative ways of overcoming these difficulties. The following outline is a starting point for nurses involved in evaluating palliative care.

• First, any evaluation of palliative care must be multidisciplinary. Palliative care is a multidisciplinary specialty and as such should be evaluated by the teams providing the care. Although it can be argued that it is important to determine the nursing contribution to effective care, in reality, because of the inseparability of the different contributions of health care professionals, the tools and methods available at the present time make this task virtually unachievable. Moreover, as little evidence exists on the effectiveness of any service, surely the first priority must be to evaluate the total contribution of the multidisciplinary team? In a discussion of quality management in nursing, Koch & Fairly (1993, p. 139) underline the importance of collaboration with other disciplines, stating:

> *Given the opportunity, it can produce a synergistic result: a positive outcome that no one discipline could have attained alone.*

• Second, nursing has a unique contribution to make to the process of collaborative evaluation – not least in our understanding of alternative (i.e. qualitative) methods of evaluation. Bowling (1997) comments that a consequence of multidisciplinary activity is that a wide range of both descriptive and analytical methods become available. In the past the temptation has been to rely solely on the experimental methods, at the expense of utilising multiple methods, which, according to Bowling (1997), can lead to questionable findings and a limited understanding of the area of interest. Corner (1996) points out that we must be creative in our approach to researching palliative care. This creativity should be pluralist, in that rather than treating the qualitative and quantitative approaches as competing and opposite methods, we should try to combine methods. The previous example of an evaluation study into hospital palliative care uses both qualitative and quantitative research methods (Farrer et al 1998) and, as a structure for evaluating palliative care, was acceptable (to the funding body) when a randomised controlled trial was not possible.

• Third, in demonstrating the effectiveness on palliative care, both audit and research have an important role to play. The aim of audit should be to highlight and improve areas of practice that fall below the expected standard. It is a reflection of the emerging nature of the specialty of palliative care that little is known about the ideal and best methods of delivering care. It is for this reason that further research is required to both measure and describe new services. This applies to services, such as hospice day care, and community and hospital nurse specialists in palliative care. Although the purposes of audit and research in health care evaluation are different, they are inextricably linked, as audit is dependent on research findings to illustrate what is the best practice. To this end palliative care, if it is going to make progress in highlighting its important contribution within health care, needs to integrate both audit and evaluation research into its quality management programmes. Through closer integration of these we can begin to prioritise what are the most appropriate methods and tools to evaluate care and highlight areas that need further research before standards regarding aspects of care can be agreed.

- Finally, it is important for palliative care nurses to become more aware of the complex issues involved in evaluation of their work. If we are to begin to meet the challenge of demonstrating our worth within the health care system then we must become well educated and be increasingly critical of the theoretical and methodological aspects of the evaluation of palliative care. Nurses are in the ideal position to lead methodologically rigorous and relevant evaluation research, which so often in the past has been the hallmark of nursing research.

■ **REFLECTIVE PRACTICE 11.5   Thinking about research?**

Having been motivated to consider the value of research and audit in palliative care, why not now compare your own and your colleagues' priorities for research within your own practice?

REFERENCES

Aaronson N K, Ahmedzai S, Bergman B et al 1993 The European organisation for research and treatment of cancer. QLQ-C30: a quality of life instrument for use in international clinical trials in oncology. Journal of the National Cancer Institute 85: 365–375

Abramson J M 1990 Survey methods in community medicine, 4th edn. Churchill Livingstone, London

Addington-Hall J, McCarthy M 1995 Dying from cancer: results of a national population-based investigation. Palliative Medicine 9: 295–305

Aitken L H 1986 Evaluation research and public policy: lessons from the national hospice study. Journal of Chronic Disease 39: 1–4

Aranda S 1995 Conducting research with the dying: ethical considerations and experience. International Journal of Palliative Nursing 1: 41–47

Black N 1990 Quality assurance of medical care. Journal of Public Health Medicine 12: 97–104

Bliss J, Johnson B 1995 After diagnosis of cancer: the patient's view of life. International Journal of Palliative Nursing 1: 123–133

Bowling A 1997 Research methods in health. Open University Press, Buckingham

Bruera E, Kuehn N, Millar M, Selmer P, Macmillan K 1991 The Edmonton symptom assessment chart (ESAS): a simple method for the assessment of palliative care patients. Journal of Palliative Care 7: 6–9

Cartwright A, Hockey L, Anderson J L 1973 Life before death. Routledge & Kegan Paul, London

Clark D 1993 Whither the hospices? In: Clark D (ed) The future for palliative care. Open University Press, Buckingham

Clark D 1997 What is qualitative research and what can it contribute to palliative care? Palliative Medicine 11: 159–166

Closs S J, Cheater F M 1996 Audit or research – what is the difference? Journal of Clinical Nursing 5: 249–256

Cormack D 1991 The research process in nursing, 2nd edn. Blackwell Scientific Publications, London

Corner J 1996 Is there a research paradigm for palliative care? Palliative Medicine 10: 201–208

Daut R L, Cleeland C S, Flanery R C 1983 Development of the Wisconsin brief pain questionnaire to assess pain in cancer and other diseases. Pain 17: 197–210

De Haes J M, van Knippenbery F C E, Neijt J P 1990 Measuring psychological and physical distress in cancer patients: structure and application of the Rotterdam symptom checklist. British Journal of Cancer 62: 1034–1038

Deming W E 1988 Out of crisis. Cambridge University Press, Cambridge

Department of Health 1994 Clinical Audit in Nursing and Therapy Professions. HMSO, London

Donebedian A 1980 Explorations in quality assessment and monitoring. Health Administration Press, Ann Arbor, Michigan

Donnelly S, Walsh D 1996 Quality of life assessment in advanced cancer. Palliative Medicine 10: 275–283

Ellershaw J E, Peat S J, Boys L C 1995 Assessing the effectiveness of a hospital palliative care team. Palliative Medicine 9: 145–152

Farrer C K, Hockley J M, Fallon M, Sandridge A 1998 An evaluation of a multidisciplinary palliative care team (study ongoing) funded by the CSO, Scottish Office, Home and Health Department

Fitzpatrick R 1984 Satisfaction with health care. In: Fitzpatrick R, Hinton J, Newman S, Scambler G, Thompson J (eds) The experience of illness. Tavistock, London, pp 284–342

Glaser B, Strauss A 1965 Awareness of dying. Aldine, Chicago

Greer D, Mor V, Morris, Sherwood S, Kidder D, Bimbaum H 1986 An alternative in terminal care: results of the national hospice study. Journal of Chronic Disease 39: 9–26

Higginson I 1993a Palliative care: a review of past changes and future trends. Journal of Public Health Medicine 15: 3–8

Higginson I 1993b Clinical audit in palliative care. Radcliffe University Press, Oxford

Hinton J 1979 A comparison of places and policies for terminal care. Lancet i: 29–32

Hockey L 1991 The nature and purpose of research. In: Cormack D (ed) The research process in nursing, 2nd edn. Blackwell Scientific Publications, London, pp 3–12

Hockley J M, Dunlop R, Davies R J 1988 Survey of distress symptoms in dying patients and their families in hospital, and the response to a symptom control team. British Medical Journal 296: 1715–1717

Holmes S 1989 Use of a modified symptom distress scale in assessment of the cancer patient. Internal Journal of Nursing Studies 26: 69–78

Hunt M 1991 Qualitative research. In: Cormack D (ed) The research process in nursing. Blackwell Scientific Publications, London, pp 117–128

Kane R L, Wales J, Bernstein L, Leibowity J, Kaplan S 1984 A randomised controlled trial of hospice care. The Lancet April 21, 889–894

Kitson A 1988 The dynamic standard setting system. Nursing Times 84: 25

Koch T 1992 A review of nursing quality assurance. Journal of Advanced Nursing 17: 785–794

Koch M and Fairly T 1993 Integrated quality management: the key to improving nursing care quality. Mosby, St Louis

Kristjanson L 1986 Indicators of quality of palliative care from a family perspective. Journal of Palliative Care 1: 8–17

Lawler E 1971 Pay and organisational effectiveness: a psychological view. Belmont, Wadsworth, CA

Leininger M 1985 Qualitative research methods in nursing. Grune & Stratton, London

Linderman C 1976 Measuring quality of nursing care, part 1. Journal of Nursing Administration June, 16–19

Macleod-Clark J, Hockey L 1989 Further research for nursing. Scutari Press, London

Maden A P 1991 Research or audit? Network – King's Fund Centre 1: 1

Malby R 1992 The process of change on nursing audit. British Journal of Nursing 1: 205–207

Maxwell R 1984 Quality assessment in health. British Medical Journal 288: 1470–1472

McCorkle R, Young K 1978 Development of a symptom distress scale. Cancer Nursing 1: 373–378

McWhinney I R, Bass M J, Donner A 1994 Evaluation of palliative care services: problems and pitfalls. British Medical Journal 309: 1340–1342

Morgan C, Murgatroyd S 1994 Total quality management in the public sector. Open University Press, Buckingham

Morse J M 1991 Qualitative nursing research: a free for all. In: M, M.J. (ed) Qualitative nursing research: a contemporary dialogue. Sage, California, pp 14–22

National Association of Health Authorities 1987 Care of the dying. NAHA, London

O'Hendley A, Curzio J, Hunt J 1997 Palliative care services and settings: comparing care. International Journal of Palliative Nursing 3: 161–167

Oxford Illustrated Dictionary 1974 Oxford University Press

Parasuraman A, Zeithamsi V A, Berry L L 1985 A conceptual model of service quality and its implications for future research. Journal of Marketing Fall: 41–49

Polit D, Hungler B 1991 Nursing research: principles and methods. Lippincott, Philadelphia

Rathbone G V, Horsley S, Goacher J 1994 A self evaluated assessment suitable for seriously ill hospice patients. Palliative Medicine 8: 29–34

RCN 1993 Standards of care: cancer nursing. Royal College of Nursing, Middlesex

RCN 1993 Standards of care: palliative nursing. Royal College of Nursing, Middlesex

Royal College of Physicians 1991 Palliative care: guidelines for good practice and audit measures. A Report of a working group of the Research Unit of the Royal College of Physicians and the Association for Palliative Medicine, London

Schipper H, Clinch J, McMurray A, Levitt M 1984 Measuring the quality of life of cancer patients: the functional living index – cancer: development and validation. Journal of Clinical Oncology 2: 472–483

Seale C 1991 Death from cancer and death from other causes: the relevance of the hospice approach. Palliative Medicine 5: 12–19

Secretaries of State for Health 1989 Working for patients (White Paper). Her Majesty's Stationery Office, London

Shaw C 1989 Medical audit – a hospital handbook. King's Fund Centre, London

Simpson K H 1991 The use of research to facilitate the creation of a hospital palliative care team. Palliative Medicine 5: 122–129

Smith R 1992 Audit and research. British Medical Journal 305: 905–906

Spitzer W O, Dobson A L, Hall J, Chesterfield E, Levi J 1981 Measuring the quality of life of cancer patients: a concise Q1 index for use by physicians. Journal of Chronic Disability 34: 585–596

Sternwald J 1995 Lessons from the symposium on palliative medicine held in the College on 8th March 1995. Proceedings of the Royal College of Physicians, Edinburgh, 25: 569–573

WHO 1990 Cancer pain relief. World Health Organization, Geneva

Zigmond A, Snaith R P 1983 The hospital and anxiety depression scale. Acta Psychiatrica Scandianaviea 67: 361–370

FURTHER READING

Clark D 1997 What is qualitative research and what can it contribute to palliative care? Palliative Medicine 11: 159–166

Closs S J, Cheater F M 1996 Audit or research – what is the difference? Journal of Clinical Nursing 5: 249–256

Corner J 1996 Is there a research paradigm for palliative care? Palliative Medicine 10: 201–208

Higginson I 1993 Clinical audit in palliative care. Radcliffe University Press, Oxford

Koch T 1992 A review of nursing quality assurance. Journal of Advanced Nursing 17: 785–794

McWhinney I R, Bass M J, Donner A 1994 Evaluation of palliative care services: problems and pitfalls. British Medical Journal 309: 1340–1342

Rathbone G V, Horsley S, Goacher J 1994 A self evaluated assessment suitable for seriously ill hospice patients. Palliative Medicine 8: 29–34

Index

Numbers in bold refer to illustrations and tables

Randomised study, specialist palliative
care service, 283–284
Recurrence, fears about, 97
Reflective practice, 36, 37
Reflexology, 181–184
benefits, 183–184
limitations and contraindications, 184
performing, 183
Regional study of the care of the dying
questionnaire, **289**
Rejection by others, 102, 103
Relationships
effect of massage on, 174
homosexual, 158–161
in terminal illness, 204
threat to, 100–101
see also Nurse–family relationships;
Nurse–patient relationships
Relatives
completing quality of care measurement
tools, 286
establishing trust, 64
facilities for, 6
identifying and prioritising problems, 65
needs assessment, 68, 70–71
night sitter services, 76
overprotective, 106
case history, 127
partners concerns about sex, 149–150
promoting support from, 109
see also Bereavement; Grief; Support
study, carers and family
Relaxation, 166–172
activities, 168–169
case histories, 171–172
coping with emotions during, 170–171
deep relaxation, 170
self-help
for the nurse, 186–187
for the patient, 187
tapes, 165
visualisation, 169–170
Reliability, measurement tool, 285
Religion
and spirituality, 116–119
assessment of needs, 131
and suicide, 261
Research, 271, 292–293
demonstrating quality of care, 279–281
measurement tools, palliative care,
285–286, **287–289**
past trends and future directions,
281–285
Resources, 38
spiritual issues, 135–136
see also Literature, palliative care
Respect, 254–255
Respite, for relatives, 76, 199
Role
of nurse, 11–14
in hospice, 20–21
research studies on, 14–17
overlap, team members, 50–51
of palliative nursing, 2

Roper, 'Activities of living model', 150–151
Rotterdam symptom checklist, **287**
Royal College of Nursing (RCN)
Cancer Nursing Society, 22, 29, 32
Complementary Therapies Special
Interest Group, 188
'Dynamic standard setting system', 276
indemnity insurance, complementary
therapies, 188
Nursing Update programme, 38

S

St Christopher's Hospice, 3, **4**
bereavement support, 234, 235
day centre, 8
St Thomas' hospital, 6
Sample sizes, audit and research, 280
Satisfaction surveys, 280, 284
Saunders, Cicely, 3, 196
Scars, showing mastectomy, 145–146
Schon, reflective practice, 36
'Scope of professional practice',
UKCC, 33, 252
Scottish Partnership Agency for Palliative
and Cancer Care, 28
Screening assessment, 73–75
Secular definition, spirituality, 119–121
Seedhouse's ethical grid, 257–258
case history, 258
analysis using grid, 258–260
discussion, 260–261
Self, learning about, 142–143
Self-awareness, communication skills, 54
Self-concept, 91, 92
Self-help
bereavement programmes, 236
for nurse, 186–187
for patients, 187
Senses, environmental stimulation, 164–165
Sensitivity, measurement tool, 285
Setting the scene, needs assessment, 82
Sex counsellors, 158
Sexual
concerns, patients' attempts to
discuss, 150
needs, 141
problems
effects of illness and treatment on
libido, 144–148
Plissit model, behavioural treatment,
157–158
problem-solving approach, 153–155
Sexuality
as component of patient care, 148–152
initiating discussion, 155
and confidentiality, 155–157
expressing in serious illness, 143–144
learning about self, 142–143
threat to, 98–99
Silence, use of, 90
Sleep difficulties
assessment, 76

About the
PROFESSIONAL DEVELOPMENT RECORD

The United Kingdom Central Council (UKCC) PREP regulations require you to maintain a personal professional portfolio, in which you record evidence of your professional development.

This book provides you with excellent educational material to assist your study and develop your practice. Reading all or parts of it can contribute to your professional development.

The *Professional Development Record* (overleaf) is designed to help you record your study activity in your portfolio and show how it has enhanced your practice. To use the Record, you can do either of the following:

- photocopy the Record and place it directly into your portfolio, or

- use it as a basis for your own individual entry.

The aim of the Record is to help you plan how this book assists your professional development, to the benefit of yourself, your colleagues and your patients/clients.

Further information:

- If you do not have a portfolio and would like to purchase one, please contact your local bookseller or, in case of difficulty, phone our Customer Services Department on 0181 308 5710.

- If you need further information about PREP, you should contact the UKCC on: 0171 333 6550.

PROFESSIONAL DEVELOPMENT RECORD

Book (fill in author, title, year of publication, publisher):

Date of completion of book (or selections from book):

Duration of study time:

Reason for reading the book:

Intended learning outcomes:

Evaluation of material read:

Planned influence on practice:

Evaluation of influence on practice:

Learning outcomes achieved: